D0810258

FACE
CHANGE

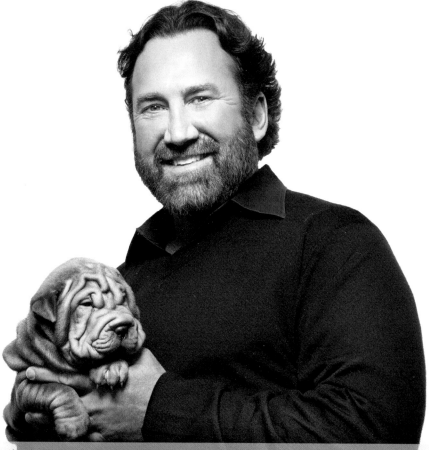

METHODS FOR LOOKING
AND FEELING YOUR BEST

By Harvey "Chip" Cole, III, MD, FACS

FACE
CHANGE

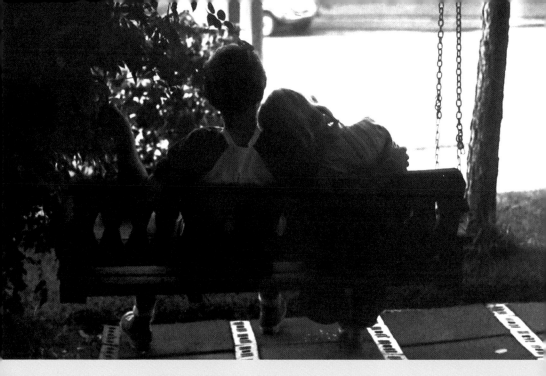

"To me, fair friend, you never can be old.
For as you were when first your eye I ey'd,
such seems your beauty still."
— *Shakespeare*

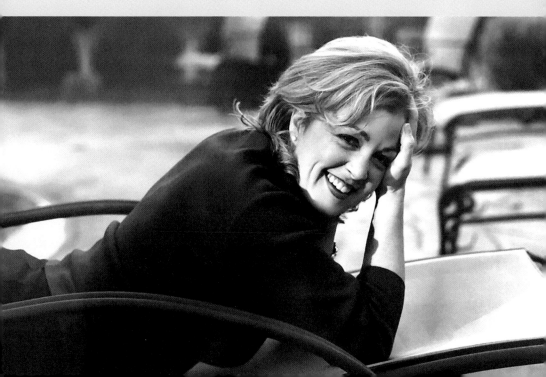

ISBN 978-0-9912143-5-8
LCCN 2014936879

DESIGNED BY
Ruffin Gillican, LLC
www.ruffingillican.com

first edition

FACE
CHANGE

INTERNAL AND EXTERNAL
METHODS FOR LOOKING
AND FEELING YOUR BEST

By Harvey "Chip" Cole, III, MD, FACS

12 NONSURGICAL SOLUTIONS

Procedure		Investment	Lasts	Recovery	Healed
1. BOTOX/DYSPORT		$300/syringe	3-4 months	Immediate	100%
2. HA FILLERS	Restylane, Perlane, Juvéderm, Belotero	$550/syringe	6-12 months	Immediate	100%
3. SCULPTRA		$850/vial	1-2 years	Immediate	100%
4. RADIESSE		$650/syringe	1-2 years	Immediate	100%
5. LASER HAIR REMOVAL		$250/area	Series	Immediate	100%
6. MICRODERMABRASION		$175	Series	Immediate	100%
7. IPL TREATMENT		$300	Series	Immediate	100%
8. CHEMICAL PEEL		$210	Sessions	3-5 Days	100%
9. FRACTIONATED CO2 LASER		$1,200	2-3 years	4-7 Days	90%
10. LASER LEG VEINS		$1,500	Sessions	Immediate	100%
11. SCLEROTHERAPY		$325	Sessions	Immediate	100%
12. LASER TATTOO REMOVAL		$375	Sessions	Immediate	100%

12 SURGICAL SOLUTIONS

Procedure	Investment	Treatments	Recovery	Healed
1. BLEPHAROPLASTY	$2,700	1	1 Week	85%
2. ENDOBROW	$2,800	1	1 Week	85%
3. CHEEK LIFT	$4,500	1	7-10 Days	85%
4. LASER EYES	$1,200	1	4-7 Days	90%
5. FACE LIFT	$6,200	1	2 Weeks	80%
6. NECK PLATYSMAPLASTY	$3,300	1	2 Weeks	85%
7. LASER FACE	$2,400	1	1 Week	90%
8. CHEEK IMPLANTS	$4,700	1	7-10 Days	85%
9. CHIN IMPLANT	$2,600	1	2 Weeks	85%
10. FACIAL LIPOSUCTION	$2,400	1	7-10 Days	85%
11. NECK LIPOSUCTION	$2,600	1	7-10 Days	85%
12. LIP AUGMENTATION	$2,100	1	1 Week	85%

Page #	Best Candidate
69	Frown lines, crow's feet, brow asymmetry, forehead rhytids
54	Nasolabial folds, forehead wrinkles, smile lines, lips and tear trough
96	Volume loss, skin-surface changes
96	Nasolabial folds, temples, prejowl, cheeks
131	Unwanted hair on face or body
54	Fine lines, crow's feet, age spots, acne scars; helps creams penetrate
98	Reduce wrinkles, sun spots, acne, rosacea, and vascular lesions
53	Sun-damaged or unevenly pigmented skin
53	Sun-damaged skin, wrinkles, acne, pigment changes
98	Spider veins, varicose veins, swelling
114	Spider veins
77	Unwanted tattoo

Page #	Best Candidate
192	Excess fat, wrinkled, drooping skin of upper eyelids
194	Sagging, low, unstable brow, frown lines, hooding
196	Lower lid hollow, bags, tear trough, midface descent
198	Wrinkles, crepiness, dark spots, loss of elasticity
202	Displaced tissue, loose skin, jowls, deep folds around mouth
204	Neck bands, turkey gobbler, poor texture, jowls, loss of jawline
206	Sun damaged skin, wrinkles, acne scars, dyspigmentation, fine lines
208	Poor midface volume, lower lid hollows, cheek volume collapse
210	Receding chin, poor neck definition
212	Excess subcutaneous fat, poor facial definition, isolated fatty regions
214	Loss of jawline, obtuse side view, multiple neck folds, isolated fat sites
216	Thin lips, poor definition, asymmetry

DEDICATION

There are two things in my life that I am most proud of: my family and my surgical practice.

I had the good fortune to grow up in Louisiana under the roof of two hard-working parents, Penny and Mugsy, who valued family above all else. I have felt their love as long as I can remember and have tried to exemplify and amplify it with my own family. When I was in eighth grade, I met a brace-faced blonde with bangs and a magnetic personality (and exceptional putt-putt skills). Now 41 years later, married for 33 years, with three grown kids and three grandchildren, I'm certainly a very proud G-pop! We all have a wonderful, loving relationship.

I have always been drawn to people and precision. Whether it was playing pixie sticks, the game "Operation," or, later, participating in a state competition for mechanical drawing, I have always enjoyed creativity and perfection. My mom was the artist and my dad the insurance salesman, or "people person." My specialized practice of both ophthalmic surgery and facial plastic surgery has allowed me to excel in a world of millimeter precision, all while effecting the overall improvement of another human being. This reward of helping a family from start to finish is simply the most rewarding aspect of my life, besides my own family.

I close by thanking my "office family," because they are such a huge part of my life. The Oculus team members are a highly trained group of professionals who constantly strive "beyond excellence!" Our dedication to each others' lives and our patients' and clients' well-being shines powerfully each day and with the contact our practice has with each person.

My goal in writing this book is that you will feel the sincere interest in your future well-being as you negotiate the process of Face Change. My additional interest is that your personal investment will directly provide help to a temporarily troubled teen, some of whom may play an important part in our country's future.

— H.P. "Chip" Cole, 2014

Acknowledgments

To my sister Kim, whose unyielding support, love, and friendship have brightened my spirits on many occasions.

To John and Bettie Sands, for their love, support, and tolerance for putting their baby girl through so many long years of school, kids, and over a dozen moves.

To my close friends Gene Kansas and Tom Bledsoe, who planted in my mind the grand delusion that I could write a meaningful book about Plastic Surgery.

To my three grandsons — Cannon Cole, Gavin Perkins, and Harvey Cole — who make me feel that my investment in my kids and my practice have all been worth it.

To my good friends Meg Reggie, Richard Eldridge, Felicia Feaster, Barbara Scott, and David Scott, whose untiring enthusiasm, hard work, creativity, and collaboration helped me focus my message to attain my desired literary and philanthropic goals.

To my practice partner, Brent A. Murphy, MD, whose unyielding friendship and support have helped me through many challenging personal and professional endeavors.

To my anesthesiologists, Elise Tomaras, MD and Lisa Drake, MD, for always going "beyond excellence" in the safe and nurturing anesthetic care they provide to our surgical patients.

To my mentor, Ralph E. Wesley, MD, whose superior surgical, nonsurgical, and many life lessons have helped guide me in a successful journey, intertwining family, faith, community, and medicine.

Most importantly, to my Oculus patients and clients, from the Southeast and abroad, who allow me the privilege of caring for you and your family to accomplish your individual facial plastic-surgery goals.

ABOUT THE AUTHOR

An innovator in the cosmetic-surgery field, Harvey "Chip" Cole, III, MD, FACS, has performed more than 25,000 surgeries since opening Atlanta's Oculus Plastic Surgery in 1994. Selected by his physician peers, he was named in *Harper's Bazaar* as one of the country's top 10 cosmetic eye surgeons, and *Town & Country* placed him among the top cosmetic surgeons in North America. In 1992, he gained vital early information regarding the cosmetic applications of lasers while learning from laser pioneer Dr. Sterling Baker. A groundbreaker in his own right, Dr. Cole has advanced the use of less invasive endoscopic surgery with minimal incisions, combining laser resurfacing, in his patented brow-lifting ABC technique (see Chapter 5).

Quadruple board certified by the American Society of Ophthalmic Plastic and Reconstructive Surgery, the American Board of Ophthalmology, the American Board of Cosmetic Surgery, and the American Board of Laser Surgery, Dr. Cole has also taught at some of the country's most prestigious medical institutions, including Harvard Medical School, UCLA, Stanford University, Cleveland Clinic, Tulane University, Emory University, and Vanderbilt Medical School. He serves as an invited board examiner for the American Board of Cosmetic Surgery, the American Society of Ophthalmic Plastic and Reconstructive Surgery, and the World Board of Cosmetic Surgery. He completed his ophthalmic surgical residency at Tulane, which was followed by a prestigious two-year fellowship in OculoFacial Plastic Surgery at Vanderbilt, where he received the specialty's highest honor, the Marvin H. Quickert Award. He now serves as a facial plastic surgery preceptor for both Vanderbilt and the Medical College of Georgia.

Among his many professional honors, Dr. Cole was named one of America's top facial plastic surgeons by the Consumers Research Council of America for the past 18 consecutive years. He received the Southern Medical Association's Most Outstanding Research Award; the C.S. O'Brien Professorship; and the American College of Surgeons' Golden Scalpel Achievement Award for surgical excellence. As a multiple-board-certified ophthalmic microsurgeon, Dr. Cole combines his expertise in highly refined millimeter-precise eye surgeries with his work as a facial plastic surgeon, offering an even greater degree of precision and knowledge to his surgical practice.

He has been an invited medical expert on Fox, CNN, ABC, NBC, *Good Day Atlanta,* and several regional and national radio shows. Dr. Cole has coauthored over a dozen medical books, has been invited to give numerous keynote-presentation speeches, and has given over 100 lectures around the world as an educator and surgical pioneer in his medical field. He attended Tulane Medical School, graduating in the top 10 percent of his class; he then did his surgical internship at Ochsner Clinic in New Orleans, where he was chosen Intern of the Year.

In addition to his clinical practice, Dr. Cole founded the nonprofit Face Change, which helps temporarily troubled teens. Learn more at www.FaceChange.info.

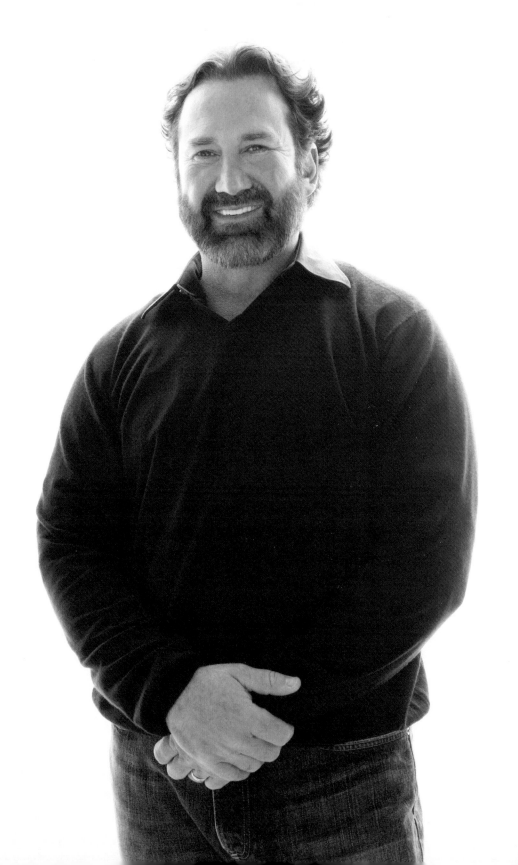

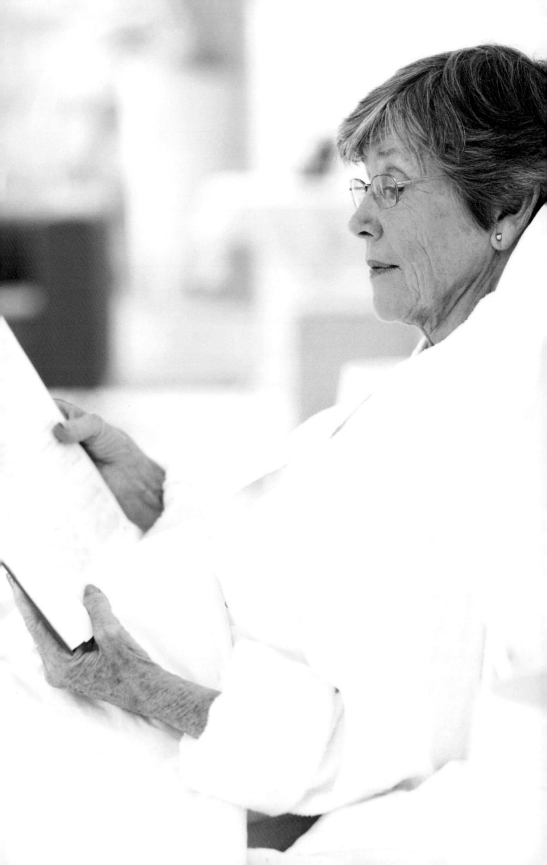

TABLE OF CONTENTS

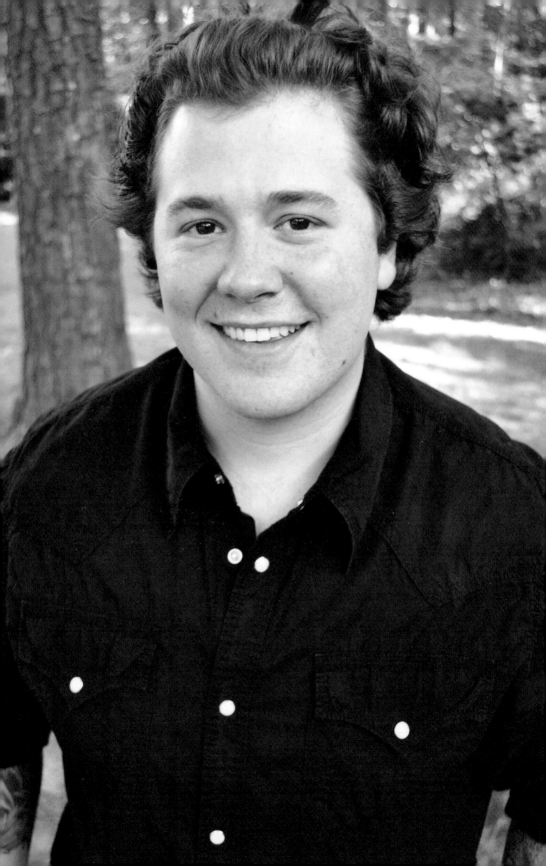

FOREWORD

* * *

BY CHRIS COLE

I want to start out by saying how very proud I am of my Daddio for writing this book, and for fearlessly engaging some of cosmetic surgery's tough existential questions — this while offering himself as a real human being first and a plastic surgeon second.

I'm often asked about my father's profession, and there was a time when I demurred, focusing only on the philanthropic aspects of his practice — how he saves people's lives and psyches by reversing the effects of burns, car crashes, dog bites, disease, or by building an eye socket where there wasn't one.

But as a seeker working toward a vision for spiritual, physical, and social wellness, I've learned that spirituality and the pursuit of physical beauty need not be on opposite ends of the spectrum. Perhaps a rich inner life and external beauty are two sides of the same coin.

This idea is reflected in Dad's dearest philanthropic venture, his formation of the nonprofit **Face Change Foundation** — dedicated to providing assistance to troubled teenagers — and I'm grateful to be a part of its mission.

If it weren't for his cosmetic practice, Dad would be unable to perform pro-bono surgeries for the community, having made it his mantra never to turn down a reconstructive patient based on the lack of financial resources. He has performed countless pro-bono procedures throughout his career, and he continues to do everything he can to put his unique skills to charitable use. Paying it forward has always been part of his mission, and it has become central to mine.

And part of that mission is to help us embrace our true power — to own the emotional and creative expression within all of us. We want our children to know they're free to be whatever and whomever they choose. And it's in service of this ethos that Dad has pledged *100% of this book's profits*, along with *10% from all cosmetic facial surgical procedures*, toward the **Face Change Foundation**.

I hope you find as much inspiration in these pages as I have, along with the power to cultivate health and beauty in every aspect of your life.

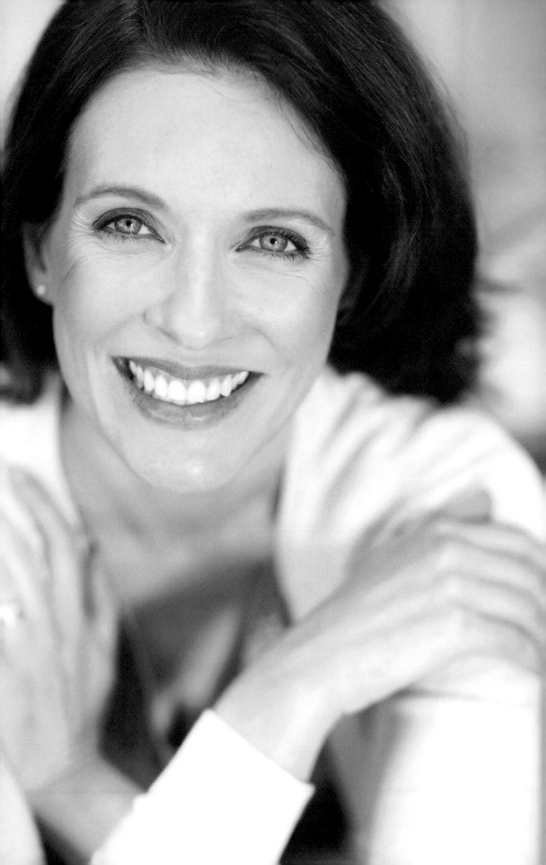

CHAPTER 1

* * *

GETTING STARTED:
WHY ME, WHY NOW?

To say there is a great deal of psychology involved in the practice of plastic surgery would be a serious understatement. When a patient comes to me with some concern about his or her appearance, it's often about more than just dissatisfaction with their face or body. Beauty is a very intimate business, connected to the totality of a patient's experiences, anxieties, childhood, and sense of self.

It's a privilege to feel so connected to my patients' lives and the stories they share with me. But there is also an enormous responsibility when so much of our emotional and psychological life is deeply embedded in the physical. The ability to positively affect a person's sense of self-worth is what makes plastic surgery such a satisfying specialty. I wouldn't trade my job for the world.

All doctors — but especially those who deal with issues of appearance, beauty, and aging — are connected to the most intimate dimensions of people's lives: what they long to be and what they fear. Patients share deeply personal details about their lives when telling me how they hope surgery will address their concerns with their appearance. Everything from not being invited to their high-school prom to being teased as a child, from a straying husband to a judgmental mother or father. Looks are so closely tied to identity that it is fundamental to understand where a patient is coming from and where they hope plastic surgery will take them.

So let's talk about my own experience and how I came to the field of plastic surgery. Born in Bossier City, Louisiana, to a mother who was a nurse and a father who was an insurance salesman, I learned early on the value of professions that are meant to serve people in times of need. Through my father's work, I discovered that life insurance was really death insurance that assisted families at the most vulnerable time in their lives. My parents' example was a lesson I took to heart.

The small-town doctors I knew, and the ones who helped me overcome childhood asthma, instilled in me a sense of medicine as a profession dedicated to nurturing.

My wife, Susan — whom I met in junior high and who beat me at a game of putt-putt on our first date — is a nurse. I don't deny that I'm attracted to people whose profession involves putting others' comfort and well-being ahead of their own. It is a higher calling.

Some of my most formative experiences involved watching my mother care for her patients, which taught me the nobility of empathy. I incorporate her example in my policy never to deny a patient medical care because they lack financial resources. Medicine, at its most profound level, is about offering the best care possible, no matter the circumstances. I received an important education in that core principle while volunteering at Charity Hospital in New Orleans, while attending Tulane Medical School. Caring for people injured in knife fights, the poorest of the poor, and people in truly desperate circumstances opened the eyes of a small-town kid to the various levels of need in the world.

I founded my practice, Oculus Plastic Surgery, in 1994 on those values and experiences, and I've never lost sight of them. Though some might view plastic surgery as a superficial profession, I'm proud of the improved quality of life it brings to my patients, from those seeking temporary fixes for a more youthful look to those requiring dramatic, medically necessary eye and facial surgery. Need is need, whether perceived or practical, and I do not make judgments about why people come to see me. As someone who treads the line between the beauty and health-care professions, I understand that one can influence the other and that aesthetics — whether the beauty of nature or a well-made suit — can enrich one's life and make it more satisfying.

HISTORY

The origins of the medical specialty in which I work are fascinating, and I believe they're worth sharing. Though tentative forays into plastic surgery occurred in India as early as 800 B.C., as well as in ancient Egypt and Rome, the introduction of anesthesia and hygienic surgical methods greatly advanced the cause of repairing disfiguring injuries. In late 19th- and early 20th-century America, doctors experimented with introducing foreign substances like paraffin into the face to correct the telltale deformity produced by syphilis — a saddle nose.

But the advent of modern plastic surgery and the real inroads in the field came, tragically, in wartime. Innovations in body-destroying weaponry necessitated improvements in the surgery that deals with shattered facial bones and gaping wounds to soldiers' faces and skulls. World War I and its catastrophic, life-altering damage to soldiers' bodies provided a significant laboratory for surgeons to develop techniques to help these men cope. Doctors who had treated disfigured soldiers banded together in 1921 to form the American Association of Plastic Surgeons (AAPS), and enormous progress was made in understanding the link between appearance and self-esteem.

Today, plastic surgery (taken from the Greek word *plastikos*, which means to mold or give form to) includes both reconstructive and cosmetic branches. Times have certainly changed, as plastic surgery has evolved from a way to treat congenital defects, injuries, and disease to become a commonplace method of enhancing one's appearance — the essence of cosmetic surgery. Both practices are still crucial, though one is necessary for survival and the other is for the most part elective.

The business of looking good is thriving. According to the American Society for Aesthetic Plastic Surgery (ASAPS), Americans spent nearly $11 billion on cosmetic procedures in 2012. Of that total, almost $6.7 billion was spent on surgical procedures. In 2012 alone, 1,594,526 surgical cosmetic procedures were performed. Of the most popular, in order, the number of procedures included: 1, breast augmentation (286,274); 2, rhinoplasty (242,684); 3, eyelid surgery (204,015); 4, liposuc-

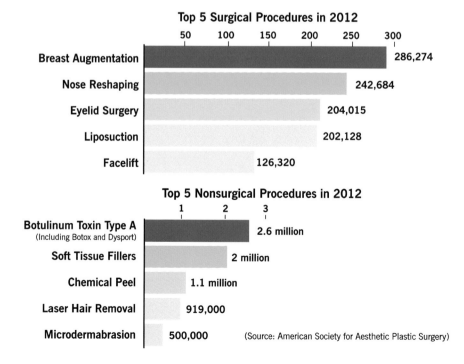

Top 5 Surgical Procedures in 2012

Breast Augmentation	286,274
Nose Reshaping	242,684
Eyelid Surgery	204,015
Liposuction	202,128
Facelift	126,320

Top 5 Nonsurgical Procedures in 2012

Botulinum Toxin Type A (Including Botox and Dysport)	2.6 million
Soft Tissue Fillers	2 million
Chemical Peel	1.1 million
Laser Hair Removal	919,000
Microdermabrasion	500,000

(Source: American Society for Aesthetic Plastic Surgery)

tion (202,128); and 5, face lift (126,320). Since 1997 there has been an incredible 250 percent increase in the number of elective plastic surgeries performed.

But the drive to make a buck sometimes undermines a sense of responsibility and aesthetic perspective. All too often, cosmetic surgery sets out to make patients look *better*, but instead makes them look *altered*. I'm pleased to have been featured in two national publications that asked physician peers who they would choose to perform cosmetic surgery on their family members. *Harper's Bazaar* named me one of the country's top 10 cosmetic eye surgeons, and *Town & Country* placed me among the top cosmetic surgeons in North America. That my fellow physicians offered that vote of confidence to my abilities is incredibly gratifying, but I'm also confident that my patients' beautiful results speak for themselves.

MISCONCEPTIONS

One of my many reasons for writing this book is to correct some basic misunderstandings about the business to which I have dedicated my life. There is a misconception, for instance, that cosmetic surgery is the domain of the wealthy and the vain. In reality, cosmetic surgery has now entered the mainstream, increasingly becoming a middle-class pursuit. In a 2010 study conducted by the American Society of Plastic Surgeons, only 10 percent of patients considering cosmetic surgery had annual incomes above $90,000. In fact, the majority of potential patients reported annual incomes of $30,000 to $90,000 a year.

The majority of people who come to me are not movie or TV stars or socialites who depend on their looks for career or social advancement, but ordinary people hoping to make improvements to their lives — improvements that are often physically subtle but psychologically quite dramatic. My practice is focused on discreet, natural changes to one's appearance, as opposed to the dramatic alterations apparent in Hollywood (for more on that, see Chapter 11). My focus is small restorations that turn back the clock. I don't wish to change a woman's appearance so drastically that she needs to buy a copy of the plastic-surgery picture book *My Beautiful Mommy* to help her toddler cope with the effects of "Mommy's new look."

My focus is on the sensible and, in my view, more female-friendly natural approach (the antithesis of the plasticized, obvious, and faddish West Coast look). Your shoes and hairstyle can be trendy, but your body and your face? Maybe not the best places to try out the latest trends. That scooped-out '60s "ski jump" nose, once the acme of modified female beauty, now looks obvious and distinctly altered. What was once a "style" of improved nose   as if ordered from a catalog — has been replaced by thoughtful plastic surgery in which the new nose is tailored to the patient's face. A unique, "tailored" nose made just for them is better than trying to meet some inflexible cookie-cutter beauty standard du jour.

If the shifting tides of fashion — from Nefertiti to Botticelli's *Venus,* from Twiggy to Cindy Crawford and from Pamela Anderson to Gwyneth Paltrow — have taught us anything, it is that our sense of beauty changes dramatically over time. Better not to be caught with "last year's breasts" but instead find the look that fits your frame and personality. Even the entertainment industry, that bastion of extreme surgery and lockstep beauty trends, is coming around. A 2010 article in *The New York Times* described the recent backlash among casting directors who are rebelling against the too-taut and filler-plumped faces of the actresses they see auditioning for roles. Ironically, all of the cosmetic intervention meant to make them more beautiful, youthful, and marketable can have the inverse effect. An immobile, overly Botoxed forehead can also impair an actor's ability to emote and express. "What I want to see is *real,*" says casting agent Mindy Marin.

It might seem counter-intuitive, but 10 percent of the time I find myself talking a patient out of a procedure. My objective is a happy patient, and an end result that speaks to the subtlety of my approach.

How is my approach different? If another plastic surgeon wanted to correct an older patient's dropped cheek pad, he would likely insert a cheek implant. My approach would be to reposition the cheek pad back onto the cheekbone. Instead of camouflaging the anatomy, I'm correcting it. The aim is to restore youth without altering your appearance. It's possible to revitalize and refresh your looks, to return them to the way they used to be. Skin will only stretch so far before it takes on an unnatural appearance. Unfortunately, too many plastic surgeons still stretch and cut. The results are dramatic (the patient is altered) but the effect is anything but natural. The goal of skilled surgery is to retain the central oval of the face. This is your true self and the key to keeping the essential *you* intact.

It's not a coincidence that we all find a baby's newborn skin appealing. We have a nearly primal response to that plump volume of fresh skin and a new life that subconsciously speaks to us of promise, potential, and the urgent human desire to nurture and protect. Scientists have observed a major component in our perception of feminine beauty termed "paedomorphism," which is the retention in adults of childlike traits, such as large, wide-set eyes, small noses, and full cheeks.

As we age, that coveted volume and satiny freshness inevitably changes and shifts. It's a natural progression, but one that small adjustments to eyes and mouths can mitigate. The result is a face that still looks like yours, but it's an improved, refreshed version. An approach defined by the artifice of the movie industry differs somewhat from the Southern approach, which is characterized by understatement and a subtle arsenal of feminine charm. In a city like Atlanta (where I practice), discretion is favored. You're unlikely to find a complete stranger in line next to you at Starbucks inquiring about where you had your lift done. I like to joke that Southern women don't lift and tell. Elsewhere, different rules apply.

It strikes me as interesting that in our culture cosmetic surgery is probably one of the most-performed procedures but one of the least discussed. Though our culture is driven by youth and beauty, there's a taboo about appearing too vain or too wrapped up in one's own appearance. People act as if nobody is doing it, but the number of patients I see from all walks of life show me that many people *are*, in fact, doing it.

As those ASAPS statistics attest, plastic surgery is more prevalent than ever in America today. But too often, when evidence of cosmetic enhancement does cross our paths, it sends a negative message about my profession. We've all been confronted with the telltale signs of too much surgery performed too dramatically: impossibly taut, stretched, and shiny skin; unnaturally downy lips; a hardened or perpetually dazed expression. In other words, a mask of beauty cloaks the essential gleam of humanity, concealing emotions and personality behind an immobile surface. Those people don't look more beautiful; they look unnaturally altered, and that's unfortunate — and unnecessary.

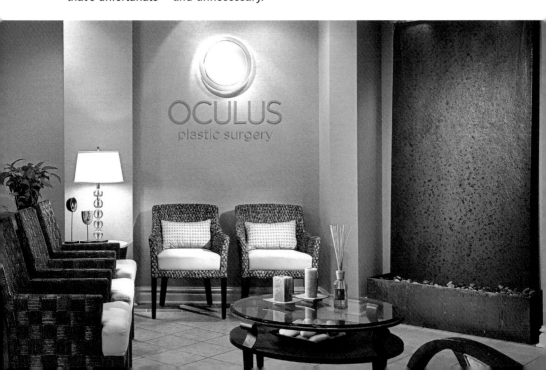

Thankfully, that's the exception rather than the rule. Most plastic surgeries are done so well that they fly under the radar. For me, that's the biggest injustice. Plastic surgeons don't always get credit for all the good work that's out there, but we're all blamed collectively when the work is bad. In reality, bad work is a rarity. It might seem counterintuitive, but 10 percent of the time, in my practice, I find myself talking a patient out of a procedure they think they need. My objective is a happy patient and an end result that speaks to the subtlety of my approach.

My aim is to treat every patient who crosses the threshold of my office as I would a family member. I treat them as I would want to be treated. In fact, though many surgeons would never consider operating on a family member, I have operated on my mother, father, wife, son, and in-laws. To my way of thinking, who could better take care of them or use better judgment? I want my loved ones to be treated by a true advocate — someone who is deeply concerned for their well-being. And I strive to extend this same spirit to *all* of my patients.

I've learned a great deal about human nature in my line of work — for instance about the stark differences between men and women when it comes to appearance. Though an increasing number of men are having cosmetic surgery and tend to be satisfied with small improvements, women seem to live in an alternate world when it comes to their looks. Women dwell in a pervasive, unrelenting beauty culture in which they are inundated with images on TV, in film, and in magazines that remind them of the centrality of looks. They're encouraged to be vigilant about their appearance at all times.

Too often, their sense of self is defined by the mirror others hold up to them, but often they are their own worst critic. Popular culture is filled with Photoshopped images of already-beautiful women transformed into perfect ones — an increasingly pervasive and troubling trend. There is no better evidence of just how judgmental our culture is when it comes to women's looks than the scathing, often cruel commentary that erupts in the media and on the blogosphere when a pop star like Jessica Simpson, an actress like Kate Winslet, or a model like Tyra Banks dares to gain a few pounds. If this is the condemnation that lies in wait for beautiful women who waver from the beauty standard, what about the average (or merely pretty) women among us?

MISSION

Regarding self-image, I find the psychological double standard between men and women both fascinating and revealing, and oftentimes a sad commentary on the culture in which we live. It's profoundly hypocritical, too. Women are expected to care for and tend to their appearance 24/7; but if they appear to be vain or spend too much time and money on such pursuits, they are judged harshly. I think we could all stand to be more forgiving when it comes to cosmetic surgery, because looking good is often linked to feeling good. And we could all use a little help in that department.

The pace of progress in the cosmetic-surgery industry has picked up dramatically. This often leads to lingering questions after that first meeting with a patient. What I hope this book will offer, in part, is an extension of the time I spend with my patients. I hope it will answer any questions that still remain — that one pressing question you always forget when you're with your doctor but recall the second you're back home. This book is my attempt to be as clear, concise, and transparent as possible, ultimately to help people look and feel better. This includes current patients, potential patients, and people who might never come into my office but are simply looking for some good advice.

I hope to help those who are considering cosmetic surgery to determine the procedures that will best address their concerns, but also to give them a way to look beyond the superficial and address the totality of self. It is important to me that patients understand that good health, emotional well-being, and a sense of satisfaction in life are vital to our progress as human beings.

Writing this book is a way for me to share some of the knowledge I've gained over the past 25 years, in a rapidly changing business in which advances in surgical and nonsurgical procedures have meant exciting progress in the array of services plastic surgeons can offer their patients. I envision the book as a private and candid conversation between a doctor and his patient, in a less rushed atmosphere than the typical 30- or 40-minute initial consultation. This is my opportunity to dispel myths, to offer beneficial information (some of it involving surgery and some just relating to good health and self-fulfillment), and to share a bit of what I've learned in several decades working in beauty, medicine, and wellness. You may be surprised by some of the things you'll read, but pleasantly so, I hope.

I believe beauty is emblematic of total health, involving one's superficial appearance, to be sure, but also reflecting one's emotional, psychological, and physical fitness. I will offer guidance about the foods we eat, the substances we should avoid, and the vitamins and minerals we ought to embrace.

For many patients, I am their mirror. They come to me and implore me to tell them what they need. But the best results happen when patients who are invested in the outcome do more than ask me to recommend enhancements. Education is the key that I hope readers will use to unlock a state of superior well-being and health.

CHIP'S TIPS

1 Learn as much as you can about your possible future plastic surgeon. You will share your hopes, dreams, and expectations with him, and you need to make sure you are in skilled, caring hands.

2 Make sure your surgeon is not only board certified by the ABMS (American Board of Medical Specialties) but is a specialist in the type of surgery you are contemplating.

3 Make your goal to have plastic surgery reflect your innermost thoughts and feelings. Plastic surgery should not define you but merely help complete you.

4 Do your homework and consider all your options. Ask questions and challenge yourself until you get that "gut feeling" that this doctor and staff are the right fit for you.

5 Your face is not the place to cut corners, use a coupon, or buy something that "tastes like Coke." Invest in the real thing.

6 Make sure your surgeon has done hundreds, and preferably thousands, of the procedure you are contemplating. You can't hide your face underneath your clothes.

7 Plastic surgery has been around for centuries; make sure your surgeon is taking advantage of modern techniques like lasers and endoscopes.

8 Review the before and after pictures of several patients who are similar to you with respect to age, gender, ethnicity, and procedure choice. You want your surgeon to do several of these surgeries each month — not over a longer period of time — which helps indicate that he is a true specialist in his field.

Author's note: *Please forgive my use of the gendered pronouns he, his, and him. While there are many qualified female cosmetic surgeons, there is no gender-neutral pronoun to describe us all. So for the sake of easing the reader's experience, I will use masculine pronouns.*

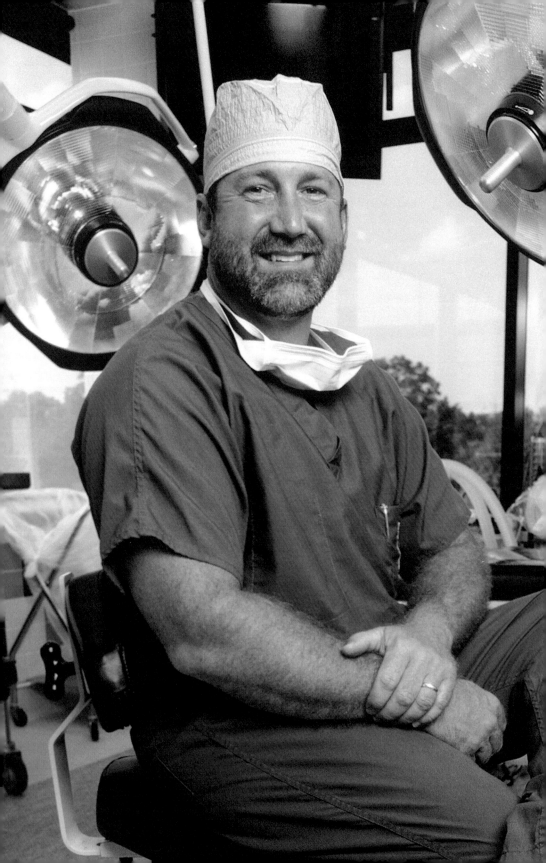

CHAPTER 2

* * *

CHOOSING WISELY:
MAKING SURE YOUR DOCTOR AND SURGICAL PROCEDURE ARE THE RIGHT FIT

"Women now mistakenly think that having a cosmetic procedure on your face is the same as having your hair or your nails done. But a bad cut can grow out. A nicked cuticle will heal. But damage to your face? That's permanent. It was an ugly lesson I learned the hard way, to the tune of about $90,000 and untold damage to my physical and mental well-being. I'm living proof that every one of us has to do our homework beforehand." — *Rhonda (see page 38)*

The doctor-patient relationship is one of the most complex, intimate, and special in the world. People share concerns with me to which even their husbands, wives, and children are not privy. Any good doctor will tell you that he takes that relationship very seriously. Which is why trust is so essential.

This is doubly true when you're looking for a cosmetic surgeon, and entrusting something as personal as the appearance of your face and body to a doctor. You are entering into a partnership based on honesty and mutual respect. That's why finding the right doctor is so vital. You want to entrust your care to someone reputable and skilled, but also someone you can communicate with and who listens to your concerns.

REFLECT ON YOUR REASONS

Motive is often the least discussed factor in cosmetic surgery — possibly because it seems too private or is considered a given. I urge my patients to take all the time they can for reflection, prior even to scheduling a consultation. After our initial meeting, I caution them repeatedly to consider and ruminate on their many options.

Don't rush into cosmetic surgery because you want to look your best for an upcoming wedding or high-school reunion. The results of this work will be with you for a significant portion of your life, but that social event will be just one of many moments in a full and rich life. So don't give your surgery a deadline.

Once you've clearheadedly considered your motives for surgery, and measured your willingness to enter into an open and forthright relationship with a doctor, it's time to start looking for a cosmetic surgeon.

TAKE YOUR TIME

Take the time to find the doctor who best fits your needs. Your search for the right cosmetic surgeon is not the time to comparison shop, find a bargain, and sacrifice quality. You aren't shopping for a car or comparing grills at Costco and Target. This is your face we're talking about, the gateway to your thoughts, your life, your personality, your soul. A grill? Well, it's just a grill, easily replaced when it breaks down. A cosmetic surgeon should not be viewed as a one-stop shop, but as an important person in an ongoing relationship who will help you to make gradual changes that correspond with the way you age. Your surgeon's office is not like the nail salon, where you go for a quick, temporary, psychological boost. You are investing in long-term results, rather than splurging on a one-time quick fix.

Take the time to shop for a doctor who understands you, respects you, listens to you, and acknowledges what you're asking for. But also make sure to find a doctor who shares his expertise and knowledge — someone who will make sure you're well-informed and making the best choices for your unique situation. You want someone who has been around for a while, has done hundreds — even thousands — of the surgeries you are considering, and who is a long-standing and respected member of the medical community.

RESOURCES

Use all the resources you can for finding the doctor who best suits you. Your first resource in choosing a doctor should not be the phone book, which only measures a surgeon's ability to pay for ad space. Somewhat more reliable are national magazines that vouch for skills or rely on certain doctors as experts in their fields. My more informed patients know, for instance, after reading the 73rd magazine article in *Vogue* or *Elle* citing Manhattan dermatologist Patricia Wexler, that she is undoubtedly a top-tier doctor and an authority in her field. Seventy percent of doctors interviewed in national magazines are leaders in their chosen fields. Reputable regional magazines with a long history and trusted journalistic practices can also be great resources for finding a quality physician.

Many such magazines with long-standing reputations, such as *Atlanta* magazine and *New York* magazine, feature annual surveys of the best doctors in each field. These publications survey doctors within the community, asking them which physician they would choose to treat them or their families. You can trust the results because the top docs are chosen by their peers, not by how much they spend on advertising. Where readers can get into trouble is putting their trust in less reputable magazines with suspect editorial practices, many of which will exchange editorial space for advertising dollars. Doctors place an ad somewhere inside the magazine's pages, and the magazine agrees to write about them in what appears to be objective reporting. So be wary of your local lifestyle magazine touting its list of the top plastic surgeons in the area: those surgeons may have paid for that prominent placement, which is not exactly a guarantee of surgical excellence.

A better approach is to ask your friends, neighbors, and people whose opinion you trust for their recommendations. Another great option is to ask a nurse who works in any of the doctors' offices you normally visit for his or her recommendation. There's a reason nurses are often a reliable and unacknowledged resource for patients: Doctors, especially those in the same field, can be very competitive and disparaging of other doctors. But nurses tend to have the inside track on area doctors; they see a lot but aren't motivated by professional jealousy or competition. They can give you a good idea of a doctor's reputation and standing in the medical community.

Another great resource is a high-end hair salon, because good stylists recognize good work when they see it. There are a dozen stylists in town whom I have never met but who send me patients all the time, because they see my work and feel confident recommending it. Think about it: what other person besides your spouse has such an up-close and personal view of your face? Stylists are in your hair, looking behind your ears. They see everything, and from every possible angle. I recommend asking one or two high-end stylists in your area if they've seen any great work, or any bad work. This is, of course, with the caveat that occasionally a doctor — knowing

that stylists are often trusted beauty consultants whose clients solicit their advice —
has been known to offer kickbacks to stylists who refer potential patients.

If you have more than one doctor on your list of recommendations, consider
visiting all of them to see which one best meshes with your personality and your
core values. It is often only through visiting more than one doctor that you can
weigh the differences in style, demeanor, values, and expertise.

But if your first visit to a recommended doctor is great and you feel like his and
your philosophies are a good fit, you can generally stop there. It's not necessary to
shop around unless you're having a hard time finding a doctor who resonates with
you. I was recently on a panel of plastic-surgery experts. Out of the five of us, I was
the only doctor who didn't charge for an initial patient consultation. Everyone was
shocked. The reason I don't charge to consult with a new patient is that I want them
to compare me to other docs. Even though someone is willing to spend $20,000
on a procedure, they're often not willing to spend $150 for each of four consultations.

As Rhonda states in the epigraph at the beginning of this chapter (and you
can read about her case at the end of this chapter), taking any cosmetic procedure
lightly is a bad idea. Doing copious research on the procedure you're interested in,
as well as the doctor who will be doing it, is imperative. Armed with information,
patients are far more likely to find happiness, rather than heartbreak, at the end
of their self-improvement journey.

GET A FEEL

It is very important to get a feel for any doctor's environment. Once you've con-
cluded preliminary interviews and decided on a cosmetic surgeon, your next step
should be to schedule a consultation at the doctor's office to see if you feel confident entrusting him with your care. Although the primary consideration is how
the doctor relates to you and vice versa, also take into account factors outside the
exam room, which can give you equally valuable information.

Much can be learned about a doctor just by crossing the threshold into the
office, which can reflect the aesthetics of its occupant. Pay attention to the surround-
ings as you wait for your appointment to begin. Does the office look established or
like it was just recently occupied and could be packed up in an instant? Is the
reception area clean, orderly, and inviting? Or are *Reader's Digests* stacked up from
five years ago? Was the office decorated with care, or does it look like someone
hastily assembled the remainders from a hotel sale? Is it located in an established
building in a reputable part of town, or is it in a space that seems dingy or temporary?

A doctor who can't afford a decent building and office space, or doesn't care
about the aesthetics of where he does business, should make potential patients

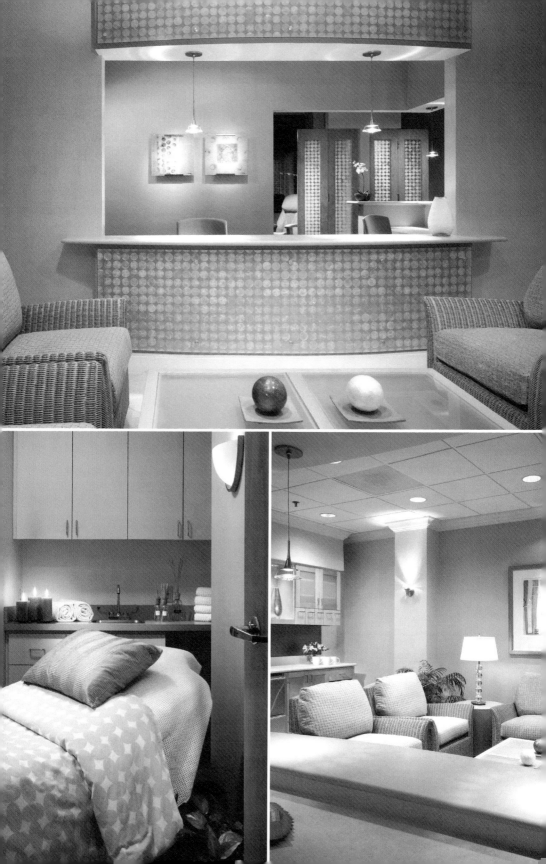

wary. If the building or the office are subpar, he is not thriving in his practice for some reason — and he is certainly not sweating the details. I'm a details person, and I tend to think that any cosmetic surgeon should be. I think it's important to welcome my patients with coffee or tea, filtered water, and fine chocolates to offer comfort and relaxation (as well as guilt-free antioxidants, of course!). Doctors who overlook what might appear to be "small" things in their office space may be the ones who overlook small things in their surgical care.

Beyond the office ambience, another crucial marker in appraising a doctor's office are the people who work for him. Are you greeted by the staff at the front desk when you approach, or do they seem disinterested in your presence? I can't stress enough how vital the attitude of the staff is to a doctor's practice and a patient's experience. Are they helpful and courteous? Or are they belligerent and uncaring? Are they professional, cheerful, and energetic, or do they seem unmotivated and careless? Whether we admit it or not, we instantly judge people by the company they keep. If a doctor hasn't trained his front-office team, people who answer the phones and schedule appointments, to be courteous and caring, what can you possibly expect from his more clinical staff — the nurses and aestheticians who will play a more essential role in your care? Medical-office team members are a direct reflection of the attitudes of the doctor they work with.

So many times, I have encountered someone in the service profession, a cashier or a department-store clerk, who was so unhelpful or downright rude that it soured my perception of that company forever. When you are dealing with something that can make you feel as vulnerable as surgery does, you don't need that kind of negative attitude marring your experience and making you feel like the people who should be caring for you don't.

The fact is, anytime we enter a medical setting, we feel like children again — exposed, uncertain, putting ourselves in someone else's hands. A doctor who doesn't get this and doesn't train his staff accordingly is not worth your time. I don't care if you're carrying a Hermès Kelly bag and wearing a softball-sized diamond or carrying a Target Marc Jacobs knockoff: everyone deserves the same courteous treatment, whatever their social station. It's really not up to the doctor's staff to do a little economic triage to sort the "worthwhile" patients from the "not worthwhile" ones. A doctor's office shouldn't make you feel like you're shopping at a snobby department store.

Other readily apparent but subtle clues at that first office visit that can reveal the kind of doctor you're dealing with. You can tell a lot from the body language of the staff when they interact with the doctor about what their relationship is like. As with so many things, there is a trickle-down effect from doctor to staff; if they seem surly or uncomfortable in the doctor's presence it could be because they don't take their work seriously, don't feel appreciated, or don't respect their boss. If the staff seem unhappy, you will most likely be unhappy, too.

All of these warning signs indicate that this is not a caring, productive, compassionate office. Think about it: if the doctor doesn't show concern for the staff he sees and works with every day, what is his attitude going to be toward patients, whom he sees far less frequently? The fact is, most doctor's offices, whether the doctor is male or female, are staffed by women: if the doctor sees his female staff as inferior and not worthy of his consideration, those prejudices may extend to his patients; he may see his female patients' concerns as petty, shallow, or trivial.

Another key element of your potential doctor's practice is maintaining staff loyalty. What is the turnover rate? I always advise patients considering major surgery to do a little reconnaissance. Get a feel for the office. Try out some skin-care services or perhaps Botox to see — without too much risk — what you can expect from the doctor as well as from his staff. Because if you are going in every few months or so and you notice a lot of new faces, they may be having trouble keeping personnel, which ought to be a red flag. This is probably not the best place to get your face lift, with a doctor who is perpetually training a new nurse to assist him.

Then there's the first meeting with the doctor himself. Does the doctor listen to you? Does he seem rushed? Does he keep you waiting a long time? Is he condescending, or does he take the time to explain the differences between the procedures you're investigating? What is his attitude toward nurses and assistants? Is he brusque, or pleasant and professional?

A good doctor will give you a comprehensive skin-care plan and let you know how he thinks you will respond to the surgery or procedures you're interested in. He'll let you know your options for your particular issue of concern. What are the quick fixes (are there some minor, nonsurgical options, like lasers or filler)? Are you interested in an expedient camouflage or a longer-term corrective procedure? What about more enduring solutions, like surgery? What are the risks associated with surgery, which can involve everything from infection to asymmetry?

To me these big-picture/little-picture conversations are a lot like remodeling your house. You can take different approaches. You can fix up the kitchen or bathroom piecemeal, or you can redo the whole house. There are advantages and disadvantages to both options. A doctor should be able to give you a sense of what you can expect from simple maintenance in contrast to a real overhaul. He should be able to tell you about the recovery process for whatever procedure you choose. Both surgery and less invasive procedures have advantages and drawbacks, and your doctor should offer frank appraisals of both without trying to promote the most invasive or expensive option. If you ever get the sense that he's trying to sell you on a procedure, you should strongly consider walking away.

I feel that the days of "trust me, I'm a doctor" are over. I frequently tell my patients that, while they may not have the surgical skills to enter the operating room and actually perform the procedure, they need to understand each procedure and know why they're choosing it. If you don't take the time to educate yourself, then you can't make the best decision. Your doctor is there to provide you with information and to assess each procedure as it relates to facial harmony; but ultimately, you must make the decision about which procedure is right for you based on all the factors the two of you have discussed. The improvements you select will be with you forever, whereas your doctor only gets to see them in the office — a mere snapshot in time.

EMANCIPATE

Try to shed past experiences so you can approach your cosmetic surgery or procedure with an open mind. Perhaps you've had an unpleasant experience with a doctor in the past and have since become fearful or cynical about doctors. If you have deep-seated trust issues with the medical community, you might want to examine whether an elective surgery is in your best interest. If you still think it's the direction you want to go, treat it as a new experience and be open to the possibilities, instead of fearful of the outcome.

SURGERY OPTIONS

Compare and contrast outpatient and inpatient surgery. Ideally a doctor should have hospital privileges for every procedure performed in an outpatient setting. This can be confirmed easily by calling the hospital(s) where the doctor has privileges and asking which procedures he has privileges to perform. To obtain those hospital privileges, doctors must go through peer assessment and peer board review, which ensures that they are competent to do that procedure. Because while board certification measures physicians' written and oral skills — or how smart they are — it doesn't measure how good a surgeon they are or how well they take care of patients. Without hospital privileges, if a doctor is working in his own surgery center, who's going to tell him whether or not he actually has the talent to perform a certain procedure? Who will critique him and confirm that he's well-trained?

There are, of course, benefits to an outpatient surgical setting. Patients are afforded a consistent level of care when a doctor has handpicked the staff attending each patient. An outpatient surgical setting ensures more privacy and a more intimate approach to each patient. Also, there are often lower costs and less bureaucracy in having outpatient surgery in a doctor's accredited surgery center, rather than a hospital.

If a doctor has only an outpatient setting and no hospital privileges, you should ask whether he is proctored by a peer physician in the community, who approves him to do surgeries in his own facility. There has to be a system of checks and balances to make sure doctors are qualified to do the procedures they are offering, and unfortunately the onus is often on you, the patient.

Another important consideration here is the anesthesia. Any surgery that lasts more than three hours, or requires the use of general anesthesia, should have a board-certified anesthesiologist in attendance. For surgeries lasting less than three hours and those requiring mild sedation, an on-staff CRNA (certified registered nurse anesthetist) is suitable. Remember that at an outpatient facility, unlike a hospital, there isn't the full complement of medical staff to assist in an emergency.

Make sure that in the event of a complication or unexpected emergency, the doctor and his staff are suitably trained to handle those situations. It's very important for a physician doing surgery in an outpatient setting to have ACLS (advanced cardiac life support) certification. If there is any adverse event, you want your surgeon to be trained in emergency and lifesaving skills.

Routine safety drills in an outpatient facility might seem like a minor exercise, but they suggest a certain thoroughness in a doctor's approach. An office where surgeries are performed should conduct all emergency safety drills — including lifesaving drills and fire-safety drills — at least once a quarter. The facility also should have a written protocol and agreement with a nearby hospital for emergency transfer, so the staff knows how to proceed in an emergency situation.

PRACTICE DUE DILIGENCE

After you've visited the doctor's office and experienced a sense of his approach, or even before you make that initial office visit, look into his credentials. Make sure you understand his qualifications and what surgeries he's able to do. As cosmetic surgery has become a more lucrative business, doctors from other specialties have begun to dip into the field. So you have general surgeons performing breast augmentation and dermatologists doing face lifts. It can be very difficult to distinguish between a doctor who is truly qualified and one who is merely a dabbler. Scenarios of doctors from other fields delving into cosmetic surgery aren't necessarily bad; you just want to make sure that the surgeon doing breast augmentation, for instance, has received advanced training. Make sure he has enough experience to do a procedure that, because of its ubiquity, may seem straightforward but is really quite specialized and complex.

The most valuable information you can have is a working knowledge of board-certification basics. The American Board of Medical Specialties, or ABMS (www.abms.org), which is composed of 24 member boards, is the first place to check on a doctor's board certification. Call 1-866-ASK-ABMS or search their website to make sure a prospective doctor is board certified in the relevant field. Realize, though, that proper credentials don't end there: If a board-certified surgeon, for example, gets some rudimentary cosmetic training — and not a full fellowship — to get into the lucrative business of breast augmentation, he won't have the experience in breast reconstruction that a plastic surgeon with advanced fellowship training might have. It follows that he also won't have the equivalent experience. So definitely look into your doctor's board certification and any advanced training.

You can also check the American Medical Association's website, at https://extapps.ama-assn.org/doctorfinder, to get some basic information about a doctor's licensing and education, and to see if they are a member of the AMA. Clearly, if a doctor says he went to Harvard Medical School, and you find from a web search of the AMA or other sites that he went to medical school in Guadalajara, you should run, not walk, away from that office. The AMA requires that its doctors adhere to its Principles of Medical Ethics, another important safeguard in checking a doctor's legitimacy. The key tenet of those principles is "responsibility to patients, first and foremost."

Some experts will tell you that potential cosmetic surgeons must be certified by the American Board of Plastic Surgery (ABPS) — the only board certified by the ABMS for plastic and reconstructive surgery. There are other qualifications that are more important in determining whether a doctor is qualified to do the surgery you are considering. Having the right credentials does not mean a doctor is skilled in the specific surgery you are having performed. And a doctor who has merely done some training in cosmetic surgery is not necessarily the best qualified for the job.

First a little background: When the ABPS first came into existence, plastic surgeons were dealing with injuries caused by car wrecks, wounds, burns, and other traumas that required reconstructive surgery. Plastic surgeons were not in the business of offering aesthetic improvements to healthy patients. Today's plastic surgeons are similarly not always well-versed in aesthetics. Those who have completed a fellowship in aesthetic training are more aptly trained and well-qualified.

So while it is crucial to have ABMS board certification, it is not an absolute requirement that the certification be in plastic surgery, which means the surgeon can be very far removed from cosmetic surgery. A plastic surgeon, for instance, might work with skin and muscle, but perhaps entirely on burns. Does that qualify him to perform a face lift or liposuction? Perhaps not.

Accreditation is another safeguard that helps you ensure that the medical facility in which the doctor operates is part of a larger community and has been monitored and declared safe by a knowledgeable board. You need to make sure that the facility where the doctor does surgery is state licensed and accredited. The accreditation should be from one of three well-recognized groups: The Joint Commission (formerly JCAHO), which is the gold standard used by every hospital; the Accreditation Association for Ambulatory Health Care (AAAHC); and the American Association for Accreditation of Ambulatory Surgery Facilities (AAAASF). To achieve accreditation, an office must meet stringent requirements for its staff and equipment, as well as its doctors, who must also have privileges at accredited hospitals.

I also urge you to check in with your state medical board to see if a physician has been disciplined. In Georgia, where I practice, you can call 404-657-6494 or check www.medicalboard.georgia.gov to see if your doctor has been disciplined since 2005. In California you would go to www.medbd.ca.gov. Every state has a searchable database where disciplinary action is noted and where you can see if a doctor's medical license is active or lapsed. For even more information about a doctor, consult the Federation of State Medical Boards (fsmb.org), which allows you to check, for a fee, that the doctor you're seeing in Georgia is not simply someone who was disciplined in New York and fled south to practice.

It gets a little more complicated to check on current lawsuits or those in which a judgment was made against a physician. You will most likely need to go to the individual court location in the county where the physician may have been sued. Each year, 8 to 10 percent of doctors working in this country are sued, and unfortunately, frivolous lawsuits are a fact of life in our litigation-happy country. According to a recent story in the prestigious *New England Journal of Medicine,* a high-risk specialist has a 99 percent chance of being sued by the time he's 65. Those high-risk specialties include neurosurgery, thoracic surgery, general surgery, orthopedic surgery, plastic surgery, and gastroenterology. So if you hear that your doctor has been sued, or find out for sure that he has, it might be instructive to ask your doctor for the details rather than automatically discounting him. What was the nature of the suit and the outcome? More than anything else, you're looking for a pattern in which a doctor is sued again and again for repeated instances of negligence or poor results.

Of course a basic Internet search of your doctor is also a good way to check on his reputation. In addition, there are a number of online health-care websites that offer ratings of doctors. *The following page shows a list of some of the best resources, along with some of our client's thoughts about our practice.*

One caveat: many of these websites allow posts from anonymous reviewers who have the luxury of protecting their own identities while savaging someone else's reputation. And many of these medical-review sites are skewed toward a certain type of customer. Generally it's the angry, dissatisfied customers who flock to these sites and not the happy, satisfied ones. So temper your findings with this understanding.

DOES YOUR DOC MEASURE UP?

Perhaps the greatest measure is the doctor's standing within the medical community. How your doctor is perceived among his peers is one of the best indicators of his level of professionalism and the medical community's regard. Ask your doctor if he does any teaching or publishing. You want someone with a sense of curiosity who partici-pates in ongoing education, including his own, and who's interested in more than just making money. This kind of engagement indicates a professional who cares deeply about excellence in the field of cosmetic surgery, and not just his own practice. It's an honor to be invited to lecture or share one's skills, a sign of respect that comes only to those who have the most to contribute. It's yet another yardstick by which to mea-sure a doctor's accomplishments. An invitation to lecture one's fellows or to publish one's findings in a medical journal is evidence of both the professional community's recognition and a doctor's credibility. These opportunities demand that professionals stay current in their field, using state-of-the-art practices.

You don't want a dinosaur who's stuck in the past, doesn't keep up with the latest advances, and still does face lifts in exactly the same way he learned in medical school 35 years ago. I can tell some physicians' work from two tables away at a restaurant because they haven't updated their techniques and are still leaving tell-tale traces of outmoded methods on their patients' faces — for instance, crossing thick skin into thin skin to create a stair-step effect that doesn't heal well. I know a certain physician, for instance, who has been doing the same nose for 25 years. Whether the patient is young or old, has a heart-shaped face or round one, they all get the same nose. It's obvious that such doctors have not kept up with the times. I like to say that this type of surgeon learns for one year then repeats for 24 more. Therefore, those 25 years of experience need to include growth in both updated techniques and current literature.

www.vitals.com *"I've had BOTOX and fillers by several different doctors in Atlanta including a dermatologist and another plastic surgeon. Dr. Cole is hands down the best in town. I won't go to anyone else ever again! Love my results!"* — B.B.

www.sharecare.com *"Dr. Cole is such a wonderful doctor and a really good person. He was so kind and caring when I saw him, he made me really feel at ease, even though I was so nervous to see him! My surgery turned out just beautiful! God bless you, Dr. Cole!"* — C.M.

www.kudzu.com *"Dr. Cole did such a beautiful job on my son's eyes. We had been to another doctor who did his first surgery and it was a disaster! Thank God for Dr. Cole! He is a very kind and caring man, and we couldn't be happier with him and his office!"* — R.H.

www.angieslist.com *"Several years ago I had Dr. Cole as a surgeon. I regard him as one of the best in his field."* — C.S.

www.yelp.com *"I saw Dr. Cole for eyelid and brow lift surgery. I live in N.C., so we stayed at a hotel 11 miles from the facility the night before surgery. Everything went so well — never felt any pain and slept all the way home. The entire experience was easy, the staff was so helpful, and Dr. Cole did a beautiful job. I'm 65 and feel so good about my appearance now! He gave me back 10 years."* — T.B.

www.ratemds.com *"I absolutely could not be happier with my skin after what Dr. Cole did for me. Strangers compliment my skin, and people who know me ask what I did — after they comment on how awesome I look! Every month my results just get better and better. The longer I go the better I look. I go without makeup, and my dark eye circles are gone; the collagen is obviously boosted, and at this point, all my desires have been <u>fully</u> addressed. I feel and look amazing!"* — P.H.

www.healthgrades.com *"I am extremely pleased with Dr. Cole about the results of this last operation/laser surgery procedure. I can truly say that this is the first time in years that I have felt good looking in the mirror."* — M.N.

www.makemeheal.com *"...since the devastating mutilation done to my eyes years ago from another surgeon (who is no longer in business), I couldn't have had a more talented surgeon than Chip to finally fix this, and I would never take a chance with anyone else in the future."* — C.M.

www.drscore.com *"Wonderful staff — excellent experience."* — E.L.

A good question for a patient to ask the doctor is, "How do you do surgery X differently now than you did ten years ago?" He should be able to explain and justify his technique.

MATCHMAKING

Ensure the doctor's experience fits the procedure you want. It's imperative to check credentials, but equally important is practical experience. Take for example a procedure called blepharoplasty, more commonly known as eyelid surgery. Most general plastic surgeons have performed roughly two dozen blepharoplasties to complete their training. A dermatologist would typically complete 30 by the time he finishes his dermatology residency. An ophthalmologist has probably done 150 to 200. Then you take someone who's finished a cosmetic fellowship, and they've typically done five hundred. Someone who's completed an oculofacial plastic-surgery fellowship, because it's completely focused on the face and eyes, has performed closer to 1,000.

As an example for comparison, over my 25 years in practice I've performed more than 25,000 surgeries. And because of my ophthalmic microscopic surgical training, I work in a world of millimeters rather than inches. When dealing with an area of the face as delicate as the eye, precision is key.

So look at your doctor's specialty and gravitate toward someone who pays extreme attention to detail. An ear, nose, and throat specialist, for instance, may exercise much more precision than, say, a general plastic surgeon, who may not have that same experience with minutiae since most of their work involves large flaps of skin and expanses of the body.

Though medicine shouldn't always be reduced to a numbers game, in this case the numbers are very important. As we know intuitively, there's an enormous difference between a 15-year-old with a learner's permit behind the wheel and a 40-year-old driver with years of practice and experience. The same is true in cosmetic surgery. Over time doctors develop a finesse and fluidity in their work that only comes from a breadth of experience. You want to be the two-thousandth patient for breast augmentation, not the third.

The frequency with which a doctor has done a certain procedure is important, too. Has the doctor you're considering done 20 face lifts over the past eight years or 20 over the past two months? This makes a huge difference, so ask about frequency as well as numbers. There's a reason we call the medical profession "a practice," because (perfect) practice makes perfect.

SEE THE EVIDENCE

Check the doctor's work and references: credentials and experience are important, no doubt, but you should also check the physical evidence. Ask your doctor to provide pictures of actual patients who have had a procedure exactly like, or very close to, the one you're investigating. This is another way to make sure your prospective doctor has done many of the type of procedure you are considering: he should be able to provide multiple images of that procedure.

Sometimes doctors will try to pass off a manufacturer's picture as their own. Not good. What you don't want to see are photos supplied to the doctor by the advertising and marketing departments of filler manufacturers and medical-supply companies. For a deeper perspective, and knowing that most doctors will only show photos of their best work (sometimes known as their "brag book"), you might ask your doctor to show images of a patient who was unhappy with her results.

When requested, your doctor should also be able to provide you with multiple references of patients who have undergone the procedure you're considering. If patients are happy with their results, and the doctor has kept in touch and has a good rapport with his previous patients, those are encouraging signs.

Over my 25 years in business I've performed more than 25,000 surgeries. And because of my ophthalmic microscopic surgical training, I work in a world of millimeters rather than inches. When dealing with an area of the face as delicate as the eye, precision is key.

I don't recommend that you talk to former patients right off the bat, but if you're a potential patient and you've looked at images, taken the time to think about the procedure, verified credentials, and still want to make sure this doctor and procedure are right for you, then talking to a few patients is perfectly appropriate. In my own practice I keep a rotating list of about 30 patients who are very happy to talk to prospective patients who are considering their procedure.

Now that you've done your due diligence in making sure your doctor is right for you, it's probably time to consider what you can bring to the table. Following are some of the things you can do to make sure that you've done everything you can to ensure good results.

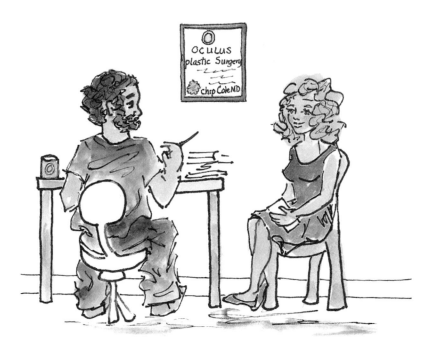

"I like the mini-lift idea…but I want the maxi-result."

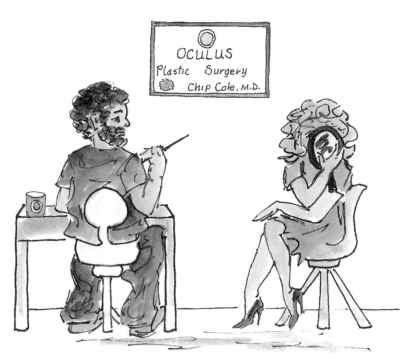

"Fix my eyes and neck, I meet a rich man,
get (re)married, and have two vacation homes."

DO YOUR HOMEWORK

I've mentioned quite a few things for patients to consider when auditioning a potential doctor (a lot of which could apply as easily to finding a good OB/GYN or dentist), but it's equally important to know what you, the patient, need to consider regarding your own role in the process. It is your responsibility to do your homework, come prepared, disclose pertinent information, and enter into a transparent relationship with your doctor. Because ultimately, the relationship between a doctor and his patient is an interdependent partnership. Each person must do his or her part to make sure the outcome is successful.

Some people mistakenly think that because cosmetic surgery is elective and deals with aesthetic issues that it shouldn't be taken as seriously as other medical procedures, or that the same degree of candor and seriousness you would bring to a visit with, say, your urologist, is not as important when dealing with a plastic surgeon. But that is simply not the case. As a 2011 story in *Forbes* reported, cosmetic surgery is a serious business worthy of real consideration. I couldn't agree more with Anne Wallace, the chief of plastic surgery at the University of California San Diego Health System, who is quoted in the article: "People think it's like going out to lunch. Like any surgery, it needs to be taken seriously."

It's startling to me how flippant certain people have become regarding cosmetic surgery, and it's frustrating when they don't want to hear about the risks associated with it. But now is not the time to omit any pertinent information. For instance, that stroke you suffered a year ago. Or the fact that you smoke, drink, or use illicit drugs. You may think these are private matters; but if you're having surgery, they quickly become very relevant (and dangerous) if the surgeon has not been previously made aware of them. Before you submit to any surgery or cosmetic procedure, take the time to have a conversation about preëxisting medical conditions, previous surgeries, health issues, allergies, sensitivities to key ingredients, alcohol and drug use, and family medical history. Communication is essential. Taking the time to exchange this valuable information could literally save your life.

The reason patients should divulge these things is because this surgery is elective, and your life should not be elective. So while issues like drug use and blood clotting are biggies, it would be wise to disclose to your doctor even minor issues, including sensitivity to certain cosmetics, food allergies, daily use of low-dose aspirin and over-the-counter anti-inflammatories, diet pills, herbal medications, and habits like smoking, exercise, or frequent sunbathing. You also need to know the dosage and strength of any prescription medicines you are taking. If you've been prescribed a number of medications, bring in a list for your doctor so you don't forget anything. What may seem inconsequential to you is of great consequence to your doctor. Also key is making sure your cosmetic surgeon has your complete and up-to-date medical records so he is well aware of your medical history. If your medical history is extensive, the best thing to do is send your records along before your doctor's appointment so he doesn't have to speed read your information during your consultation.

It's also useful to do a little research before seeing a doctor. Launch a fact-finding mission into the procedure that interests you. Do this in the same way you would do some preliminary research on a company before interviewing for a job there. I like it when my patients have a baseline level of information when they come to see me. The more intelligently someone can discuss a procedure, the better decision they're going to make, because they're not coming into my office feeling overwhelmed or uninformed. During consultations, I'll sometimes sense hesitation or confusion on the part of a patient, because they may have little familiarity with the sorts of procedures they are requesting.

This can be avoided with a little research. It's helpful for someone interested in fillers, for instance, to know the difference between a volume filler — which I liken to putting a pillow under a sheet, allowing you to walk out that day with improved volume — and a stimulatory filler, which uses an agent to stimulate your body to make more collagen to thicken your skin. The latter is great because it looks so natural and develops over a three- to six-month period. But if the patient wants to go to a reunion in two weeks, they clearly don't have time for a more gradual stimulatory filler. The difference between those two procedures makes more sense to patients if they walk into the conversation with a foundation of knowledge.

In terms of plastic-surgery results, it's important to set realistic expectations. If you think a cosmetic procedure will make someone fall in love with you, transform your life, or guarantee happiness, then surgery may not be for you. Plastic surgery can improve your appearance, but it may not significantly alter your life. So don't ever enter into a face lift or breast augmentation to make someone else happy. Your plastic surgery should be for you. When someone who says (or even implies) their love for you hinges on a change to your appearance, perhaps it's the relationship that needs to be examined, not your looks.

There needs to be a lot of soul-searching involved in cosmetic surgery, and I think it's helpful to do some emotional homework long before you make that first appointment to visit your prospective doctor's office. The worst thing you could possibly do is make a fix to your exterior when there are deeper issues at play, either in your relationship or in your own sense of self, that need more immediate attention.

It's also helpful for patients to bring in pictures from ten years earlier. Why? Because it gives the doctor a good feel for the rate at which the patient ages. People assume that aging progresses each year at the same pace. But aging is like a lot of things; it comes in spurts. A stressful event, weight changes, and other factors will give you a little burst of aging. So it helps to see where someone was ten years ago. Plus, I like to talk to patients about their expectations regarding aging, so they're not doing procedures that work against their natural anatomy or to conform to some aesthetic ideal.

Pictures can be a big help in that regard. I've found that pretty much everything is relevant when it comes to the face: the whole complex network of a patient's psychology, history, and present state of mind come into play when striving to achieve great results. An open dialogue between patient and physician about expectations for results guides the physician to use those pictures to gauge the patient's concept of self.

I'll give you an example. I had a patient who had an issue with her eyelids that she wanted to have corrected. The photos she brought in were full-body shots from her competitive bodybuilding days. You couldn't even see her eyelids in the images. But what I could see was a woman who had the sense that fixing that one issue with her eyes could possibly restore the youthfulness, vitality, and athleticism she had exhibited in the past. Those images were a way for me to gain some insight into her expectations and self-image.

The pictures you choose will tell your doctor so much, reinforcing the idea that it's up to you, the patient, to be reasonable in your expectations. I've had women in their 70s come in with a picture of themselves from when they were in high school. That's when I know I need to have a conversation about realistic expectations and explain, as diplomatically as I can, that surgery can turn back the clock but it can't bring back that 17-year-old girl. Unfortunately, there's no cure for aging. That's another reason I like to put a 10-year limit on photos.

I also advise patients to listen to what their doctor tells them. Don't go in with a fixed idea and refuse to trust the experience and wisdom of your doctor. He may be able to suggest alternatives and things you haven't thought of. I, for one, am all about educating people. I'm a big believer that if you're educated properly, what you learn will resonate with your soul. Often, older patients will come to me when their spouse has died, or one of their children has gotten divorced, or because they've received an insurance settlement. I'm always cautious recommending a procedure when the attendant emotions (anger, confusion, elation) are at play. I tend to suggest that they wait until things settle down a bit, that this is not something we want to rush into.

Which brings me to my next point about patient awareness: Don't rush. Take your time. Don't make the decision until meditating on it for a month or more; you don't want to be impulsive. I recommend that if you're getting ready for an event that's slated for the next quarter or two, consider fillers and Botox. Six months later, you can perhaps think about doing the full monty. Timing is everything.

I like to see patients two months after a significant birthday or event. Because by then, they've settled down and they can plan. Sometimes patients need a reality check when it comes to timing their desired surgery. If, for instance, a patient is thinking about a face lift in preparation for a major event like a wedding, I try to be the voice of reason. I remind them that they aren't preparing just for that wedding date. They are going to have parties, see friends, be photographed, and they don't want to be recovering and making excuses.

Patients need to prepare themselves for the realities of surgery: the investment, downtime, recovery period, any possible complications from surgery, and the real possibility that they may need a follow-up surgery (aka "a touch-up"). It's best to find out how your doctor handles such follow-up procedures should they become necessary.

THE MATTER OF MONEY

All this brings us to the subject of money and the consideration of your finances. You may think a certain procedure is absolutely necessary, but is refinancing your home really a suitable way to make your dream come true? You might be considering borrowing money or tapping into your savings for a procedure. But if follow-up surgery is required, or if complications arise, do you have the financial safety net to handle that contingency? As I mentioned, I don't turn patients away for inability to pay, but for most doctors this is not the case. When the money is gone, so is the care. But the onus is truly on the patient to make sure he or she has a financial safety net to handle any complications that could arise.

Some people would advise you to ask your physician about the breakdown of costs for a particular procedure. But that can be a problematic question. When discussing doctor's fees, my typical response is, "My assistant is taking detailed notes so that when you meet with my scheduler, she can enter the procedures into the computer and give you the various costs to consider. My focus right now, though, is on your medical care. Let's not backward-engineer an approach based on budget, but rather focus on what procedure will be the best for you."

But it is important when assessing fees to make sure you're being quoted the total fee. When you are quoted a fee by the doctor's staff, make sure it includes not just the surgeon's fee but the operating room facility fee, anesthesiologist costs, and any other related expenses.

PREPARE YOUR FAMILY AND FRIENDS

If you are planning extensive, invasive surgery — like a breast augmentation, rhinoplasty, or a face lift — prepare the people closest to you. You don't need the trauma of others' surprise, not to mention their own negative issues, when going through recovery. If you're the only woman in your peer group who has had a breast augmentation, for example, prepare yourself for possible issues of jealousy and the judgment that can result (which usually extends from others' own body issues). Women are often the worst critics of other women, and you should prepare yourself and possibly your friends for the possibility that while *you* may end up loving the results, *they* may not. If they are true friends, you might ask them to demonstrate that fact by keeping their negative comments in check. After all, you're hoping for their *support*, not just their *approval*.

Prepare your spouse, too. Let them know that the surgery is for you and does not reflect negatively on them or on your relationship. If you have small children who will notice the physical change in your appearance, reassurances are needed on that front, too. This applies less to things like Botox or Juvéderm or a host of other procedures that, let's face it, even husbands don't notice sometimes. But for more substantial and noticeable procedures, let your children know that — like buying a beautiful new suit or dress, or wearing makeup — you're just trying to look and feel your best.

Most children think their parents are perfect as they are, and could be dubious about the prospect of improving on perfection. Or your child might be frightened by talk of doctors or surgery if those things are associated in their minds with injury and trauma. It's probably best to spare them too much detail on that front, but prepare them for the reality of bandages or recuperation time so that it won't come as a total shock.

The most important thing is to reassure them that you're going to be OK and that nothing will change in your relationship with them. Do remind them that you love them just the way they are and that there is nothing they need to change about their appearance. This is especially important for girls, both teenaged and younger. You don't want them to get the message that acceptance and love in your family is conditional and based on the way they look. To keep them from feeling judged or found wanting because of your procedure, you may need to go a little overboard on this. After all, teenagers are already contending with the toxic aspects of an appearance-based culture.

KNOW THE RISKS INVOLVED

Surgery is surgery, whether elective or essential, and it helps to know the risks. This is a serious endeavor, and there are always risks involved. We live in a society full of disclaimers on everything from our morning coffee to our gym memberships. We tend to tune out the disclaimers because they're everywhere. But you can't afford to ignore the risks. As a primer, here's the first paragraph from every patient consent form in my practice:

> *People naturally want their results to be good, and generally believe they will be. They also tend to believe that possible serious complications, many of which are rare, will not happen to them. But despite the best care, complications can arise. Although the overall incidence of a given complication may be low, if it happens to you, the incidence is then 100 percent in your case.*

Ask your doctor about complication rates, but understand that complications are difficult to quantify. I think a reasonable question is, "Have your patients ever experienced complications?" Ask the doctor how those complication were resolved. What you should be looking for is the way in which the doctor responds to that question. If they're defensive, if they say they never have complications, if they're dismissive of the question, be wary.

You can learn a lot about a doctor by their demeanor when responding to a question about complications. They should be forthcoming and honest, and if they have had a complication (and most doctors who practice with some frequency have), they should openly admit as much.

Finally, if you've had a bad experience with another cosmetic surgeon, I would advise you to first take the time to fully recover before changing to a new doc for a redo. But before you seek one out, if at all possible return to your original surgeon and give him the opportunity to resolve your issue. I have found that if the patient maintains a united front with the original doctor, and they both work together to manage the case, most often the outcome is positive.

In the end, the relationship you have with your cosmetic surgeon is vitally important to your physical and psychological well-being. If at any point in the process, you end up losing respect for or rapport with your doctor, you need to find another one—but only after you've attempted to reconcile your differences. You owe it to yourself to be forthright with your opinions and honest about your dissatisfaction. Your doctor knows the extent to which time heals all wounds; you may not.

Look at that discussion as an opportunity. If it indeed becomes a failed relationship, then you will feel so much better knowing that you made every effort. It will serve your psyche well during the upcoming redo surgery, with its prolonged recovery and added expense. Needless to say, try to find and use the best surgeon to minimize the chances of a postoperative complication.

I can honestly say that I've never seen a complication that could not be resolved by working together rather than against each other. Make sure you protect your health by thoroughly investigating the doctor to whom you are entrusting your face and body. But by the same token, consider your own responsibility in that arrangement and make sure you're doing everything you can to be honest, realistic, and fair when dealing with your doctor.

Despite the best care, complications can arise. Although the overall incidence of any given complication may be low, if it happens to you, the incidence is then 100 percent in your case.

ASK THE RIGHT QUESTIONS

A key question to ask your potential doctor is, "What will happen once I am undergoing the operation?" Ask him if he will do the entire surgery himself, or if he will use any assistants to help suture, or for other tasks. Some doctors will allow surgery residents to watch them perform surgery, which is common, and a good way for new doctors to educate themselves on procedures. It's also positive for patients: it shows that your doctor is a trusted, involved, and consulted member of the medical community, rather than some rogue surgeon working in isolation. Of course, if a patient objects to having other professionals observe, I would respect their wishes.

What you don't want is your doctor using residents to assist. It happens all the time, especially at university hospitals, that a doctor may do one side of a patient's face and allow a resident to do the other side. You want to avoid this scenario at all costs. I've seen patients in my office (and I can tell this before even examining them) who've had two different surgeons work on them.

The fact is, plastic surgery is a subtle, sensitive art, and two doctors doing the identical procedure will almost invariably not achieve the same results. Certain intuitive qualities that are intrinsic in surgery — tension, pressure, thickness — constitute the art of medicine; everything you can't teach but can only learn over time. There's a lot of "proprioception" (from the Latin, meaning "one's own") involved in the delicate art of cosmetic surgery. Proprioception is that sense of the position of parts of the body relative to neighboring parts of the body. A patient with a mass in his cheek feels that mass from the inside as well as the outside, whereas a doctor can only feel it through touch, and only from the outside. What comes with experience and technique is a doctor's ability to understand those connections between the part and the whole of a patient.

TAKE RESPONSIBILITY

Finding a great cosmetic surgeon is a two-way street. It's not just about you interviewing a potential doctor. It's also about taking responsibility for your role in this partnership and being a good patient who divulges important information, is informed, does not set unrealistic expectations or come to the doctor's office with a hidden agenda. Establishing trust with your doctor requires absolute honesty from the get-go. You're putting your skin, musculature, blood, and bones in this doctor's hands.

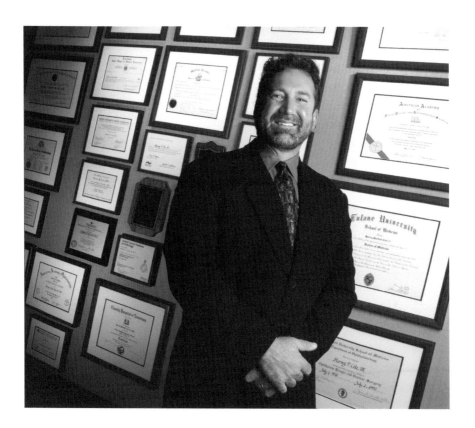

Be careful not to be coy or selective with the information you offer. If a doctor is going to do his best work for you, he has to know everything about your situation. You can hold a little in reserve for your psychiatrist or for your significant other — give them something to work for, a mystery to unravel. But a consultation with your doctor? This is the time to unburden yourself of all those mysteries. You (and your doctor) will be glad you did.

When considering plastic surgery, honesty is key — both with yourself and with your doctor. I'm shocked again and again by the information patients withhold from me that could have a disastrous effect on their surgery and its outcome. I am a trained professional with over 25 years' experience in my line of work and copious additional specialized training. I treat surgery as both an art and a science. I don't like a jack-in-the-box that jumps out at me when a patient is lying on the table. I often think, for instance, of the woman contemplating major surgery who failed to tell me about a stroke she had suffered years earlier that had left her with still-sluggish motor skills and without full mobility in her arm. Or patients who fail to disclose previous surgeries, or the fact that they smoke, use recreational drugs or drink frequently — all highly contributive to the surgical outcome.

A WORD TO THE WISE

Computer imaging has afforded great advances in the field of cosmetic surgery. Patients can see, with the aid of realistic images, what their likely results will be. But pay attention to the way your doctor uses this technology. Is it used as an educational tool, or for the "wow factor," to coax you into a procedure with the promise of dramatic improvements? My personal goal is that more patients come back to me after surgery and say they look better than their imaging predicted. If your doctor instead feeds all your pixelated fantasies, you may be disappointed by your actual results. Additionally, a doctor should be able to share image sets from former patients, to demonstrate how closely the final surgical outcome matched the computer rendering — another useful tool for assessing his results.

Be wary if a doctor is offering huge discounts not associated with bona fide companies that frequently team up with doctors to offer such specials. For instance, a supplier will often approach its leading injectors and offer them Botox at reduced prices, to incentivize them to bring in more Botox patients. This is very different from a doctor promoting 50 percent off of his services on Living Social or Groupon. If a doctor is offering a filler deal on Groupon, it looks more like an act of desperation than anything else — like Walmart putting deeply discounted peanut M&Ms up front to lure you into the store.

WHEN CONSIDERING A DOCTOR...

1 Ask friends, trusted health-care professionals like nurses, other doctors, and even hair stylists for recommendations.

2 Pay attention to the office. Does it look like a fly-by-night operation, as if things could be packed up at a moment's notice? Notice the ambience of the office space, its cleanliness and location.

3 Pay attention to staff behavior and attitudes. Are they efficient and friendly or brusque and unhelpful? Is there a lot of staff turnover?

4 Ensure that your doctor is really there for you. During your exam-room visit, is your doctor prompt? Is he an active listener who gives you the big picture about a procedure you're considering or does he try to hammer home his own ideas?

5 Check the doctor's credentials. Is he board certified by the American Board of Medical Specialties?

6 Make sure the facility where your operation will be performed is accredited by one of three organizations: The Joint Commission (TJC); the Accreditation Association for Ambulatory Health Care (AAAHC); and the American Association for Accreditation of Ambulatory Surgery Facilities (AAAASF).

7 Choose a doctor who teaches or publishes regularly, which demonstrates active engagement with the medical community and a commitment to keeping abreast of developments in his field. Both are positive signs of a doctor's competence.

8 Research your doctor on one of the many medical rating boards. You'd Google a prospective first date to find any available information; you should do the same for a prospective doc.

9 Find out about licensing and disciplinary action taken against a physician by consulting your state medical board.

10 Ensure that your experience will be as safe and comfortable as possible. A doctor should have hospital privileges for every procedure he does in an outpatient setting.

11 Make sure your doctor will be doing the surgery without assistance from a resident or other attending physician.

12 Check how often, and over what span of time, your doctor has performed the procedure you're considering.

13 Ask to see photos of actual patients and, if still in doubt, speak to a patient who has had the surgery you're considering.

14 Examine your doctor's motives. Does he use computer imaging to educate and show realistic results? Or does he use the "wow factor" of the technology strictly to peddle his services?

15 Get a realistic sense of the cost of the procedure that you are interested in.

16 Be wary of discounts and advertised specials.

YOUR TO-DO LIST

1 Disclose all pertinent information about your medical history, prescription and over-the-counter medications, lifestyle, and drug and alcohol use to your doctor.

2 Understand that cosmetic surgery is a serious business, with risks and possible complications, and it should not be entered into lightly.

3 Research in advance the procedure you're considering, so you can walk into your consultation with some awareness of suitable treatments.

4 Set realistic expectations about what a surgery can do for your life. It will not make someone love you, and it may not transform your life.

5 Bring in photos of yourself from 10 years ago. It helps the doctor assess the rate at which you age, as well as your self-image.

6 Listen to your doctor. He should have ample experience in the procedure you are considering and be able to offer realistic and reasonable advice.

7 Don't rush into surgery, especially not with an event in mind, like a wedding or a milestone birthday (ending in zero). Consider it carefully.

8 Make sure your finances are in order. Don't undergo surgery if you have to refinance your house and if you really can't afford it. Make sure you have a financial safety net, should complications arise.

9 Prepare those closest to you for the unveiling, especially if the changes will be noticeable or dramatic.

10 Assess the general risks from the procedure, but also those that apply to you personally.

11 Familiarize yourself with the American Medical Association's Code of Medical Ethics, which was devised to protect you. Be on the qui vive for doctors who veer from these established codes.

Four years before she came to see me, Rhonda had impulsively decided to have a quickie filler procedure during a weekend shopping trip with girlfriends in Washington, D.C.

"I was in my early 40s and had a few fine dry lines I wanted to take care of," Rhonda recalls. "The doctor injected me with the wrong filler and I ended up looking like a freak."

Rhonda admits she didn't do her homework prior to the procedure.

"With all the magazine and TV ads and all your girlfriends throwing at-home Botox and filler parties, where you stand around and sip cosmos, the risks associated with these procedures are being completely ignored," warns Rhonda. "Women now mistakenly think that having a cosmetic procedure on your face is the same as having your hair or your nails done. But a bad cut can grow out. A nicked cuticle will heal. But damage to your face? That's permanent. It was an ugly lesson I learned the hard way, to the tune of about $90,000 and untold damage to my physical and mental well-being. I'm living proof that every one of us has to do our homework beforehand."

One refund in D.C. and four follow-up surgeries later, Rhonda was back home in Louisville, with pulled-down eyelids and severe lumps beneath her eyes. Doctors had removed the filler and subsequent scar tissue, but they couldn't take away the pain. For four years, every time Rhonda looked into the mirror, she would jam her index finger into the two miniature speed bumps under her eyes, silently willing them to submerge forever into her face.

It never worked.

"I looked hideous," she recalls. "Every time I looked in the mirror, it hurt my self-esteem and my very soul. It was a constant reminder of how stupid I had been. After a general plastic surgeon at Duke recommended Dr. Cole, I flew to Atlanta and consulted with him, toting along my 70 pages of medical records," says Rhonda. "At the end of the session, I finally heard what I hadn't heard from any of the other doctors I had been to. It was just six little words, but they meant the world to me: *'I think I can help you.'*

"He had a confidence that none of the other doctors had demonstrated. With those six words, he had instilled hope in me again. I remember thinking, 'He's a nationally known teacher on this, he's quadruple board certified, and he has a decades long resume.' That doctor in Washington, D.C., incidentally, is now out of business. So, I signed on for surgery number five.

"Before the surgery, I called my surgeons in Louisville to describe the procedure Dr. Cole had recommended. They told me, 'We've never even heard of that!' He was even able to re-sculpt my cheekbones the way they used to be," marvels Rhonda.

Outcome: I wish I could tell you the need for a redo like Rhonda's is a rarity, but unfortunately it's all too common in my line of work. Here was a woman who had opted to have a procedure without doing adequate research and then had a far from optimal result. It's so important to stress that one-third of my medical practice is devoted to redoing surgeries of other doctors' work from all over the world. Through the years, I've acquired a pretty extensive national and international reputation as the "eye guy" for doing repair work on many patients.

The sad truth is this: People will spend twice as much time researching an automobile purchase than a plastic surgeon, to whom they are granting access to their face or body. For most body surgeries, such as breast augmentation, you can certainly hide any asymmetries, for the most part. You can hide an unflattering haircut under a hat until it grows out. You can change your brand of makeup or your wardrobe if you make a poor decision; it's a much more serious prospect to change your face if a mistake is made. When something goes wrong, fixing it can be costly and devastating.

Remember this: It's far easier to go to the right doc the first time around than it is to restore your looks after you've had less-than-optimal surgery. Restorative surgery means dealing with scar tissue and blood-flow issues, which complicates and compromises follow-up efforts, no matter how skilled the surgeon.

Unfortunately, Rhonda was a representative example of that scenario. She had a lot of contour changes, scar tissue, excessive skin that was removed, and volume deficits that were challenging to correct. She also had an unnatural, surgical look and a harsh appearance to her eyes. As her doctor, seeing those eyes made me truly sad, because Rhonda is such a sweet person and she has a huge heart.

I recommended a leading-edge restorative procedure that entailed surgically going up through Rhonda's mouth to the upper gum line, about an inch above her teeth, to remove scar tissue and any remaining filler from previous procedures, as well as to restore volume where it was needed. Because she had already undergone four previous surgeries to correct the problem, I encountered significant scar-tissue and blood-flow challenges. But I was able to get her back to where she had been, appearance-wise, before that first ill-advised procedure in Washington, D.C.

Following her corrective surgery, Rhonda spent the night in an Atlanta luxury hotel and returned early the next morning for a follow-up visit with me, before her father drove her back to Louisville.

"Dr. Cole's staff held my hand every step of the way," she says. "I think they knew, given my history, that I required a little more attention because my faith in doctors was shaky at best. Either Dr. Cole or his staff checked in on me routinely in the days following my surgery and were always available when I called them. The staff understood my fears about the swelling on my face and reassured me that the outcome would be different this time. I even got a reassuring phone call from Dr. Cole a few days after surgery."

Rhonda had photos taken of her post-op progress and emailed them to my nurse, who showed them to me. I closely monitored Rhonda's recovery from hundreds of miles away in Atlanta. In subsequent photos she regularly took from her home in Louisville for me to evaluate, I could tell the surgery had been a success (I could also tell from the smile on Rhonda's face!). When she told me her old confidence and spirit had returned and that she felt renewed energy and drive in her career, I knew her positive results were everything we had set out to accomplish together, and more. After four long years, Rhonda's sweet personality was back and she was smiling at people again.

"Even though we weren't in the same city, the level of patient care was amazing," Rhonda reflects. "As I recovered and the swelling began to subside, I saw my old face reëmerging. I'm a professional woman who travels for work. I'm the president of my local Humane Society. I have to look my best. I'm not one of these ladies of leisure, spending her day at the spa. How I look has a huge impact on my career. Slowly, for the first time in years, I felt my old confidence and self-esteem returning. I went from looking like a bloodhound to having eyes that are beautiful again. I get emotional even now, talking about it. I'm not going to sugar-coat it: Dr. Cole is a miracle worker."

"Be who you are and say what you feel,
because those who mind don't matter
and those who matter don't mind."
— Dr. Seuss

CHIP'S TIPS

1 You have a legal right to your medical files. Retain a copy for your records and bring them with you whenever you see a new doctor for the first time.

2 Before your visit, give a lot of thought to how you feel about the way you look; make specific notes regarding the areas you're dissatisfied with so you'll remember to bring them up during your consultation.

3 When making a major purchase such as a car, you take the time to carefully weigh your options. Your face and body deserve far more cautious consideration.

4 There are many resources available to find the plastic surgeon who is best for you. Two of the best are nurses and stylists. They know great work when they see it.

5 You pride yourself in knowing what is best for you. Follow your instincts — you have spent many years developing them through many experiences — both good and bad.

6 Modern technology alone is not a guarantee of great results. Discuss the pros and cons with your plastic surgeon and review his before-and-after books. Be sure the pictures are his — not an instrument company's or another doctor's.

7 When you are undergoing surgery and trying to minimize all risks possible — always lean toward M.D. anesthesia, preferably at a ratio of one anesthesiologist to one patient.

8 Discuss your surgical goals with your closest friends and family before surgery. It is very stressful to keep dodging those who are closest to you.

9 The best and most natural-looking way to counteract gravity ("the big G") is to restore your own natural anatomy. The number-one thing I recommend is volume correction.

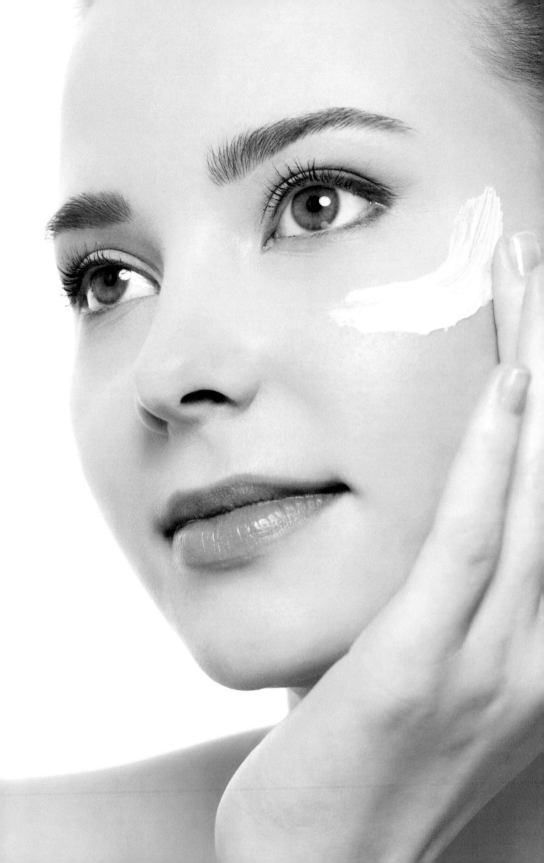

CHAPTER 3

*** * * ***

THE KIDS ARE ALL RIGHT:
LOOKING YOUR BEST THROUGH
THE TEENAGE YEARS

It's undeniable that teenagers are thinking, even obsessing, about looks much earlier than they did in the past. In the world we live in — filled with preening pop icons, celebrity supermodels, and paparazzi-hounded movie stars — they may have no choice.

In my day, long before the advent of metrosexuals and cougars, people cared about their appearance; but it was considered unseemly, even a little vulgar, to be preoccupied with your looks. I like to refer to those days as the development of "Catholic guilt"! Those days are long gone. You need look no further than the latest newspaper shocker about an eight-year-old beauty contestant getting Botox or a 16-year-old pop star undergoing breast augmentation to realize that some of us have lost our grip on reality. Unfortunately, impressionable children and teenagers are often those hit hardest by the toxic beauty culture that tells them looks are *the* most important thing.

When even adults show questionable judgment in their relentless pursuit of perfection, how are kids supposed to get a rational perspective? Driving to work recently, I was listening to a radio show about a woman who had lost 50 pounds and still felt unattractive. She believed, even with her dramatic weight loss, that her friends still got more attention from men. Her mirror-mirror-on-the-wall response to that anxiety? To post photos of her friends on the station's website and ask radio listeners to vote for the most attractive among them. These are adult women, mind you. Just the fact that in 2014 grown women are asking to have strangers rate them does not exactly set a great example for children and teenagers, who could probably use a better class of role models.

Today's teenagers live their lives so much more out in the open, on Facebook and Twitter or in posted videos on YouTube. They have become exceedingly public and increasingly vulnerable, exposed and dependent on the judgment of others in the process. And this is often before they've even developed a sense of self. When you care too much about how others see you, you stop focusing on what makes you happy. Teenagers today swim in a more visually oriented ocean, and that pervasive indoctrination to look better, even perfect, is relentless and damaging to kids still formulating their identities. Once upon a time, the magic of Disney was limited to movie theaters or Sunday-night TV; now it's in their face 24/7 and even available as an app for their smartphones.

It presents a quandary for someone in the beauty business, which is founded on the idea that alterations to one's appearance can improve quality of life. On the one hand you want to take the concerns of your teenage patients seriously. On the other, especially as a parent, you want to tell them not to grow up too quickly, not to let looks define their lives.

My objective — both in my practice and in this book — is to give young people useful, realistic advice about the beauty issues they face, while helping them gain that elusive quality of perspective. Perspective is probably the most useful thing adults can hand down to their kids. But it is often very hard for kids to swallow when they see adults as hopelessly clueless, old, and out of touch. Nevertheless, I feel it's part of my job to remind kids that the things they find so important at 16 — their nose, their weight, their dimples, you name it — probably won't be what they're obsessing on at 26 or 36. Education is a key part of what I do, and it's not just kids I'm educating. I want anyone considering a surgical change to their appearance to think "long term" and not "quick fix." I encourage them to examine the root reason for their visit and whether surgery is really the best way to fix it.

My whole reason for writing this chapter about teenagers is twofold. As the father of three children who have successfully navigated the various minefields of their teenage years, I feel protective of this age group. Teenagers are endless sources of fascination but also repositories of fear for older Americans. They often get a bad rap in our society, and adults tend to stereotype them as brainless or sex-crazed, shallow or out of control. We tend to worship babies, adore children, then become wary when they mutate from obedient, parent-admiring creatures into parent-questioning, willful teens. But I love the sense of discovery and questioning, and the formation of personalities, that continue as kids transition into adolescence. I think parents need to respect and honor this time of transition — instead of vilifying it — and help teenagers navigate the treacherous waters of our often superficial, instant-gratification culture.

The other reason for my interest in helping teenagers and doing something positive to improve their lives, both through skin care and through other causes, is more personal and painful.

When my youngest son was growing up, he had issues with drugs and alcohol. It was a scary time, and things became so bad that we actually had him escorted to a wilderness program that turned his life around. To this day, he is so grateful for this rather dramatic intervention; it showed him that his parents loved him and would do anything to make things right. He learned that through hard work and endurance he could overcome anything.

But one of my son's closest friends at the time suffered from social anxiety and also struggled terribly with drugs. Unfortunately, his was a very different, tragic outcome. He used drugs to self-medicate — the same way you often see adults using alcohol in social situations to feel at ease and treat their own anxieties. He wasn't as lucky as our son. His parents did everything they could to help him — they even sold their house to help fund his therapy. They are the most loving and family-centric parents I know — "perfect parents" by anyone's definition. For a time, their son managed to quit drugs. But what many don't realize is that people who use hard drugs develop a physiological tolerance. After they quit the drug and have been away from it for a while, if they relapse and return to using the same amount as before, their body loses its tolerance and isn't prepared for the shock. And so, at 21, he accidentally overdosed. I can't imagine a worse thing for a parent to go through than to lose a child in such a violent, heartbreaking way. His name was Cody.

It made me think: if that could happen to a teenager whose parents could afford to give him everything in terms of love and supportive involvement, and to pay for therapy or detox to help their child, what happens to kids who don't have those resources?

I want these extremely sensitive kids to realize their worth, turn their situation around, and become productive, contributing citizens in society. That is the reason I founded the nonprofit **Face Change**, which has become a way for me to help make a difference. Face Change is dedicated to helping teenagers find their way through what can be a very painful, difficult time in their lives. It expresses my belief in the importance of the teenage years in shaping the person to come. Today's teenagers will be tomorrow's world leaders.

Through my experiences with my own children and their friends, I have recognized that there are a lot of kids who could use education or counseling to get through difficulties in their lives. In starting the nonprofit, my goal was to create a program to address real-world problems faced by teenagers. I decided to earmark 10 percent of my surgical fees from every Oculus Plastic Surgery facial procedure and 100 percent of all profits earned from this book, to provide scholarships and counseling for teens going through a whole host of difficulties — from anxiety disorders to bullying to drugs — whose parents don't have the financial resources to pay for professional help. I want to help them, in the best way I know how, to transition from their teenage years to adulthood, letting them know that there are adults out there, even strangers, who care about them.

To me it seems a win-win for all the well-intentioned people who want to have a cosmetic procedure but feel guilty or embarrassed about putting their money toward something elective when there is so much need, suffering, and financial hardship in the world. I wanted to somehow allay those reservations by making it possible for them to have the improvements, while knowing that a portion of their money was "paying it forward" to help a kid in need. To learn how you can help, go to ***www.FaceChange.info*** for more information.

In the meantime, understanding what a huge role skin plays in a teenager's self-image is a good start. Knowing the difference between when a young person needs help, and when they are merely convinced they need it, is an art — one shared by patient, doctor, and parent. Below are some very real issues teenagers face:

ACNE

The most pressing skin concern for my teenage patients is, of course, acne. Acne is a shortened term for the bacterium that commonly causes surface skin changes: *Propionibacterium acnes*. And the most in-demand cosmetic procedures for this age range are chemical peels and microdermabrasion.

Acne is a nightmare for teenagers; parents should be sensitive to its effect on self-esteem and do everything in their power to help. It just isn't fair that at a time when kids are at their most self-conscious — and dependent on the approval of their peers — this social scourge starts to crop up. Acne is not just a physical malady, it's a psychological one, undercutting self-esteem and keeping its sufferers from enjoying life. It can engender loneliness, isolation, and sometimes even deep depression. Don't let this happen to you. Get help instead of suffering with it.

Fortunately there are a number of treatments that can keep acne in check and diminish the aftereffects of scarring, both prescription and non-prescription. These

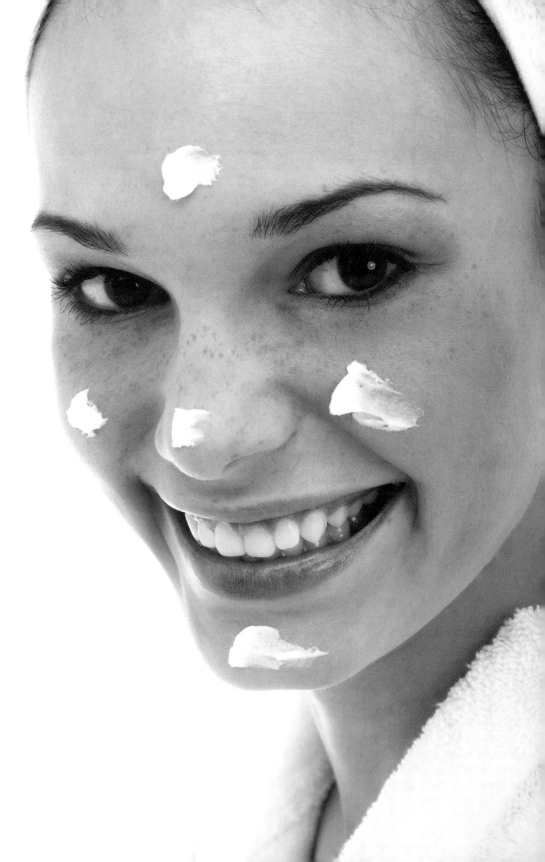

include oral antibiotics, retinoids, and topical antibacterial treatments like benzoyl peroxide. I advise teenagers who suffer from acne to consult with a plastic surgeon, dermatologist, or medical aesthetician right away — especially if over-the-counter treatments aren't helping and their acne is interfering with their social life, making them feel anxious or isolated. There is no reason to live with it. Remember that the majority of teenagers get acne, so you should never feel like it's just you. After all, you're special, but not *that* special.

Before I offer solutions, here's a little background on the how and why of acne, a condition that comes in several different forms: Deep under the surface of your skin are beneficial sebaceous glands, the oil-producing factories that keep your skin hydrated. Acne begins when the surging hormones of adolescence cause an increase in the production of oil (sebum). When that sebum mixes with bacteria and dead skin cells in our pores, it leads to a blockage in the pore, most often a blackhead (in which the surface of the pore remains open) or a whitehead (where the surface of the pore is closed).

Cystic acne forms deep beneath the surface of the skin and produces painful red sores — mini-lakes of infection under the skin — making this the most serious and damaging form of acne. The infection is so deep under the skin that there is no way to drain or "pop" the pimple to hasten its departure, so patients are advised not to pick at cystic acne. This can cause it to get even more inflamed, as the infection spreads beneath the skin's surface. Cystic acne is more likely than its more benign counterparts to leave scars, so it's important to find a good treatment to clear up this kind of acne.

Beyond prescribing antibiotics or topical treatments, a doctor can use cortisone injections to get rid of a new pimple when you have a big date or an important event coming up.

The most important thing to remember when dealing with acne is to keep your skin clean and make sure the oils and dirt that can clog pores don't have a breeding ground. One of the most basic but crucial things to remember is not to touch your face — at all! That means no cradling your chin in your hand or allowing your fingers to drift thoughtlessly to your face, as your teacher drones on and on about history (those who fail to learn from history are doomed to repeat it in college). Avoid hair gels and oils that can seep from your hair into your skin and cause irritation along the hairline.

I also recommend a rigorous regimen of ruthless cleanliness when it comes to all the things your face comes into contact with: pillowcases, towels, washcloths, and so on. Change your pillowcases at least twice a week. Change your washcloth with each cleansing. And keep a dedicated towel on hand just for your face — one that doesn't accumulate all the hair-care product, toothpaste, and soapy buildup that can gunk up your workhorse towels. Change that face towel at least a couple of times a week. The whole point is to keep free of all the bacteria and hitchhiking dirt and oils that can jump from those linens onto your face.

SKIN CARE

Among the most valuable things I provide teenagers is help with skin care. The Oculus Skin Care Centre offers everything from the cleansers that will keep their skin clear to the makeup that will make them look subtly beautiful instead of slatternly. (Look it up; it could be on the SAT.) Ten percent of my patients are teenagers and, besides the occasional medically necessary procedure, such as correcting blepharoptosis (drooping eyelids that can affect vision), most of them want to find out how to take better care of their skin, inside and out.

CLEANSERS

For teenage patients susceptible to acne, I recommend cleansers with the anti-inflammatory ingredient salicylic acid, alternated with a pore-purging cleanser with benzoyl peroxide (like Oculus MH Cleanser) and a spot treatment like Oculus BlemErase touch stick with sulfur and resorcinol. Sulfur and resorcinol are usually found together in acne products. Resorcinol helps prevent comedones by removing the buildup of dead skin cells. Sulfur has been used for more than half a century to treat acne, although exactly how it works is still unclear.

I am a firm believer in spending adequate time cleaning the face, rather than the usual soap-on, soap-off routine. A great tool for making sure the skin gets scrupulously clean, and one that's also great for exfoliating, is the Clarisonic brush, which forces you to stand at the sink for two minutes washing your face while the sonic frequency removes makeup, oil, and dirt with a thoroughness manual cleansing can't. You can pick up a Clarisonic brush up at a number of retailers or at the Oculus Skin Care Centre.

Toners can also be useful as a way to remove any makeup or dead skin cells that remain on the skin after cleansing and can give a refreshing, super-clean feel to your face. Toners are ideal for those with very oily skin. Super-hydrating toners are a wonderful option for dry skin because they allow serums to penetrate deeper into the skin. They are more of an optional step, so if you like the way they feel and your budget allows, go for it.

MAKEUP

A common mistake young people make in using cosmetics is to apply too much.
A thick, heavy concealer can clog your pores and mask your problem rather than
allow your skin to breath. Often all you need is a tinted moisturizer, a cover-up stick
for individual blemishes, maybe some translucent powder, some great eye makeup,
and a light gloss. These should all be noncomedogenic, meaning they won't clog
your pores. Your goal with makeup should be to enhance what you already have
rather than cover it up.

For teenagers beginning to use makeup, I recommend they see their dermatologist or visit a physician-supervised skin-care center like Oculus. Here they can
find help in tailoring products specifically to their needs (rather than experimenting
willy-nilly or rushing to the department-store counter, where the makeup artists
are just going to try and sell their products). A doctor or aesthetician will likely
steer them away from irritating or pore-clogging makeup.

I also tell my adult patients that individualized, boutique skin-care service will
help them more in the long run than the generic experience of going to a department
store for advice. When our aestheticians do makeup applications for teenagers,
they emphasize subtle, flattering, less-is-more makeup. Products like foundations
and concealers that claim to be oil-free are not enough to keep pores clear.

**Earlier I mentioned noncomedogenic makeup. I recommend the Jane Iredale line
of cosmetics to my teen patients.** Iredale makeup contains ingredients that are so
good for your skin, some of my aestheticians tell me that young people can
occasionally sleep in the makeup and not wake up with a terrible breakout the next
day. (Although I would never recommend that to a teenager.) I like this line because
it is free of oil, talc, dyes, parabens, preservatives, and fragrance, all of which can
irritate the skin. The powders and foundations also include sun protection, a great
value add. And Jane Iredale Disappear is a concealer that contains green-tea extract
to help treat blemishes while hiding them.

It's also good to change out your makeup regularly — especially eye products
like liners and mascara, which can lead to infection when they get old, but also any
foundations or concealer sticks, which can harbor bacteria. If you are worried
about acne, the best approach when using mineral makeup or powder is to clean
your tools every day. Your brushes or your sponge applicators — whatever tools you
use — need to be cleaned with soap and water and allowed to completely dry
before you use them again.

LET'S GET SERIOUS

When those over-the-counter Clearasils and Oxys aren't working anymore, it's time to break out the big guns. Over-the-counter products can only do so much, because the strength of their crucial ingredients (like benzoyl peroxide or salicylic acid) are so low. The benefit of working with a doctor or a medical spa is that you can find products with higher strengths — a moisturizer with 15 percent AHA/BHA (alpha hydroxy acid and beta hydroxy acid), for instance, versus a measly 2 percent over-the-counter formulation. The 15 percent AHA/BHA from Skin Medica, available at Oculus and other doctors' offices, is a good moisturizer that will help keep your skin clear.

PHYSICIAN-STRENGTH PRODUCTS

In addition to an array of higher-strength cleansers, moisturizers, and toners that can improve your skin, your doctor can offer prescriptions of topical treatments, injections, or antibiotics that can considerably improve the skin's condition.

While Retin-A might seem like something for women worried about wrinkles, this topical prescription retinol is actually useful in speeding up cell turnover, that very important process that keeps gunk out of your pores. You can probably expect some redness, irritation, and flakiness when you first begin using this product; but with time, most of those side effects should go away. I always tell my teen patients, if you are going to use Retin-A to clear up your acne, then you need to use products with a reasonable SPF during the day and be extra vigilant about avoiding the sun. Caution is advised, because Retin-A will increase your skin's sensitivity to the sun, and you will be more likely to burn.

Many female patients who suffer from acne also respond well to birth-control pills (Ortho Tri-Cyclen, Yaz, and Estrostep), which contain the hormones estrogen and progestin, and decrease the amount of the acne-spiking androgen hormone. Side effects include an increased risk of stroke and blood clots, so women of any age should definitely not smoke while using these pills. Come to think of it, they shouldn't smoke at all. It will wreck their skin, and it leads to the kind of bad breath most teenage girls who are interested in relationships want to avoid.

The drugs Sotret, Claravis, and Amnesteem, which contain the potent ingredient isotretinoin (also found in the once discontinued drug Accutane), offer a last-resort medication for patients with severe cystic acne. Female patients who are on these medications must be on birth control to avoid pregnancy, since the drug can cause severe birth defects. They also should check in with their doctor every month, so side effects such as depression can be monitored.

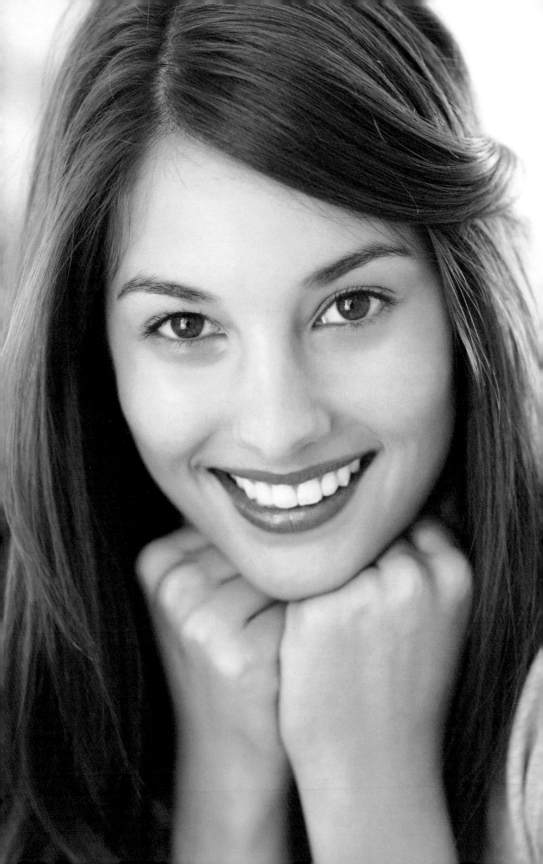

LIGHT CHEMICAL PEELS

Parents tend to hear the word "chemical" and usually say, "Not my child." But chemical peels are minimally invasive procedures in which a mild acid such as glycolic, lactic, salicylic, or malic acid is applied to the skin to allow dead skin to slough off. They can have a big effect on acne and acne scars, helping the skin to clear rapidly. My preferred peel is a light 45 percent glycolic-acid peel, where there is no downtime, or an Illuminize Peel, both of which work wonders in removing the ravages of acne, as well as brightening the complexion. The peel can be repeated at regular intervals until the optimum results are achieved. Risks include hyperpigmentation and infection; but as long as you discuss your skin and medical history with your doctor, he should be able to tell you if the procedure is right for you. You will likely experience some stinging, redness, and irritation following the peel. This "therapeutic buzz" is a desirable temporary effect that will quickly subside.

FACIALS

Regularly scheduled facials can work miracles in keeping skin clear, especially when they are tailored to acne-prone skin. A deep pore-cleansing facial that uses steam and extractions can do wonders in cleaning the skin and clearing pores of debris. If you have acne-prone skin, just be sure to tell your aesthetician (if it isn't obvious), so they can be sure to use products that won't aggravate your condition.

LASERS AND FILLERS AND DERMABRASION, OH MY!

LASERS
A great option for treating acne scars is the Fractional CO2 laser, which is used for skin resurfacing. The process essentially boosts the skin's collagen production. Collagen is the substance that makes your skin plump and healthy looking. The Fractional CO2 laser uses beams of light energy to bore tiny holes into the skin, which speeds up the skin's collagen formation as part of the natural healing process. There is minimal recovery time, with redness and swelling tending to last only a few days. However, the results can be incredible.

I always recommend that patients considering procedures that produce noticeable changes to their appearance do them during transitional times in their lives. One of the best times for teenagers to do such a procedure, so as not to attract unwelcome attention during high school, is the summer before they start college.

I'll never forget the young patient who had developed fairly extensive acne scars and came in for laser resurfacing between high school and college. After undergoing the Fractional CO2 laser treatment, the difference in this young woman's appearance, confidence, and improved quality of life was just incredible. It's this kind of sweeping transformation in someone's outlook that makes me so glad I went into this line of work.

FILLERS

Another good choice for more limited acne scarring is a Hyaluronic acid filler, which is a temporary option to fill in scars. Hyaluronic acid is a natural substance already found in your body in soft connective tissue, cartilage, joints, and skin. Commonly known under the brand names Belotero, Juvéderm, Perlane, and Restylane, these fillers are non-permanent and reversible, so if the outcome is not what the patient wants, it can be dissolved with an enzyme injection.

DERMABRASION

Though I tend to prefer laser resurfacing, which offers more predictable results and a more controlled, precise delivery system, I have found remarkable improvements with dermabrasion — not only in teenagers' deep acne scars but in their self-esteem. This involves a controlled surgical scraping that carefully sands the outermost layer of skin, using a rough wire brush containing diamond particles attached to a motorized handle. The process leaves skin red and swollen for a few days to a week, and your skin can remain bright pink for several weeks. I liken it to the childhood experience of falling and skinning your knees: a scab forms and then falls off eventually, and underneath is new pink skin. The skin essentially heals from the inside out, so one shouldn't pick at it, but allow it to float away without any extra encouragement.

Because there is so much potential for scarring, uneven skin pigmentation, and a greater downtime with dermabrasion, I recommend that anyone considering this procedure do extensive research to make sure the doctor has strong expertise in this technique. In the wrong hands, dermabrasion can do more harm than good.

MICRODERMABRASION

I typically recommend microdermabrasion as the first step for patients who are looking for a nonsurgical approach for getting rid of dead skin cells and to speed skin-cell turnover, which is essential for healthy, clear skin. A more intense form of exfoliation that uses a minimally abrasive instrument to gently sand the skin, microdermabrasion removes skin cells at a more superficial level than dermabrasion. This procedure can be wonderful for treating acne, correcting uneven skin tone from sun damage, or treating light scarring. There is no real downtime involved in microdermabrasion, which is a definite plus for patients who eschew the more intensive recovery time involved in dermabrasion. Another advantage of microdermabrasion, which is generally performed as a series of treatments, is that afterward, skin-care products will penetrate the skin more effectively and makeup will go on more smoothly.

BLUE-LIGHT LED TREATMENT

In this procedure, non-ultraviolet light (wavelength 405-420 nanometers) is used to destroy acne-causing bacteria (called *Propionibacterium acnes)* and repair skin cells damaged by inflammation. The light causes the bacteria to die, and the body's natural healing properties then shrivel away the pimple — or cystic pustule — on the surface of the skin. During the treatment you will rest with your eyes protected while a blue light is applied for 15 to 20 minutes. The treatment does not hurt, there is no downtime, and you can often experience noticeable improvement after the first treatment. This approach normally calls for treatments every four to six weeks, but you can opt for a more intense rate of treatments, seven to ten days apart, when a big occasion is coming up and your skin needs to clear up fast (like yesterday).

VITAMINS AND NUTRITION

You Are What You Eat. In Chapter 8, I go deeper into some of the best vitamins you can take to improve your skin and contribute to your health, but here's my "CliffsNotes" version: To decrease the inflammation of acne, I advise teenagers to avoid shellfish and other foods that contain iodine (eggs, sushi, milk, and dairy products), which is linked to breakouts. And make sure you put the following acne-fighting foods in heavy rotation to help your skin stay clear: Seek out foods high in zinc, such as lean red meat, kidney beans, and lentils. Lentils have lens-shaped seeds, usually two per pod, and have the third-highest level of protein of any legume or nut, after soybeans and hemp. Foods containing zinc, which is also an anti-inflammatory, are important in stopping the growth of acne-causing bacteria. Omega-3 foods are also inflammation-busters and include tuna, salmon, and trout, as well as flaxseed, tofu, almonds, and walnuts. Other foods that have been shown to improve acne are turmeric, ginger, green tea, deep-red foods like berries, and leafy green vegetables. Vitamin supplements that can improve acne are vitamin A, vitamin E, zinc and evening primrose oil.

Even though folk wisdom (aka "Mom said") has long held that greasy foods and chocolate could cause acne, medical literature has denied the claim that fried foods and chocolate cause breakouts. But while those old bogeymen of chocolate and grease may not cause acne, there are growing indications that some foods will. Studies have found that raised insulin levels often result from high-glycemic foods (meaning foods like white rice and white flour that quickly convert to sugar in the body), sugary foods (including that teenage favorite, soda and a Snickers), and diets high in dairy. These insulin spikes flood the body with hormones and in turn cause pimples. Doctors, nutritionists, and patients themselves have seen a link between the high blood-insulin levels that result from eating too many sugary foods and the increased sebum production that comes from the proliferation of dead skin cells.

While I don't recommend my teenage patients give up dairy altogether, the hormones in dairy and the insulin spikes that milk create are a concern. If you can, make sure your parents pick up organic milk (which doesn't have artificial hormones added) and significantly reduce your intake of dairy (but be sure to take a calcium supplement to compensate). Such changes might prove effective in clearing up your skin. Occasionally, in place of milk, try almond or rice milk for cereal and coffee, which can be just as good as the real thing.

I also strongly advise maintaining a low-glycemic diet, which means staying away from sugary foods (including that teenage favorite, sodas) and refined grains like white rice and pasta, Danishes, croissants, waffles (which means no late-night Waffle House!), bagels, donuts, muffins, and pancakes. Also beware of the hidden sugars lurking in foods like ketchup and salad dressings. Mom always said it was the French fries, but it was really the ketchup. The body absorbs all that sugar and causes your insulin levels to skyrocket, which means increased skin-cell production, oil production, and elevated acne-causing androgen hormones. Instead, choose whole grains; but *multigrain is not the same as whole grain* so beware of this term on packaging. My best dietary advice to teenage patients is to stick with lean protein, lots of veggies, and lots of fruit—and avoid processed, packaged foods with long lists of unpronounceable ingredients.

Lastly—and this advice applies to every age—*drink water.* Water is crucial to keeping your skin clear and glowing while also keeping your brain alert.

> My best dietary advice to teenagers is to stick with lean protein, lots of veggies, and lots of fruit — avoid processed, packaged foods with long lists of unpronounceable ingredients.

EXERCISE

What you do is not as important as doing *something* to get out, move around, and get your heart rate going. Exercise can decrease your risk of stroke and heart disease in adult life. Exercise is a huge stress reliever and keeps skin clear by boosting your circulation and nourishing skin cells. Plus, the resulting stress release can be huge for teenagers struggling with school, relationships, and skin problems. The increased blood flow brings oxygen and nutrients to the skin and also helps carry away free radicals and waste products.

I recommend exercising without wearing makeup, so sweat and dirt don't clog pores. If you're working out in the morning, wash your face before heading out; if you're working out late in the day, wash off your makeup first. Even if you aren't wearing any makeup, you should wash your face to remove the accumulated dirt and oil from your skin before you begin. If you are working out or running outdoors, be sure to wear sunscreen and avoid exercising during the peak sun hours of 10 a.m. to 4 p.m. If you can, wear a hat for extra protection as you sweat, since perspiration can decrease the effectiveness of your sunscreen. Be careful when wiping your face with your hands, or even a towel, during your workout: blotting perspiration is always better than wiping, because this can also lead to breakouts. And be sure to shower right after exercise for even more prevention.

GUYS GROOM, TOO

Most guys' grooming routines are probably fairly minimal, but the metrosexual trend and the media have definitely made them more aware of their appearance than they were in my day. The guys who come into Oculus (or have their mothers bring products home for them) are often most concerned about acne.

There are other things to think about that are unique to guys. For one thing, shaving their faces. Guys are lucky because the constant exfoliation provided by shaving can mean they don't wrinkle as soon as women do. But be sure to change your razor blades regularly to prevent cuts. I think the best place to shave is in the shower when your pores are open. Use a shaving cream or soap to make things easier. And don't be such a "manly man" that you can't imagine using a moisturizer. If your skin is super dry, use one. There are a ton of products made just for guys that weren't around when I was a teenager. And they have the kind of non-girly packaging that means you won't have to hide them under all the groceries in your shopping cart.

On the grooming front, if odor is an issue, try one of the clinical-strength deodorants and body sprays (but not too much). And don't overcompensate with cologne. There's nothing worse than B.O. masked with Polo. To avoid garbage-feet, always wear socks with your shoes, wash your sneakers occasionally, and try some Gold Bond Powder on your feet to keep the stink at bay. For breakouts on your body, use a body wash with salicylic acid. You can thank me later when the girls start beating a path to your door.

Did I mention that girls don't like kissing a mouth that smells like an over-flowing ashtray? Stay away from the cigarettes.

HAIR COLOR

You might not believe this coming from a cosmetic surgeon, but I actually think natural is better. It's a philosophy that applies to surgery, too: I don't think patients should pursue a look that goes against their anatomy and bone structure. In the same way, I think teenagers, and really most people, tend to look better when they keep their hair color at a shade that works with their complexion. Many young men and women with dark hair are especially tempted to go blond, because it creates such a dramatic change. But I would advise against it. Dying dark hair blond can be very damaging, creating brittle, more stressed hair. You're also looking at a very expensive and ongoing schedule of maintenance to keep those telltale dark roots from showing. And unless you're really disciplined and have time and money to burn, you'll likely regret ever trying it in the first place.

By the same token, going from blond to a darker color entails a lot of work and is best handled by a colorist who can make sure the color doesn't work against your skin color or look flat. Better perhaps is to work with highlights to add rich-ness to your blond hair. For both dark and light hair, highlights — especially around your face — can really open up your face and add a halo effect of brightness.

GLASSES

I think having to wear glasses was probably much more traumatic in my day than it is now. Back in the '70s, the options were pretty limited and unappealing: heavy black glasses for boys, maybe some semi-funky cat-eye glasses for girls. But today teenagers shouldn't have any reason to lament glasses. You see celebrities wearing glasses all the time — whether prescription or not — to look hip, indie, or intellectual. I think the best approach for those who wear glasses is to treat them as fashion items. They dramatically increase your options for changing your looks — and what teenager, male or female, doesn't want to experiment with their appearance? If the family budget allows, get a few different pairs for daytime — maybe something bright and something more reserved. For nighttime, you could choose a really dressy or subdued third option, when you want your clothes and makeup in the limelight.

PUBLIC ENEMY NUMBER ONE: THE SUN

Sad to say, but it's true. That glowing orb we once worshiped, that parents shoved their little children into unprotected so they would have a little color in their cheeks, has become like a Greek god that was formerly worshipped by the world, but now is rendered false and obsolete. Once beloved, now shunned.

Look at the lines, brown spots, and wrinkles on your parents' faces. Pretty gruesome, right? Well, unfortunately, with the depletion of the ozone layer, by the time you reach their age — I can hear you denying it'll ever happen to you — chances are your skin is going to look even worse without the proper protection. Unfortunately, sun damage is more prevalent in the younger generation than it was in mine because of damage to the ozone layer, which has increased the sun's ability to reach the earth with its harmful UV rays.

Sunscreen is a hard sell, I know. You look at your unlined, undamaged skin, which springs back from everything you throw at it, and can't imagine anything as elderly and unthinkable as skin cancer lying in wait. I understand. Really, I do. I was once a teenager too, probably as reckless and uninformed as kids today. As a member of the Coppertone brigade, I competed with my friends to see who could get to the desired walnut — or, worse still, club-chair hue — the fastest. Growing up in Louisiana, I'd lie out on a foil blanket, greased down in baby oil and iodine like a piece of tilapia prepped for dinner. In addition to being serious sun worshipers, my wife, Susan, and I were both lifeguards, so we clocked some major time in the sun.

We had our first rude awakening about the dangers of the sun when Susan was diagnosed at 28 with a basal-cell carcinoma, a very serious form of skin cancer. It was a wake-up call. It quickly led to a reëvaluation of the sun and a new embrace of sunscreen and hats, as well as the end of sunbathing. But that has turned out to be a good thing. UV light is a proven human carcinogen. We know that sunlight causes cancer, plain and simple. It was good to get our warning early, while there was still time to change our habits.

We know sunburns are bad: they hurt, they look horrible, and the damaged skin peels off in sheets. Some people associate suntans, however, with good health. Unfortunately, neither burns nor tans are doing your skin any favors. Sunburns and suntans are the same in that they indicate underlying damage to your skin's DNA.

As you probably know from science class, DNA is the building block of human life. Try to avoid damaging the part of you that's so structurally fundamental.

Some teenagers believe the sun clears up their acne, and they use tanning beds or sun tanning to help their skin. But as we have learned over time, sunbathing is one of the worst things you can do for your skin because of the increased risk of skin cancer. Tanning beds are especially dangerous because they emit primarily UVA radiation, at a dosage that's up to 12 times higher than the sun's. Scary, huh? The use of tanning beds before the age of 35 has been linked to a 75 percent higher chance of developing melanoma, the most deadly form of skin cancer. The American Academy of Pediatrics has lobbied for years (unsuccessfully) to get tanning beds outlawed for those under the age of 21.

A great tool we use at Oculus Skin, Laser, and Longevity Centre is the skin-imaging Visia Complexion Analysis machine, which offers a look at things like the bacteria level on your skin, pore size, wrinkles, and most dramatic, the amount of UV sun damage your skin has been exposed to. It's a way for never-gonna-grow-old teens to see that even they are subject to the aging properties of the sun. Not too long ago, a young lady who plays softball came into the office. She wears a ball cap, so her forehead is protected, along with her nose, which she slathers with sunscreen. But her cheeks are not protected. So when she put her face into the Visia, her cheeks lit up like a Christmas tree. The Visia machine teaches my teenage patients that even at their age, they need to take care of their skin.

So what should you do to protect your skin? For one, wear a sunscreen with at least an SPF of 30 every day and up that number to 50 if you plan to spend the whole day at the beach or on the water. In 2012, the Food and Drug Administration mandated that all sunscreens provide protection against both UVA and UVB rays. Avoid the sun during the peak hours of 10 a.m. to 4 p.m. I know what you're thinking: You mean I have to become a goth and lurk in the shadows? No, you don't have to avoid the sun completely — just be aware of when the sun is most dangerous and take steps to protect yourself, like reapplying sunscreen every two hours. When doing so, aim for about a teaspoon for your face and anywhere from two to four tablespoons for your body. Also look for a lip balm or gloss with a decent SPF, a protective step people often skip. A great option for sunscreen that doesn't lead to breakouts is Advanced Ultra Light Day Repair SPF 30 by Pro+Therapy. And if you plan to be in the sun for a long time, a hat to protect your face is also essential.

If the bronzed look is really the look you want, there are some safe, nontoxic, eco-friendly spray tans and lotions on the market that are reasonable alternatives. A number of self-tanners create a sun-kissed look without direct exposure to the sun, and a makeup artist can help you find a bronzer that works for your skin tone.

SMOKING

I'm not going to beat around the bush here. Don't do it. In addition to causing a whole range of cancers, smoking breaks down the collagen in your skin, creates free radicals, and attacks skin protein — all of which lead to premature aging. Smoking has also been said to aggravate acne, one more reason to avoid it, if the big C isn't enough.

TATTOOS AND PIERCINGS

As the parent of three grown children, my advice, naturally, is please don't. Utterly conventional and expected, right? I can't profess to be the perfect parent whose children follow my every piece of hard-earned wisdom. My oldest son is a proud member of the inked-set. But he took my advice and waited until he was 25, and he chose a half-sleeve so that if he needed to one day hide his tattoos from a future employer (or a future wife!) he could.

Often my teenage patients feel safe asking a nonjudgmental observer like me for advice, and I try to treat them just like I did my own children. I tell my patients the same thing I told my kids: wait until you're 25 for anything permanent like multiple piercings or tattoos.

Tattoos and piercings may make you cool in your crowd when you're still in high school. But will those people still be your BFFs, and will their opinions even matter, when you have that first job interview and blow it because the grown-up on the other side of the table doesn't want someone who just follows the crowd and makes rash decisions?

If you've ever been to such top-tier hotels as the Ritz-Carlton, Four Seasons, or St. Regis hotels, you'll notice that many of their employees wear long sleeves or sweat bands, even in the hottest summer weather. That's because displaying tattoos is verboten.

The thing that many kids don't understand about tattoos is that what rocked your world at age 18 could very well make you ashamed, queasy, or regretful at 28.

And tattoos are not easily removed, despite what people think. There are countless advertisements for procedures that claim to remove tattoos, but the truth is quite different. You can disguise a tattoo, as when Johnny Depp converted his "Winona Forever" biceps tattoo in honor of girlfriend Winona Ryder to "Wino Forever" once the couple split. When a tattoo is removed it leaves an ugly red mess not unlike a burn treated with a skin graft. So there's really no such thing as erasing tattoos, only camouflaging them. If you feel compelled to get a tattoo and your parents approve, try to place it where it can be easily hidden if you decide you don't like it someday. I have a buddy who has a big tattoo of his college fraternity right above his ankle. He hates it. It will be the middle of summer, everyone else is in shorts, and this poor guy is wearing a pair of linen pants because he can't stand to show his misguided (now lifelong) allegiance to Sigma Chi. I really feel for him. Imagine having all of your life's fashion choices dictated by something you did in college, under liquid influence.

I can't even envision what will happen with this whole new generation of kids getting enormous tattoos on their shoulders, full arms, or necks. Mike Tyson went from feared boxing champ to laughable movie chump in *The Hangover* series, mostly because of his poorly placed facial tattoo. Personally, I get a little nervous when I think about the nursing homes and retirement villages of the future filled with wrinkled, fading, inked-up grannies and grandpas driving golf carts and playing bingo while sporting full-back phoenixes and arms devoted to a history of comic book art.

> When a tattoo is removed it leaves an ugly red mess not unlike a burn treated with a skin graft. So there's really no such thing as erasing tattoos, only camouflaging them.

Youth may not be forever, but tattoos are. If somebody could come up with a good hemp tattoo that could last for six months they'd be a billionaire, because everyone likes to play around a little but most sensible people realize that at some point down the line, their tastes will change.

The same words of wisdom apply to piercings. Again, you think it's temporary and that you can always remove that nose or tongue piercing when you lose interest. Even though you can take the stud or loop out, the hole remains — in your tongue, in your nose, in your eyebrow — so think long and hard about the wisdom of such a permanent step. I've closed the ear grommets on more than a dozen patients who were enlisting in the U.S. military, because such piercings are not allowed under admission guidelines.

My wife and I have a close friend, a good-looking guy, who had two earrings. Right out of college he started going to job interviews, and no one hired him. He was told the problem was the earrings he insisted on wearing to every job interview. People judge you. Right now you don't care about being judged because you're expressing your individuality; but someday, when you find your dream job, you might.

COSMETIC SURGERY

The American Society of Plastic Surgeons (ASPS) has found that teens tend to get plastic surgery to fit in with their peers and to look similar to others. Adults tend to have plastic surgery to stand out from the crowd. According to the ASPS, almost 236,000 cosmetic plastic-surgery procedures were performed on people age 13 through 19 in 2012. The most popular procedures for teenagers are rhinoplasty (nose jobs), chin augmentation, liposuction, breast reduction, and gynecomastia (the reduction of excess breast tissue in males). But it's important for a teenager considering any of these major surgeries to be psychologically and emotionally ready to contend with this change. They need to be sure they're undergoing procedures for the right reasons, not to please their parents or because they think such a change will be a guarantee of happiness.

I may take a different approach from my peers when it comes to cosmetic surgery for teens. In a nutshell, I tend not to advise it for kids under 25. There is a reason car insurance companies charge teenagers higher premiums than adults. Teenagers are more likely to act before they think, to take risks and not think about their mortality the same way adults do. For the same reason, I believe that the buzzing, whirring teenage brain — which acts impulsively and doesn't think about consequences — is probably not the best one to choose a plastic surgery they may end up regretting.

There is definitely such a thing as too young when it comes to plastic surgery, although there are exceptions. If a teenager has a medical condition that creates problems in their development, a corrective procedure might be necessary. For instance, a droopy eyelid blocking a child's visual stimulation can have a huge, negative impact on eyesight. A child with such a condition might even compensate for his diminished field of vision by tilting his head back a little bit in order to see, which over time can lead to arthritis and neck problems.

Rather than the medically necessary surgeries, the ones that concern me are the cosmetic procedures performed on kids at a very young age. When girls as young as 14 or 15 are getting breast augmentation, which carries risks of rupturing, permanent scarring, and inevitable replacement down the line, it's time for a reality check. We know we've lost touch when teenagers who haven't even finished developing are seeking complicated, risky procedures before their self-image has even matured. Unfortunately, this approach is often fueled by well-intentioned but misguided parents. Physical maturity and the final look of breasts is not even in place until between the ages of 18 and 22, so I recommend waiting. The same is true for breast reduction, which should be postponed until a girl has reached physical maturity. I realize it can be a challenge to the ego when there is severe

I often think of Tammy when I see teenage patients because of what she represents: young people who see a mountain where only a molehill exists. Tammy was a freshman at Ole Miss, dying to get into a sorority at that very Greek-centric college. In what was undoubtedly a painful, psychologically devastating experience, Tammy went through rush week but didn't make it into any of her desired sororities. She was so traumatized by the rejection that she switched schools. Tammy was convinced that the reason for not making it into her sorority of choice was a barely perceptible small fold in her eyelid that became, for her, the explanation for her rejection. I could have corrected what Tammy saw as a flaw that the rest of the world didn't see at all, but it felt unethical to me. Why change something in this beautiful young woman when it might be replaced by some newly imagined fault that would explain some other instance of hurt feelings? The truth is, we all have things we may not love about ourselves, but most of them are probably not worth stressing about.

Outcome: I talked Tammy out of going through with surgery to her eyelid, which would have been perceptible only to her. Rejection stinks. Tammy was lovely and bright, and I couldn't figure out how to explain why she didn't make it into a coveted sorority except to recommend that she rent *Mean Girls* or *Heathers* and realize that maybe she was better off.

*"Nature made us individuals,
as she did the flowers and pebbles;
but we are afraid to be peculiar,
and so our society resembles a bag of
marbles, or a string of mold candles.
Why should we all dress after the same fashion?
The frost never paints my windows twice alike."*
— Lydia Maria Child

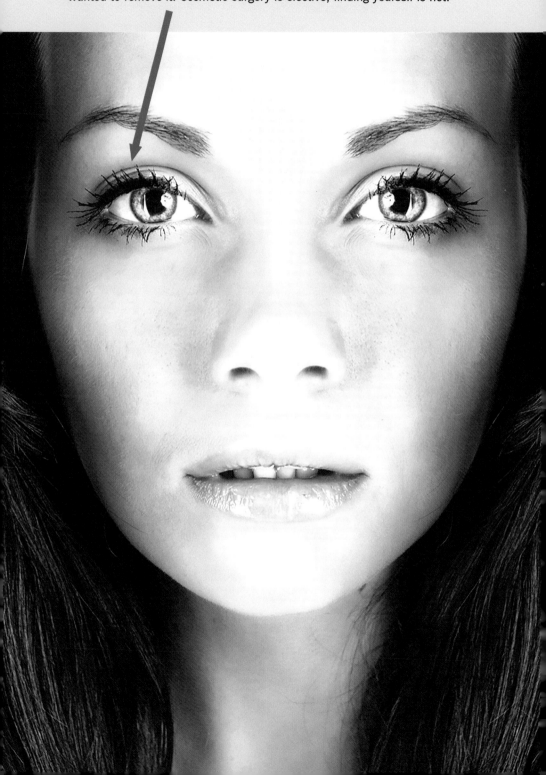

Tammy was 19 years young and still searching to define herself. This half-millimeter fold was intermittent, depending on her fluid intake and sleeping habits. I told her to come back at age 25 if it still bothered her and she still wanted to remove it. Cosmetic surgery is elective, finding yourself is not.

asymmetry (uneven size) in breasts, but I do think that waiting until your body is finished growing is the best approach.

In some situations it may be beyond just a cosmetic issue and more of a psychological one: ears that stick out too far, a nose whose shape or size makes a teenager painfully self-conscious, breasts that are asymmetrical. In many of these cases, I think it's a matter of kids growing into their own bodies. Some of these issues work themselves out; the body changes. Characteristics that were once pronounced as you were growing are no longer obvious. However, if teenagers feel that something about their appearance is keeping them from socializing, making them anxious or self-conscious, or dominating their thoughts, plastic surgery may be an option.

If cosmetic surgery is something you really want, you understand the risks, you've thought it through, and your parents agree, there are some things you can do to make it easier on yourself. The best way to go about making a change is to do it in the summer between high school and college so that you don't become the favorite topic of conversation ("Hey, have you seen Dylan's new nose?!") at school. If you're coming in for surgery to fix your prominent ears, for example, a surgery that works great for you may not register that way for your classmates. The truth is, kids can pick up on anxiety with laser-like precision. Even though you may look better, they will hone in on that anxiety and the change. This can make you feel more self-conscious than when you started, so be aware of the effect your surgery might have on your peers, and act accordingly.

> Bottom line: cosmetic surgery is best left to adults who understand the risks and whose bodies have finished growing. You have your whole life ahead of you. Enjoy your youth, be healthy, have fun, keep things in perspective.

The other thing I suggest young people can do to downplay their surgery is use an alibi, like a new hairstyle. That way if someone says, "Oh you look great," you can say, "Thanks, I love my new stylist."

Here's the bottom line: cosmetic surgery is something best left to adults who are old enough to understand the risks and whose bodies have finished growing. You have your whole life ahead of you. Enjoy your youth, be healthy, have fun, and keep things in perspective.

CHIP'S TIPS

1 Everyone needs a go-to sunscreen. If you like the way it feels on your skin, you'll be more inclined to wear it daily. Make sure it contains SPF 30 with a minimum of 7 percent zinc oxide to protect against UVA/UVB rays. Add protection by wearing mineral-based makeup that also contains SPF, but don't let this be your only protection.

2 What you eat will show up on your face. Eat healthy, exercise, and drink plenty of water. Keep your skin hydrated, and it will stay clear and glowing.

3 I recommend the Jane Iredale makeup product line to my teenage patients. I favor this line because it is free of oil, talc, dyes, parabens, preservatives, and irritating fragrance — in other words, all the ingredients that can aggravate skin.

4 I recommend exercising without makeup, so sweat and dirt don't clog pores.

5 Enjoy social media and all the great things it offers. But beware, everyone that may have access to your comments and video posts may not have your best interests at heart.

6 Stay close to your family, especially your siblings. Friends will come and go but your family will be there for you forever.

7 Physician-strength skin care is the secret to surviving the teenage acne years. A professional aesthetician can truly become your "BFF."

8 It is physiologically impossible to smoke and have good skin. It is not if, but when: it looks sallow, wrinkled, and pigmented — then turns into cancer.

9 Growing up as a teenager, I always cherished my mother's insight. "Mugsy" told me: "If at first you don't succeed, do it like your mother told you."

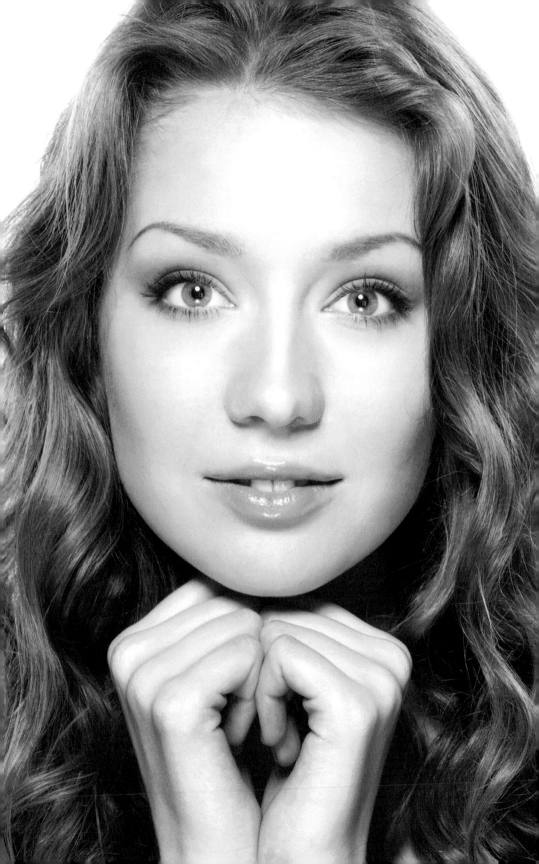

CHAPTER 4

* * *

STAY LOOKING LIKE *YOU*

There's a lot to be thankful for as you move into your 20s and 30s. If you suffered skin trauma in your teen years, you've probably come out of it and developed a skin-care regimen that yields positive results. If acne has continued to be an issue, as it sometimes does, there are numerous strategies detailed in Chapter 3 to help you cope. If I've learned anything in my practice, it's that everyone's skin is unique and responds differently. So try some of the methods recommended in this book, but also meet with a qualified cosmetic surgeon, dermatologist, or medical aesthetician if acne continues to trouble you. He or she can prescribe a special treatment tailored to your needs.

Some of the same habits you adopted in your teens should be maintained as you reach your 20s and 30s. Sunscreen, vitamins, plenty of fruits and vegetables, and exercise are your constant companions (I hope). If you make healthy living part of your routine, you will find that time really is on your side. Your 20s and 30s, if you practice good skin care, can be the best, most glowing years of your life. It's the sweet spot between the acne and oiliness of puberty and the inevitable wrinkles and loss of elasticity that comes with age.

When we think about plastic surgery, visions of face lifts generally come to mind. That's unfortunate, because the cosmetic-surgery industry offers so much more. Noninvasive and preventive skin care is an equally important, often overlooked, aspect of many plastic-surgery practices; our own Oculus Skin Care Centre, for example, prominently features skin care as part of its integrated offerings.

The focus at this point in your life should be on the preventive steps you can take to maintain your skin's health and beauty. The surgery that may come into play later will help turn the clock back, but the skin care and minimally invasive procedures you adopt while you're still young — from lasers to preventive Botox or Dysport — will pause skin aging significantly. Prevention, of course, also significantly delays the need for surgery; and when you do opt for surgery, the healthiest skin often yields the best outcome. I always tell my patients, if you can slow down the skin-aging process with sun protection and therapeutic, physician-involved skin care at this age, it can make a tremendous difference for years — even decades — to come.

Whatever your age, if you want the best results from your skin-care routine, you need to look beyond the fancy packaging and outsize promises at your local department-store counter and seek out the prescription-strength products that are really going to benefit your skin. Department-store skin care is what I like to call the sizzle without the steak. A lot of bragging and bluster, with little in the way of measurable results. Only prescription products can truly penetrate the skin's epidermis and dermis, and make a visible difference in your skin. The Food and Drug Administration has mandated that over-the-counter skin care must not penetrate beneath the skin's surface; if it can, it's considered therapeutic and must be supervised by a doctor.

> Only prescription products can truly penetrate the skin's epidermis and dermis and make a visible difference in your skin. The FDA has mandated that over-the-counter skin care can't penetrate under the skin's surface.

So keep that in mind as you read through the latest issue of *Marie Claire*, *Vogue*, or *Glamour*, with their advertisements promising miraculously transformed skin in four to six weeks. Not gonna happen. Better to consult with your plastic surgeon, dermatologist, or medical aesthetician to find the cleanser, toner, moisturizer, and age-defying serums that will improve your skin quality, texture, and tone.

TAKING IT SLOW

Though the 20s are often the years when women look their best — with taut, radiant skin and all the physical advantages of youth — ironically enough, they can be the time of greatest anxiety and insecurity about one's looks. For that reason, I recommend that young women steer clear of permanent plastic-surgery modifications. Do too much at this age and you risk the Lindsay Lohan effect: looking too drawn, harsh and old before your time.

At this age, there's a danger of patients rushing into procedures before they are emotionally ready. Many are still dealing with the tail end of their teenage years, still feeling the insecurities about their appearance that may have caused them pain in high school. They can turn to boyfriends for advice on how to look better, or they can emulate movie stars, imagining that if they only had *her* lips, or *her* nose, or *her* chin, they could be happy. But I think it's important for women in their 20s to realize that they are still in formation.

Most women at this age are still trying to figure out what works best for them, and they should not be turning to their boyfriends (who may be as temporary as those high-school friends whose opinions they once thought were so important) or be using the pages of *People* or *InStyle* as their beauty bible. Don't get me wrong. You can pick up some great advice and ideas from magazines; but be a discriminating reader and know when something is a great tip, or a sales ploy bound to build up false hopes of unachievable results.

A rising trend I've noticed in my twentysomething patients is the tendency to emulate favorite celebrities to the point of impersonation. Sometimes I feel like they get confused: they think these are people they want to *look* like, but perhaps they are instead people they want to *be*. When a patient brings in photos of a star like Angelina Jolie, but can't pinpoint the features they want to emulate, perhaps they're after the glamour they imagine Jolie's life entails. In such cases, I've often found it helpful to use computer imaging, placing that photo of Angelina side by side with the patient's own face so they can see how different they look, and how you can't just transplant someone else's features onto your own face and achieve a beautiful result.

So I try to get to the heart of the matter when a 20-year-old comes into Oculus wanting a more prominent chin, plumped up lips, hollowed out cheeks, or other procedures that may be trendy now but probably won't stand the test of time in five or ten years. Cosmetic surgery can be a remarkably faddish business, and it's important for patients to recognize that the overinflated lips that may be sexy in 2014 are potentially going to look garish and out of place by 2016. Don't let your face be the Silly Putty/Pet Rock/Beanie Baby fad of the moment.

It may not sound very good for business, but I consider it a point of pride that of my young patients, half never come back after our initial surgical consultation, or they scale back the procedure they had in mind. They decide that what they want may be unrealistic, or after reflection they change their minds. I would much rather see someone not choose a procedure than be unhappy with the one they impulsively selected. It's the spring-break mentality — that live-for-the-moment, undoubtedly alcohol-fueled certainty that a tattoo of their boyfriend's name on their forearm is a brilliant idea. Nothing presages a breakup as much as stamping your boyfriend's name onto your skin. So don't make the same mistake by rushing into a surgical procedure, because you and your face can't break up.

I advise my patients in this age bracket to think about the long-term effects of what they are considering. A procedure might seem like a good idea now, but what about in 10 or 20 years? For example, I see a fair number of models in my practice, and sometimes their agents will advise them to bring drama to their faces with a more hollow, sunken area just below the cheek bones. It's a relatively simple procedure, involving the removal of the buccal fat pad. But over time, that absence is going to make them look gaunt and older and, ironically enough, will leave them in need of more fillers to compensate for the lost volume. I feel it's my duty to let them know of those consequences, and I often suggest working with a team of skilled medical aestheticians, who are able to help with makeup techniques that can give that sculpted look without surgery.

IF YOU MUST…INCREASE YOUR BUST

Though my practice deals exclusively with the face, I have found from speaking with my colleagues in the plastic-surgery realm that a lot of women begin thinking about breast augmentation in their 20s and 30s. Once again, I recommend waiting until you are at least 25 to consider any major cosmetic surgery, but if you make this choice earlier, you can be strategic about it. As I advised in the previous chapter — that procedures done in your teenage years should be undertaken in the summer between your senior year of high school and before college — the same applies for your 20s. Try to schedule it for between college and career. And by all means don't let a boyfriend or fiancé drive this decision. This is *your* body, and you need to make sure this is something you are doing for *you*. Consider the risks, because you, not your boyfriend, will have to live with them. Risks include loss of nipple sensation, development of scar tissue, a possible decreased ability to breast feed, difficulty in reading mammograms, and hardening or rupturing of the implant. Too often, the implants need to be replaced. Implants are not forever.

Make sure you choose a surgeon who knows this procedure well, who has performed many successful breast augmentations, and who can explain the best method for you — behind the muscle or in front, saline or silicone — since many of the potential complications can be minimized in a skilled surgeon's hands.

ETHNICITY AND APPEARANCE

Another issue I often see in my practice Is younger patients requesting surgery because of some ethnic trait that makes them feel self-conscious, whether it's the absence of a lid platform (that shelf enhanced by eye shadow) in Asian eyes, or the wider nose of some African American patients. But my advice remains the same: wait until you are older, until you're certain you aren't entering into surgery too soon. Many awkward-looking teens and twentysomethings have been shown to fully grow into beautiful women or handsome men. And with patients who are considering plastic surgery to change a feature of their ethnicity, which they have in common with friends and family, even greater caution is needed.

When Asian clients come to me to change their lid platform in order to get a more Caucasian-looking eye, I generally ask them to meet with me more than once, so they can consider the enormity of their decision. Changing one's appearance to conform to a more Westernized standard of beauty happens most often in military families or in interracial couples, where a patient is straddling two cultures and feels anxiety about which culture they belong to. There can be pressure to change one's appearance to further a career or to fit within workplace norms. Plastic surgery can be a search for clarity; but if all my years as a doctor have taught me anything, it's that such issues are generally best resolved internally (before they're tackled externally).

Changing a feature you share with members of your family, one that identifies you as belonging to a certain cultural heritage and ethnicity, can be an emotional and psychological minefield if not carefully considered, because it's not just a cosmetic change. There is an almost innate cultural rejection involved in removing a distinctively ethnic feature, which probably won't sit well with your family members. Sometimes an Asian patient with a Caucasian spouse will fixate on the difference, and feel like an outsider because of it. They need to consider not just what their new community may think about their appearance but how their old one will perceive the change. Undertaking cosmetic surgery to distance oneself from one's ethnic group can inject a lot of tension into relationships within that group. It's something I often tell my clients, and I think it bears repeating: Just because something *can* be done doesn't mean it *should* be done.

Cosmetic surgery involves navigating a great deal of psychology. And it's important for patients to understand that just because they think surgery will make their lives better, there is no guarantee it will.

WORKING IT: WHEN YOUR FACE IS YOUR FORTUNE

Are there instances when plastic surgery can help in some tangible way? Can plastic surgery allow you to get ahead in work or in life? In some regards, our face is *always* our fortune. Looking pulled together, well-groomed, and attractive are positives in any line of work. It's known as the *"halo effect"* — the ability of good looks to make someone appear smarter, more competent and more appealing, simply based on their pleasing appearance. As you get older and notice the difference in how you're treated because of your looks, those advantages and disadvantages become even more apparent. It's a subtler form of discrimination than that of race or gender, and it can often affect hiring practices, promotions and overall professional success. Your parents were right when they said looks aren't everything; but there's also something to be said for paying attention to your appearance and understanding what it can convey to the world.

As you enter the workforce, certain aspects of your appearance may begin to bother you. If you have a deep tear trough (or nasojugal groove) — the area under your eyes where the lower eyelid meets the cheek that often harbors gray-blue circles — you can look tired and worn out, which can create a negative impression on the job. In instances such as this, yes, cosmetic procedures can certainly prevent your face from telegraphing that you're tired or not up to the job. Using fillers in that area can make a dramatic difference in your appearance, making you look refreshed, energetic, and far younger — a definite career booster.

If you work in a field in which appearance is paramount, such as the fitness, sales, entertainment, or real-estate industries, maintaining your looks and youthfulness can be very important in making deals and staying competitive. And certainly there are both surgical and noninvasive solutions to sharpen your edge and enhance your image.

Strong furrows between eyebrows can appear even in 20-year-olds, registering the effects of hours of studying. If you're worried about what those signs of stress say to a potential employer, you're not alone. Many young patients with these visible worry lines come into Oculus for treatment. But a new wrinkle has emerged, if you'll pardon the pun, in which patients are now able to take preventive steps to keep those lines from forming in the first place.

A big trend now is prophylactic (or preventive) treatments — with patients seeking out Botox or Dysport to nip wrinkles in the bud — often to counteract anatomy or family history. The logic is that, if Mom or an aunt has strong furrows between her eyebrows (an area called the glabella, which, by the way, is the only place the FDA has approved for cosmetic Botox use), a patient may use an injectable wrinkle relaxer to keep those muscles from contracting into the deep folds that are her genetic heritage. I have dozens of patients now in their early 20s who are doing just that.

LET'S GET PHYSICAL

Do you know the three things doctors and beauty experts say will greatly contribute to the premature aging of your skin? Two of them aren't surprising, smoking and

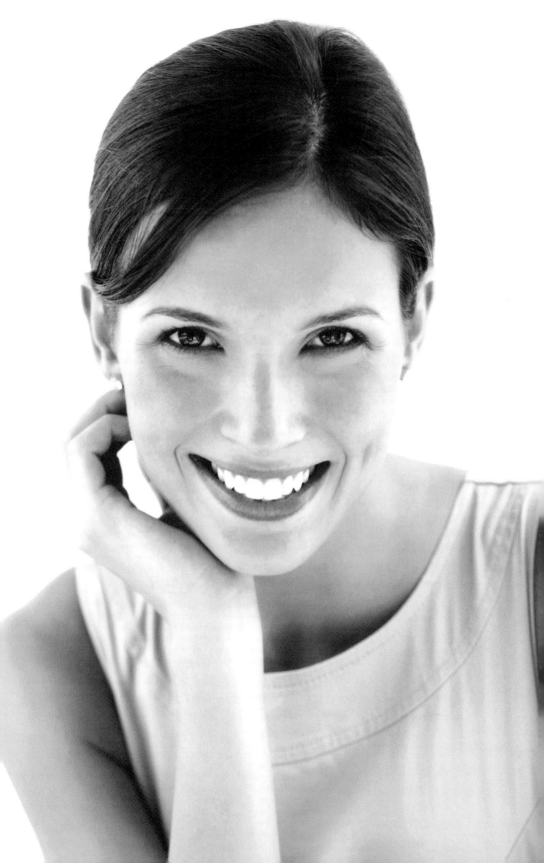

sun exposure, but the other one may be: weight fluctuation. It's a difficult issue, especially in young adulthood, given the negative effect it can have on your skin's elasticity. Let's hope that by your 20s you've found an exercise plan that suits you, and that you know about eating healthy foods and avoiding unhealthy ones.

I always think of a funny quote from the French film icon and legendary beauty Catherine Deneuve, who said, "a 30-year-old woman must choose between her bottom and her face." The reason is that you can have plump, glowing, youthful skin on your face if you let your body go a bit, but if you choose to be skinny, your face may look fatigued and less youthful. Luckily, we've come a long way since Deneuve made that observation at the tender age of 25.

A broad selection of techniques, including fillers and surgery, now allow women to maintain full, alluring features without keeping an extra 20 pounds on their frame. That said, as you get older it's crucial to maintain a steady weight, because yo-yo dieting can lead to slack and sagging skin. Getting enough protein is also key as you age, because we need it to stimulate the collagen and elasticity in the skin. With rapid weight gain and loss, your skin is stressed and becomes less elastic. So in your 20s and 30s, begin working toward maintaining an ideal healthy weight and avoiding the nutrient-robbing, skin-damaging diets so many young women try at this age.

CLEANSE

One of the most important steps in a skin-care regimen is often most neglected, because it's so basic. But a thorough cleansing routine with a great cleanser every morning and evening, preferably with the Clarisonic brush, is essential for healthy skin. The Clarisonic's best feature is that it forces you to stand at the sink for a dedicated amount of time to ensure that you're getting a really deep cleanse and removing all the layers of makeup, pollutants, dead skin and product from the day. One of the most damaging things you can do to your skin is to go to sleep in your makeup. It is during sleep that your skin has the opportunity to breathe and heal. If you leave your skin entombed in a shroud of makeup, neither of those things can happen; and if you sleep on your side, your makeup grinds even more deeply into your skin. A great cleanser for younger skin is Oculus LactiCleanse, a soap-free, non-irritating cleanser that incorporates glycolic acid for a substantial, deep clean.

For a slightly more aggressive approach as you ease into your 30s, Jan Marini Bioglycolic is a real multitask cleanser that contains lactic acid, an alpha hydroxy acid known for its gentle exfoliating and cleansing properties.

REMEMBER: PROTECTION IS THE BEST TREATMENT

The French have a great approach to skin care. They start young, recognizing that beauty is not just about makeup, clothes, and hairstyle but about really treating your skin like an asset that can pay long-term dividends.

At Oculus Skin Care Centre, we take a cue from the French in recommending that patients look for skin-care products with the following active ingredients:

1 **Hyaluronic acid**, because it holds up to 40 times its own water weight, which leads to hydrated, healthy skin
2 **Ceramides**, which assist in the skin's ability to hold water — again, key in maintaining healthy, plump skin
3 **Vitamin C** (applied topically), a great antioxidant that helps protect against future skin damage
4 **Zinc oxide**, which protects skin from UVA/UVB rays
5 **Kojic acid and hydroquinone**, skin-lightening agents that treat melasma and hyperpigmentation to give skin a smooth, porcelain complexion
6 **Human growth factors**, which produce collagen and improve fine lines and wrinkles
7 **Green tea** to reduce redness and inflammation
8 **Jojoba beads in facial scrubs**, which are perfectly spherical and therefore won't cause microscopic rips in the skin

Remember: when you shop for skin-care products at that fancy department store, you aren't necessarily getting full disclosure from behind the cosmetics counter. Take the time to scrutinize labels. Unlike the more regulated food industry, the definition of organic, for instance, is much more lax on health and beauty products. A true organic skin-care product will carry the USDA Organic seal. Likewise, there are a lot of products out there claiming to be "all natural" when they're not. True all-natural products contain no solvents, preservatives (parabens or ethanols), or artificial coloring.

We also advise patients to steer clear of products with fragrance, because frequently it irritates the skin. Lastly, products with mineral oil or lanolin create a barrier on the surface of your skin, clogging pores.

EXFOLIATE

How intensely you exfoliate in your 20s is often determined by skin type. For patients with oily or combination skin, a more intense exfoliation with medical-strength alpha hydroxy acid may be a necessity to keep pores clean and free of the dead skin, sebum, and bacteria buildup that can lead to pimples. But someone with normal skin may not need such an aggressive approach. I suggest gauging your needs according to a skin analysis by your doctor or medical aesthetician.

If you want to keep your skin looking fresh while speeding cell turnover, a scrub is a great tool — one that will help slough away dead skin cells but won't damage your skin. SkinMedica's Skin Polish has beads that are perfectly round and do not cause microscopic tearing of the skin.

By their 30s, most women generally need some kind of exfoliation to give skin-cell turnover an extra nudge. And when you move into your late 30s and early 40s, you will most likely want to switch to a chemical exfoliation with retinol or a higher percentage of alpha hydroxy acids, which begins the anti-aging process. As a rule of thumb (but again, depending on your skin type), I recommend exfoliating with a scrub in the shower two to three times a week.

PROTECT AND MOISTURIZE

Proper moisturizing is one of those daily habits that, if begun in your 20s before fine lines are even visible, can significantly delay skin aging. Like putting money into a 401K when you're still young, the benefits of moisturizer may not be immediately apparent but will yield significant long-term results. Moisturizer is a good way to keep fine lines and crow's feet at bay. The best approach is to do double duty and incorporate an absolutely essential daily sunscreen with a truly effective moisturizer, such as TNS Ultimate Daily Moisturizer + SPF 20. I also like Jan Marini Transformation Face Cream, which contains plant growth factors that are very healing to the skin but not quite as expensive as the human growth factors you'll read about in Chapter 5. On that front, I think beginning to incorporate a serum into your beauty routine while you're still young, such as SkinMedica's TNS Recovery Complex or Oculus CEGA

> Just like putting money into a 401K when you're still young, the benefits of moisturizer may not be immediately apparent but will yield significant long-term results.

serum, ensures that your skin gets that little extra repairing boost to prevent free-radical damage and significantly improve the tone and texture of your skin.

SUNSCREEN

Most important, for the kind of protection that will pay off for decades to come, protect your skin from the sun. One of the most profoundly damaging habits that will begin to reveal itself in premature aging as early as your 20s and 30s is the devastating loss of collagen and the breakdown of skin elasticity resulting from prolonged exposure to the sun. To avoid these damaging effects, use sunscreen with at least a 30 SPF every day, rain or shine, since harmful UVA and UVB rays penetrate the skin whether the sun is out or not. Find a sunscreen that feels good on your skin. If your daily sunscreen is too greasy or has a texture that doesn't work with your makeup, you will be much less likely to use it. If you adopt the daily use of a comfortable sunscreen in your 20s, you'll be able to see the benefits as you age: your skin will look far better than that of your friends who don't take this vital daily step. You can often do double duty by finding a moisturizer (tinted or otherwise) with an SPF of at least 30. If breakouts are an issue, choose a non-comedogenic moisturizer and sunscreen that won't clog pores.

If you don't believe me when it comes to the cumulative damage wrought by unprotected exposure to the sun, try looking at your skin under the VISIA machine, a leading-edge skin-evaluation technology we routinely use at Oculus Skin Care Centre. It's a real wake-up call, and often quite a shock, to look through the window into the true state of your skin, including sun damage not visible to the naked eye.

I advise all of my patients to go through a computerized skin-health review using the VISIA Complexion Analysis (see photo, page 80). When you come in as a new patient, my nurses will discuss your medical history with you and develop a personalized chart. We will normally take a series of before photos from different angles — we want you to understand what we're starting with here. Sun exposure, smoking, diet, and alcohol consumption have a cumulative effect, all factoring into the look and feel (and healing) of your skin.

We also want you to understand the fitness level of your skin. Computer imaging allows you to see yourself critically, to notice things you never saw before. Through imaging technology, you may discover there's much you can do to improve the condition of your skin, even without surgery. I assign a new skin-care regimen to patients as their homework. Just like when you were in school, you've got to do your homework before you're ready for the exam. In my practice, the exam is the procedure or the surgery.

When patients come in for that first consultation, most tend not to realize exactly how much ultraviolet damage we can receive over the years through unprotected exposure to the sun's rays. When you see an ultraviolet photo of the damage to your skin, most patients are shocked. It is often a great cautionary experience that jolts even my youngest patients into taking better care of their skin.

WHEN YOU WANT TO REV THINGS UP

Though perfect skin is really the gold standard for young adults, you may find that you need a little extra something to combat the formation of lines around the eyes. However, at this age you want to avoid doing too much too soon with aggressive products. Clearly you'd never want to substitute youthfulness for a harsher, more artificial, prematurely aging look.

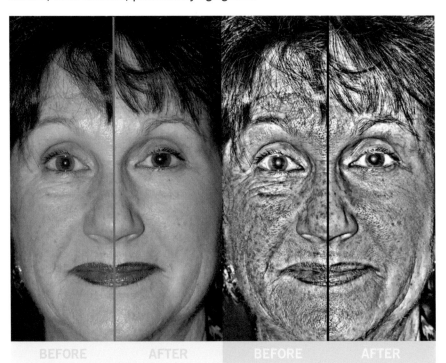

BEFORE   AFTER   BEFORE   AFTER

FILLERS
Reversibility is key at this point. If someone at this age wants to experiment with fillers, say in their lips, I advise a temporary hyaluronic acid filler like Restylane, Juvéderm, or Perlane over anything permanent. Don't fall victim to the whims of plastic-surgery fashion by pursuing something more permanent; your desire for

those superstar lips might end in a permanent look you may not want in two or three years. As you age, your lips change, and a lip implant that fits the shape of your lips at age 20 is not necessarily going to fit them at 40, so proceed with caution in this regard. A permanent lip filler may also cause significant scarring and permanently affect your smile mobility.

Dermal fillers have an additional use that can be quite beneficial at this age for patients who may have struggled with severe acne in their teens: they can be used to fill old pockmarks that are the telltale traces of previous deep blemishes.

MICRODERMABRASION AND PHOTOFACIALS

Both microdermabrasion and photofacials offer significant exfoliation for more problematic skin. Unless there is a real problem, like serious sun damage, these bigger guns are often better kept in reserve for your older years, when the effects of aging — like crow's feet and brown spots — become more apparent. However, if scarring from previous bouts of acne is an issue, then microdermabrasion in particular might be a great choice for sloughing away evidence of your skin's past.

TARGETED LASERS

I don't recommend an overall laser treatment in young adulthood, when most patients will do fine with a precision laser treatment, which targets specific areas of damage or discoloration. If you have just a small brown spot or old acne scar that's bothering you, a targeted laser treatment, rather than a much more intense full-face laser peel, might be the best solution.

CHEMICAL PEELS

The same minimally invasive, 45 percent glycolic-acid peel that worked wonders on acne-ravaged skin in your teens can also do wonders to brighten and clarify an uneven complexion through your 30s. Though downtime is minimal, you may experience some irritation and redness following the peel.

RETINOL

Retinols have been an incredible boon to modern therapeutic skin care. A form of vitamin A, retinols are the go-to treatment to achieve glowing, clear skin, because they speed skin-cell turnover, which can mean a visible reduction in pore size and fine lines. As early as your 20s, you should begin a regimen with a retinol cream and an antioxidant serum. These two products not only maintain the skin, they improve it. The advantage of a retinol cream such as SkinMedica Tri-Retinol Complex ES is that it doesn't have the irritation factor of Retin-A but can do wonders in treating the fine lines and wrinkles that can begin to crop up in your 30s.

BOTOX
Prospective patients always want to know this: at what age should I start to think about this type of procedure? Honestly, there's no hard and fast rule. A lot depends on how you feel when you see yourself in the mirror, and on your lifestyle and genetics. Botox can actually be used to prevent wrinkles from getting more pronounced (not just to relax a wrinkle, but actually to prevent them). If you're out in the sun a lot and you're frowning and starting to notice the formation of lines, you might start with Botox treatments at an earlier age.

FINAL THOUGHTS

If there's one takeaway from this chapter, it's that therapeutic, doctor-prescribed skin care is the golden ticket that will define and maintain your beauty for decades to come. While surgery can often yield instant, dramatic results, if done when you're too young it can be a case of too much too soon. When young adults pursue surgery, it's possible to lose perspective and look for more and more dramatic results and fail to age naturally. Ultimately it's possible to lose sight of who you are.

Your 20s and 30s are a time to solidify good habits, lay the foundation for great skin as you age, and count your blessings. For those lucky enough to be enjoying these charmed decades, relax, enjoy, and don't mess with perfection.

CHIP'S TIPS

1   Moisturize your skin daily, and you'll enjoy the benefits for decades to come.

2   Don't let your face be the Silly Putty/Pet Rock/Beanie Baby fad of the moment. Dramatic, trendy procedures and surgeries are a bad idea at any age.

3   Steer away from products with fragrance, because it frequently irritates the skin. Also avoid products with mineral oil and lanolin, since they clog pores and create a barrier on the surface of your skin.

4   Don't get too much work done in your 20s and 30s or you'll risk the Lindsay Lohan effect: looking too drawn, harsh, and old before your time.

5   Don't let your significant other drive a cosmetic-surgery decision. This is *your* face, and you need to make sure this is something you're doing for *you*.

6   Protect your beauty now with preventive measures. While surgery can help turn back the clock, an ounce of prevention is worth a pound of cure.

7   Only prescription-strength products (supervised by a physician) can truly penetrate the skin's epidermis (outer layer) and dermis (middle layer). The FDA has mandated that over-the-counter skin care can't penetrate under the skin's surface.

8   Department store skin care is a multibillion-dollar business. Remember the product results ("the steak") is more important than the free bag or free lipstick ("the sizzle").

9   Remember the "halo effect" and try to "dress for success," especially early in your career, when you want to make a memorable impression. After you become the boss, dress how you want.

10   During the young adult years, try to only (or primarily) make your desired improvements with reversible solutions. You will be surprised how your tastes and goals will change as you get older.

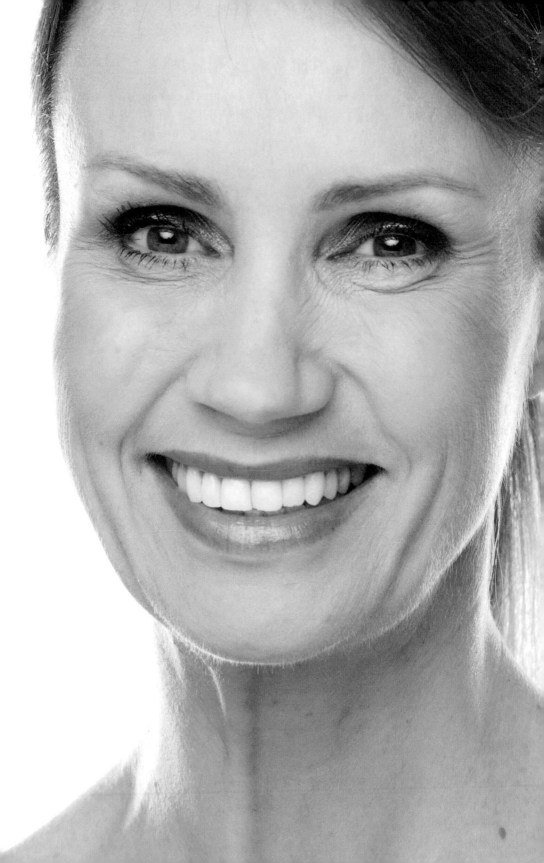

CHAPTER 5

* * *

MAKING MIDDLE-AGE
THE BEST YEARS OF YOUR LIFE

"One thing that never gets old for me is hearing from others that I look good. Now I'm saving for that touch-up in ten years!" — *Rachel* (see case study, page 118)

"If you pay attention to skin care every day, you'll never look into the mirror and see a person who looks ten years older than you want to be." — *Bethany* (page 117)

Your 40s and 50s can be an amazing time. For many women, this is the new golden age. You hear it all the time: 40 is the new 30, 50 is the new 40. Don't believe me? Look around at any fashion or celebrity magazine cover. Some of the most beautiful women in the world — Madonna, Jennifer Aniston, Michelle Pfeiffer, Elizabeth Hurley, Naomi Campbell, Angelina Jolie, Heidi Klum, Halle Berry, Jennifer Lopez, Cate Blanchett — are over 40; some are over 50 and considered style and beauty icons. It's hard to avoid the fact that right now, midlife is considered a pretty extraordinary time.

But the onset of middle-age can be a double-edged sword. Many women have reached a secure place in their lives. Work, children, marriage, friendships, and home have all fallen into place. This is life's sweet spot for many women, filled with a sense of contentment and security about their lives, with less of the anxiety that plagued their younger years. In other words, they're comfortable in their own skin.

But on the subject of skin, middle-age can bring some attendant issues, too. Wrinkles may begin to set in around the eyes and mouth. Deep nasolabial folds on the sides of the nose, and marionette lines extending from the corners of your mouth toward your jaw, can add years to the face. Skin can lose some of the luster and elasticity it once had. If the 20s and 30s are all about taking preventive action, then the 40s and 50s call for serious, doctor-approved solutions in skin care, as well as surgical and nonsurgical procedures. The face lifts women might have had done in the past when they turned 40 or 50 have been vastly improved.

Instead of the pulled-too-tight, overly stretched look so prevalent in the '80s and '90s, women in their 40s and 50s are now undergoing more subtle face lift procedures to look naturally younger.

In general, as women at this stage of their lives become dissatisfied with these signs of aging, they often take a no-nonsense approach to fighting back. My patients in this age range certainly don't feel old. They're often in excellent shape, take good care of themselves, and aren't going to let a few crow's feet or facial "parentheses" make them feel less positive about their lives when they look in the mirror. Women can develop a captivating self-confidence after they've survived their teens, 20s, and 30s. Many come in with a short (or long) list of the procedures they want. Unlike my more indecisive or anxious younger patients, most of these women have been considering cosmetic surgery for years.

It's refreshing to see that kind of certainty when so much of my work involves trying to figure out A) what the patient wants, and B) whether it's realistic and achievable. Women at this age have cast aside some of the anxious vanity of youth and tend to get down to brass tacks, as in *Fix the crow's feet, I'm going to Vegas!*

While most of my patients in this age range are pleasantly decisive, others tend to need a little more discussion. Some women are certain they will appear vain and self-centered — and be bad mothers — for thinking about something besides the health and well-being of their children. There can be a tendency at any age to put others ahead of yourself financially: sports camp for your kids, home improvements, a luxurious vacation getaway for the whole family. Women tend to be wired as givers. A lot of the women I see in my practice are used to taking care of everyone but themselves.

Those who are in this frame of mind have a tendency to dress without much care, throwing on whatever is most comfortable or functional. They haven't updated their hairstyle in years, and they feel self-conscious or embarrassed about not putting any effort into their appearance. Sometimes they're even evasive and can't talk to the nurse about why they've come to see me. They'll often speak in the third person — as if they're really more concerned about a friend with a specific complaint, rather than themselves. It's hard for some of these women even to admit their feelings.

It can also be hard to spend money on something that our society often writes off as unnecessary and self-absorbed. A lot of women feel guilty for even considering a youth-revitalizing procedure; but I tell my patients all the time that they should not feel like they're required to put themselves in last place. Just as spring cleaning gives you a feeling of satisfaction and freshness, why not think of improvements to your looks in the same way?

Here is my affirmation if you need it: It's OK to take care of yourself. You've earned it. If you need it, you have my blessing — even if the voice in the back of your head is saying a new refrigerator would be so much more practical — because I truly believe that if you take better care of yourself, it will trickle down to everyone else in your life.

SKIN CARE

At the end of this chapter you'll read more about one of my favorite patients, Bethany. I've enjoyed working with Bethany for a very simple reason: she understands the connection between looking good and feeling food. Her lifestyle is founded on good nutrition, exercise, and small improvements over time that help her look her best. She practices some of the subtle but important steps that I advise all my patients in this age range to think about. Most important, Bethany has always taken good care of her skin. In fact, a skin-care regimen — carefully guided by a dermatologist, cosmetic surgeon, or medical aesthetician — is the best way to keep your skin's healthy glow at any age.

A mistake women in their 40s and 50s frequently make is being unduly impressed with every new product, always snapping up the newest, latest, greatest. Part of the problem with that approach is that sometimes the latest and greatest doesn't justify the price if it doesn't have years of tried-and-true research behind it. It's a common pitfall.

Women at this age are even more prone to play the field with the latest miracle cream that promises wrinkle-fighting properties. They can fall prey to the seductive claims by cosmetics manufacturers' pie-in-the-sky promises of crow's feet eradication and increased "luminosity." While some women may think that spending $150 on the latest wrinkle-fighting miracle will somehow grant them access to the secrets of anti-aging, the chances are slim. I can assure you that over-the-counter miracle products are few and far between.

And cosmetics companies, while they seem to offer endless variety and resources, are actually a pretty small family. Estée Lauder, for instance, owns Smashbox, Clinique, Bobbi Brown, Origins, M.A.C., Aveda, Jo Malone, and Prescriptives. If you think there is really that much variation between your age-defying face creams, think again. Many times, high-end companies are selling mystique more than anything, an air of exclusivity and the promise of rare, esoteric ingredients.

Instead of taking a chance on an expensive cream that probably won't work, consult with your cosmetic surgeon, dermatologist, or medical aesthetician; they have access to medical-grade products that are far more effective than what can be found in a commercial setting. Medical-grade products with carefully tested ingredients actually work; they will be suited to your particular needs and they might even be less expensive than the miracle creams, serums, and treatments offered up by the beauty industry. Fashionable marketing doesn't necessarily equate to satisfying results.

If I could advise the more mature woman on just one thing, it would be this: instead of wasting your money on skin-care products that don't have the potency to penetrate the skin's epidermis, why not put that money toward products and procedures that will show measurable results? Your skin's first job is to keep things out, so the challenge is to get a product through that surface and down deep into the skin, which often necessitates a higher-strength prescription or medical-grade product. Translation: over-the-counter is not going to cut it.

Even the vice president of the American Academy of Dermatology, Dr. William P. Coleman, has been pretty blunt in his assessment of what people can expect from over-the-counter moisturizers and wrinkle creams: in effect, *not much*. As Dr. Coleman told *The New York Times,* "You have to think of cosmetics as decorative and hygienic, not as things that are going to change your skin." Prescription medicines undergo rigorous testing before they can receive approval from the Food and Drug Administration. Therefore, over-the-counter cosmetics, defined as topical products that do not alter the structure or function of the skin, do not require FDA approval.

During your 40s and 50s you need to get more aggressive with your skin care, to address the cumulative effects of sun damage, collagen loss, thinning skin, larger pores, and wrinkles. The great thing about this time of life is that most women tend to know what works for them, or are vigilant about seeking out remedies to their problems. With advances in medical-strength anti-aging skin care, their choices are boundless.

YOUR NEW BFFS FOR DRAMATIC RESULTS

With aging come more relentless attacks on collagen, skin elasticity, and vibrancy. Which is why it is so important, as you near 40, to mount a three-pronged attack: **H**uman growth factor, **A**ntioxidants, and **R**etinol — or **HAR** (as in "I laugh at your futile attempt to age me — Har!"). If you want to make things easy on yourself, you can use TNS Essential Serum, which contains all three. I can recommend some great products in each of these categories that will help you laugh in the face of wrinkles:

HUMAN GROWTH FACTOR

Originally used to aid in the healing of wounds, human growth factor originates in human tissue reproduced in a lab. Though it sounds a mite sci-fi, the potential of this new technology to stimulate collagen production in the skin is amazing. Newly repurposed for cosmetic use, anti-aging human growth factors are a great option for women in their 40s and 50s. Human Growth Factor tricks your skin into thinking it's younger than it is. It stimulates collagen production to get rid of fine lines, wrinkles, and spots. And unlike Retin-A, which can cause irritation and flaking in some patients, the nice thing about human growth factor is that it's healing and therapeutic to the skin. It's most typically used in a gel form applied twice a day, as with SkinMedica's TNS Essential Serum.

ANTIOXIDANTS

Antioxidants are substances that protect your skin from the effects of free radicals. Free radicals are the molecules created when your body breaks down food or is exposed to damaging agents like pollution, tobacco smoke, or radiation. Free radicals have been linked to cancer, heart disease, and accelerated aging. Among the many powerful antioxidants are beta-carotene; vitamins A, C, and E; selenium; lycopene; and lutein. While many of these are the ingredients of a healthy diet, a new breed of medical-grade skin care allows patients to reap the benefits of antioxidants topically. One of the most effective is vitamin C.

The antioxidant properties of a topical vitamin C serum, in tandem with an oral vitamin C supplement, are critical at this age. Known to stimulate the body's production of collagen, vitamin C can also aid healing, combat inflammation, and strengthen the skin. The best topical vitamin C is vitamin C-ester, which is more easily absorbed into the skin and will not irritate. A good option is Jan Marini C-Esta Face Serum, applied twice a day to both face and neck, to help repair sun damage.

RETINOLS

Retinols, which are a form of vitamin A, have become the go-to skin-care treatment for their ability, when absorbed into the skin, to speed skin-cell turnover.

This leads to unclogging of pores, reduction of fine lines, and an evening of skin tone — all tremendous pluses in making skin look refreshed, healthy, and glowing. Prescription-strength retinoids include Differin, Retin-A, Renova, Avage, Tazorac, Atralin, and Avita. If you haven't yet incorporated a retinol into your beauty routine, now is the time to begin a regimen with Retin-A or another retinol — ASAP. If you don't want to use Retin-A, you can try SkinMedica's Tri-Retinol Complex. If you are already using Retin-A, you can up the strength and/or frequency of your application, from every other day to every day, or from once daily to twice daily, depending on your skin's tolerance, recognizing that use of these products may lead to greater photosensitivity, peeling, and flaking.

PEPTIDES

As we age, the collagen proteins in our skin decrease. Peptides send a signal to your skin that it is damaged and needs to make more collagen. Though some over-the-counter creams promote their use of peptides, only medical-grade peptides will actually penetrate the surface of the skin and offer the best results. This is why I always advise patients to seek out medical-grade creams and serums containing peptides at their doctor's office or medical spa first before wasting time and money with over-the-counter products.

DRY BRUSHING

A great technique for removing dead cells on the skin's surface, dry brushing can enhance circulation by increasing blood flow and thereby detoxifying the skin. Natural boar bristle, plant-fiber brushes, or a loofah are preferred to synthetic brushes. The technique, which can be done once or twice a week, is relatively simple: moving from your feet upward, until you reach your back, brush toward the heart. Work the brush gently in circular motions, avoiding the delicate skin of the inner thigh, under the arms, the nipples, and face. Follow with a shower to wash away all the dead skin that results from dry-brushing, and finish with a moisturizer to protect your newly glowing skin.

MOISTURIZERS AND SUNSCREENS

As you age, the oils that keep your skin hydrated will diminish, too. Drinking water is always a good thing. If you aren't drinking enough, up your intake to eight to ten glasses a day. But just as important is finding a really great daily moisturizer, preferably with sunscreen, that works well with your skin type, so you'll enjoy the way it feels and use it every day. A moisturizer can reduce the look of wrinkles and give your skin a healthy, dewy glow. Specifically formulated with aging concerns in mind, Jan Marini's Age Intervention line is another great choice for its moisturizing properties.

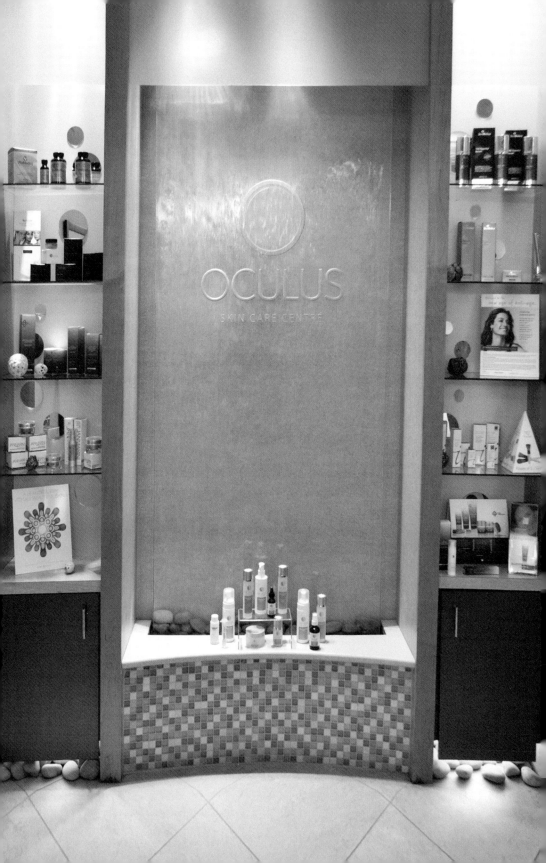

For a daily moisturizer that includes sun protection, I like SkinMedica's TNS Ultimate Daily Moisturizer + SPF 20. It's a great product for limited outdoor exposure, like running your daily errands. But for a long day at the beach or an afternoon walking the streets of Paris, you should up that SPF and use an active-wear product like SkinMedica Environmental Defense SPF 30 or SPF 50 for extended exposure.

WHEN YOU'RE READY TO GO DEEPER

In addition to HAR, that *Charlie's Angels* triumvirate of skin-care necessities, women can turn to a number of other procedures to correct the brown spots, decreased luminosity, slackness, or wrinkles that appear with increasing frequency as we age. Our patients with the fewest wrinkles and who are glowing with health — even into their 60s — generally seek out more effective skin-maintenance options to really protect their investment. Their skin is lustrous because they know the anti-aging mantra: maintain, maintain, maintain. But even perfect skin care can only go so far. Below are a number of options that take it to the next level:

MICRODERMABRASION
Microdermabrasion, or medical exfoliation, is a step up from the kind of weekly or daily exfoliation you perform at home to keep your skin clear and luminous. The procedure involves a wand containing abrasive diamonds or crystals that pass over your skin, which can smooth away age spots, wrinkles and some scars, and can even reduce the size of pores. In order to achieve the best results, I recommend a series of treatments, which can be scheduled at Oculus Skin Care Centre if your travels bring you to the Atlanta area.

LASERS
Back in the mid-1980s, I first witnessed the power of the laser. It was being used in surgeries of the sinus and tear duct, and to remove tumors. That's when I realized the potential for this technology in cosmetic surgery. As a perfectionist, it's the laser's precision that I learned to appreciate most. If you compare the work of a laser with that of a scalpel six weeks after surgery, you'll see a similar result in healing. But it's those first few weeks after laser surgery where you see the real improvement in healing, with less bruising and swelling.

Patients can get back to work faster following a laser surgery. Performing that same procedure with a scalpel, it can take you twice as long to get back to work. Let me explain why: When using a scalpel, the doctor is making an incision, which causes bleeding. He then has to put the scalpel down, pick up a cautery tool, and zap the blood vessels in order to stop the bleeding. With a laser, however, blood vessels are sealed simultaneously with the incision. Bleeding is minimal; and without that excess bleeding, you don't get the bruising and the resultant swelling.

My brain began working overtime thinking about the potential uses for this. I started looking at the things that had been done in the surgery arena. Some procedures had been tried and abandoned due to the limitations of laser technology at the time. When the technology didn't immediately meet the need, people dismissed it completely.

I didn't.

When the technology improved a few years later, it gave us an opportunity to reintroduce lasers and to develop new applications for their use.

By 1992, I was performing surgery using CO2 lasers. I spent some time, one-on-one, in Oklahoma City with laser expert Dr. Sterling Baker, who provided advanced, hands-on training and education about the potential uses for this technology. He was the laser blepharoplasty pioneer, a doctor who was far ahead of the technology curve in the early 1980s. He taught me that anatomy and concepts of disease could be approached with a laser the same way they had been with a scalpel. I saw incredible potential. One could work both inside and outside the skin without making a visible incision.

I started looking at lasers for the resurfacing and tightening of the skin. I learned that with a laser, you can actually restore the integrity of skin. Patients should realize that as they get older, their capacity to generate new skin diminishes. And with aging, the skin's integrity also changes. But the beautiful thing about lasers is that they allow you to actually rejuvinate skin to the form it had 20 years ago — a sort of laser shrink-wrapping — without cutting and without removing it.

By 1993, I was incorporating advanced laser techniques into my daily practice. By 1996, it was booming. Several things had happened. The technology had advanced, so there was a larger therapeutic and safety window for doctors and patients. Contemporary laser treatments simply weren't as high risk as those of the earlier-generation lasers. Doctors could use them on a greater number of patients, with a higher degree of safety. Before that, you could achieve a similar result, but only with a lower margin of safety.

The advent of automated, computerized pattern generators markedly reduced the potential for human error. The doctors felt more confident, the patients felt more comfortable, and things really took off. Several other laser companies (in addition to the pioneer, Coherent Laser Company) got involved in manufacturing, and the industry expanded.

As an early adopter, I was doing a lot of hands-on teaching, as well as live surgical demonstrations, for physicians and laser companies. It's something I still do. People started coming to Atlanta from all over the country to have me instruct them on laser instrumentation and advanced surgical techniques.

By the mid-1990s, we had installed fiber-optic lines in my office and accredited surgery center so I could simultaneously teach and perform live surgeries, both stateside and abroad. It became an interactive tool we could beam out to New York, Los Angeles, even Australia — all in real time.

Lasers are now used every day in my practice. Not only in surgeries but in skin care as well. We now use lasers to treat various sunspots, pigment issues, vascular blemishes and rosacea. We use them for skin tightening, resurfacing, and hair removal. With modern lasers, we can adjust every parameter, including how many microns deep into the skin we want it to go. The approach offers enormous precision as well as complete customization.

Patients these days are more educated about lasers. Today's informed patient will come in knowing that if I use a laser for a procedure, it means a smaller incision and quicker healing time, and that it typically achieves a more natural-looking result, too.

Patients these days are also better educated about lasers. The informed patient today will come in knowing that if I use a laser for a procedure, it means a smaller incision and quicker healing time, and that it typically achieves a more natural-looking result, too.

The Fractional CO2 laser can be a game changer for patients approaching middle-age, as the skin's volume and clarity begins to diminish. It reconditions the skin, which has begun to lose its integrity. By reconditioning and tightening the skin, this procedure essentially erases crepiness (crepe-paper skin) and fine lines, while the deeper wrinkles visibly improve.

The traditional way of looking at cosmetic facial surgery is that it's a bit like ironing a sheet to remove the wrinkles — but you're still working with a cotton sheet. It hasn't improved the quality of the sheet. The astonishing thing about the laser is that it can turn your cotton sheet into a satin one. Unfortunately, a lot of surgeons still haven't adopted laser technology. A typical laser costs upwards of $150,000. For those not performing a great number of laser surgeries, how can they justify spending top dollar for a laser unit? The average plastic surgeon, who isn't an oculofacial specialist like I am, is probably only devoting 5 to 10 percent of his practice to facial cosmetic work. He can't justify a $150,000 coat rack sitting in the back of his OR. Which is why I advise people, whether or not they come to Oculus, to make sure their doctor has the very latest laser technology at his fingertips. The technology has changed dramatically through the years, and if your doctor is not using top-of-the line equipment and isn't exceptionally well-versed in using lasers, you're doing yourself a disservice and risking real, and often irreversible, physical harm.

ENDOSCOPES

Dovetailing with the development of lasers and Botox in the mid-1980s, endoscopes, which are lighted telescopes, were first used in sinus surgeries. By the early 1990s, flexible fiber-optic instruments were being used in tear-duct surgeries. Cosmetically, endoscopes came into use around 1993, which was right around the time that Botox and lasers were transforming the industry. These advancing technologies all intersected and pushed plastic surgery forward in a remarkable way. The ride was fast and furious, but I enjoyed helping steer the ship.

Years ago, when I was finishing my surgical training at Tulane and Vanderbilt, we were still required to make large incisions. We would literally make an ear-to-ear incision and pull flaps of skin and muscle down while performing brow- and face-lifting procedures. Now with endoscopes, we can make a one-inch access point and insert a lighted telescope with a camera attached into a surgically created optical cavity. This allows us to look underneath the facial soft tissue, and we no longer have to pull anything down.

The patient's scalp and everything else stays in place, including the delicate blood supply and sensory nerves. When we had to make that ear-to-ear incision, the anatomy was disrupted. We were cutting through all those sensory nerves. Some of those areas remained numb forever. Things might look fine visually, but the patient never again feels like himself or herself. Now, that 20-inch incision has been reduced to one or two inches. It's dramatically better, and has made a lot of surgical procedures more acceptable to patients, because they don't mind a small incision. More important, it's safer and results in fewer complications.

Also with the endoscope, healing takes a fraction of the time compared to a procedure performed with a scalpel, because you don't have the muscle and nerve damage. It's become a deciding factor for many patients who might otherwise resist cosmetic surgery. Thanks to all these incredible advances, I'm now able to help my patients achieve a more youthful, more natural appearance with less downtime for recovery. Unfortunately, many plastic surgeons have not taken advantage of this technology.

INJECTABLES

Fillers and partially denervating agents, such as Botox and Dysport, relax tensed muscles to inhibit the formation of wrinkles. The options in such nonsurgical approaches are many — from hyaluronic acids such as Restylane, Juvéderm, and Perlane, which plump up the skin for a number of months or years, to collagen stimulators like Radiesse, which offer both immediate and long-term results. Sculptra and Selphyl, on the other hand, generate progressive volume over time through collagen stimulation. On the permanent end of the spectrum, fillers such as Artefill must be used by a well-qualified, skilled surgeon or dermatologist, since complications can be more difficult to correct and results are slightly more unpredictable.

A lot of my female first-time consults will tell me, "I'm afraid I'm turning into my mother." That provides a great starting point for us to discuss the role of genetics in their appearance. I also want you to share those photos of the younger you and I want to hear about how that younger you stands in contrast to the current you. Photos allow us to discuss what's realistic in terms of potential results. But I also want to get feedback from you on what you think is realistic. I'm listening for what features you like best about yourself, not necessarily how you felt or what you were doing or where you were in your life when the snapshot was taken. I'm listening to see if your expectations track with reality.

If you tell me, "I felt like my eyes were a very strong feature when I was younger. I used to get compliments on them but I don't anymore," that's useful information for me to have. It gives me the framework to talk to you about how your eyes have changed over the years — and more important, what we can do to restore a more youthful appearance to those eyes.

The number-one thing I recommend is volume change — to add or restore volume to your face. The second is shape. As we age and things shift, most of us go from a face shape with a base-up triangle to one with a base-down triangle. This happens when the cheek pad and jowls drop down, squaring off the chin region. It's just gravity at work, perfectly normal but not always what you want to see in the mirror. Gravity ("the big G") is a big issue. But a good plastic surgeon can help counteract the big G to restore your anatomy to its proper alignment.

BOTOX AND DYSPORT

The Botox that might have been useful as a preventive measure in your 20s and 30s can now be very effective in combating those notorious 11s that form between your eyebrows, or the worry lines that register on your forehead. If you were to come in and point out the formation of some frown lines you've noticed due to sun exposure, I might suggest that you freshen things up with Botox treatments. Botox is used as the generic term for all injectable muscle relaxers — similar to Kleenex for facial tissue.

For wrinkles on the neck, Botox and Dysport are a method of easing muscle tension. Because the eyes are among the first areas to show signs of aging, I often recommend treating hooded, saggy upper eyelids with Botox and Dysport, which inhibit the depressor muscle that pulls down the eyebrow. Both are capable of reshaping and refreshing the eye area by lifting the brow — subtly and without surgery.

Sometimes Botox can be used in conjunction with other procedures. For instance, with laser resurfacing I discovered that Botox could also be used for its secondary healing benefits. Following a laser treatment, Botox acts as a cast by immobilizing the treated area. If the area is not moving, it can heal faster and more effectively. In 1993, I first presented my ABC Technique for brow lifting at a national meeting of plastic surgeons. A is for Anchoring, to stabilize the brow; B is for Botox; and C is for CO2 laser.

Although I have been recommending Botox therapeutically as far back as 1986, I still get inquiries from patients about its safety. The truth is, I've been treating my wife, my sister, and my mother with Botox since the 1980s. I've even treated my mother-in-law with it, so you know I have confidence in the FDA-approved medication. If that doesn't convince you, it might help to consider that Botox has a better safety profile in patients than common aspirin.

The only time you hear stories in the news about Botox is when unlicensed, inexperienced individuals use it to inject people with a black-market substance that hasn't been tested. You simply don't know what you're getting, and that's a scary situation. Unfortunately these days, you can go on YouTube and watch a video on how to inject someone with Botox and then go online and order it from somewhere in Mexico. But Botox is much like any other treatment: if you take the proper precautions and use it in a controlled fashion, it's quite safe.

FILLERS
As we age, our skin begins to develop hollows around the eyes which can result in a gaunt, aging effect, nasolabial folds, marionette lines, and other indications of skin aging and volume displacement. This is especially true when women are extremely fit and have lost some of the volume in their face. That full, puffy baby-face look that signals youth begins to diminish. One of the best tools for fighting this effect is the use of dermal fillers to add volume, contour, and carefully targeted fullness. Volume control — whether adding or shifting it — can change everything. It's the beauty of addition, not subtraction.

Fillers can address a number of specific complaints for women in their 40s and 50s, though patients should remember that fillers are really camouflage; they can temporarily disguise issues that only surgery can truly correct. To add volume to the cheeks, hyaluronic acid and collagen-stimulating fillers help plump up this area of the face. For those annoying marionette lines that run downward from the corners of the mouth, hyaluronic acid fillers (which last about six months) and Radiesse (which lasts a year or longer) are great options, although really committed patients interested in a more long-term effect can opt for Artefill, which is permanent. I do not recommend permanent fillers in the face, because the facial tissues are dynamic and ever changing. New technology should have minimal side effects or none at all.

With the proper use of fillers for tear-trough, temple region, chin, and jawline augmentation — and to target nasolabial and melolabial folds — the effects can suggest something like a liquid face lift.

I consistently recommend that patients stick with reversible fillers unless they are quite certain they want to go with a permanent approach. In conjunction with this, I always advise anyone considering a permanent procedure who is in a long-term, committed relationship to discuss the idea with their significant other. You might be surprised by how many men respond viscerally and angrily to a change in their wife's or girlfriend's appearance. So it's wise to definitely pave the way before undertaking anything permanent.

The other thing to consider is how predictable a permanent filler will be, based on the area of the face you're treating. The tear-trough area beneath the eyes, for instance, is not as predictable in the way it responds to a permanent filler. You need to find a surgeon with the experience and skill to inject a permanent filler in that area with great precision. I see patients all the time who have had bad permanent fillers injected, and the results can leave them despondent and deeply distressed. Scar tissue can form, and surgery is often necessary to correct the problem. Permanent fillers are not to be entered into lightly, so make sure you are in very capable hands before making this choice.

PHOTOFACIALS
Photofacials are treatments in which pulsed light is used to treat a range of skin conditions. An Intense Pulsed Light (IPL) facial uses a high-intensity light to target the melanin that creates brown spots or the blood vessels that produce broken capillaries. IPL facials, which stimulate collagen, are most useful for treating pig-mentation issues, including melasma and other brown spots, as well as for vascu-lar issues such as broken capillaries and spider veins. They also have the ability to tighten or refine pores, although any reputable doctor will tell you that pores cannot be erased, only made to appear smaller.

SURGICAL PROCEDURES
The key to doing anything surgical at this age is to keep it natural. I advise aim-ing for small, incremental changes that preserve the core of your face (your eyes

Sheryl
Tear Trough Fillers

The tear trough is the groove or sulcus at the medial lower eyelid that shows the orbital rim below. A volume issue, it can be camouflaged by filler. The "bridge procedure" usually lasts 6-12 months.

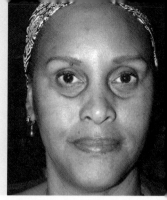

AFTER ▶   ▲ BEFORE

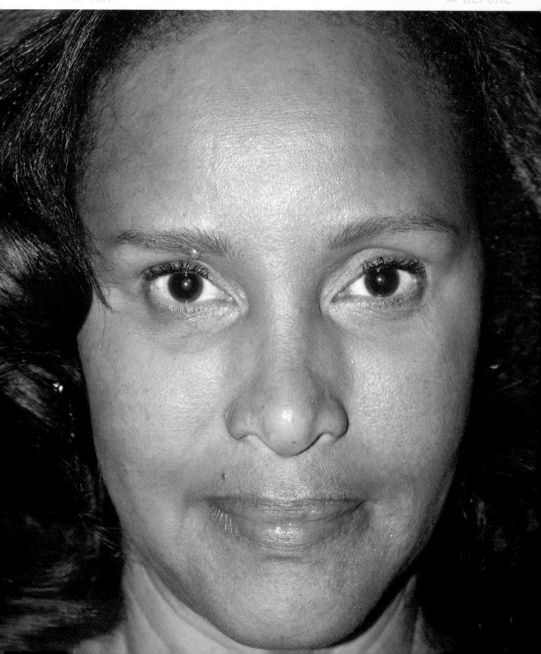

and mouth) while adjusting the framework. Though it might not be something you notice consciously when a person changes portions of their face in an exaggerated, artificial way, the brain registers that something is amiss. That's why some women who have had too much surgery look askew, even from across the room. You can't quite put your finger on why something is off, beyond recognizing that they've had too much work done, but you know. As we say in the South, "somethin' ain't right."

By the same token, when you see someone whose eyes and mouth haven't changed artificially, despite small surgical adjustments, they still look like themselves. It's imperative to focus on your face's essential framework. I use the example of movie stars Meg Ryan and Michelle Pfeiffer to distinguish between the two kinds of surgery — the regrettably obvious approach versus the more natural one. While Ryan has altered her face, lips, and eyes with what appears to be the aggressive use of fillers (to the point where she barely resembles her former self), Pfeiffer has tweaked and improved without losing sight of that core. (For more on the various pitfalls and triumphs of celebrity plastic surgery, see Chapter 11.)

I have found that when a woman reaches the age of about 40 or 50, the cheek pad migrates downward and inward. This shift in volume reveals the orbital bony rim, revealing a double bag and shadowing below the eye. The same shift also then deepens the nasolabial groove. Done endoscopically, a cheek lift often lends itself to subtle but quite rejuvenating results. Two incisions are completely hidden in the temple hair and at the gum line, so there are no visible signs. A carefully orchestrated cheek lift can take 10 years off of your appearance. It doesn't change your eyes and it doesn't change the architecture of your face — you still look like you. Madonna had this procedure, among many others, and the results speak for themselves. In her 50s, Madonna has aged slightly from the Material Girl of the '80s, but the changes are so subtle, so finely drawn, that you notice only that she looks fantastic and appears to have made time stand still.

Plastic surgery is an art founded on delicacy, and very small shifts that can discreetly transform a face. Computer imaging is a marvelous tool for envisioning how your surgical results will look and how little change is really needed to create a beautiful result. For example, if you've always had full cheeks and suddenly you want a more tapered supermodel look, with hollow cheeks and more dramatic lines, that's going to change your whole face. I think it's important for you to understand that, which is why computer imaging has become such a vital part of my practice for the last 20 years. It's an amazing tool.

In the beginning, my biggest concern was that patients see imaging for what it is, an educational tool and not a wow-factor novelty or conversation piece. At other plastic surgeons' offices, computer-imaging technology can be abused in the same way art directors use Photoshop to manipulate images for magazine covers, fashion spreads, and advertisements. Some may remember the controversy that erupted in 2009 when a photograph of Demi Moore on the cover of *W* magazine looked visibly altered. Some speculated that Moore's head had been Photoshopped onto a twentysomething supermodel's body.

The same thing can happen with computer imaging in a plastic surgeon's office: you run the risk of idealizing people's faces, then disappointing them when they see the actual real-life alteration. It's amazing technology, but I make every effort not to fall prey to its wizardry. I show my patients actual pictures of other patients whom I've treated, in addition to their own computer image. I include the pre-surgery, computer-imaged, and post-surgery photos. Seeing the stages helps them to understand the power of this essential tool but also to maintain realistic expectations about their predictive power.

Thanks to this wonderful modern technology, I can now photograph you, upload your image to the monitor, and demonstrate the changes you want to have performed. I then email the results to you, which you can print out and tape to your refrigerator door or bathroom mirror, so you can get acquainted with your new look. It's a fun way for you to live with your new self prior to actually committing to a procedure. Some of my patients have even had "face reveal" luncheons, where they print their anticipated sneak peak as placemats, inviting their close circle of girlfriends to comment before the actual surgical procedure. You might even decide cosmetic surgery is not the best option for you.

> The key to doing anything surgical at this age is to keep it natural. Aim for small, incremental changes that preserve the core of your face while adjusting the framework.

You'd be amazed how many times a patient will look at before-and-after pictures of a procedure done on other patients and request the same thing. However, that patient's opinion can radically change when I tap a few strokes on the keyboard, swirl around the mouse, and apply exactly the same changes to a computer-enhanced photo of their face. Thankfully, to this day I've never had a single patient tell me afterward, "My imaging picture looked better, and I'm disappointed." If anything, I want to underpromise and overdeliver. Minimalist architect Ludwig Mies van der Rohe famously said, "Less is more." For me, less is better.

I urge my older patients who are considering surgery to understand that sometimes when a patient undergoes a major change to their appearance later in life, they can be surprised by the results. Some patients have difficulty adjusting to the changes made in a face they've lived with their entire life. By the time you reach your 40s and 50s, your sense of self is more deeply rooted, and a dramatic alteration may not give you the happiness you anticipate. If patients enter into surgery with their eyes wide open and knowing the risks, I am confident that everyone can be satisfied with the outcome.

PIGMENTATION ISSUES

Alterations in your skin's pigmentation — which can occur with hormonal changes, pregnancy, and aging — can be treated with a variety of bleaching creams in low, medium, and heavy strengths. At our office, we have what I like to think of as a "couture" triple-bleaching cream, custom formulated at Concord Pharmacy exclusively for Oculus; it uses glycolic acid, hydroquinone, and Retin-A to penetrate the skin's surface. I also use EpiQuin Micro for skin lightening, with a typical treatment cycle of four months on and four months off. This does wonders for brown spots and for acne scarring.

FOR GOODNESS' SAKE, EXFOLIATE

Exfoliating becomes more and more critical as we age. Dead skin cells can take their time sloughing off, and as a result, the skin begins to look dull and tired. Adding alpha-hydroxy acid (AHA) or beta-hydroxy acid (BHA) products to your skin-care routine can reveal brighter, clearer skin with fewer wrinkles. These are available in cleanser or cream form.

Derived from fruit and milk sugars, AHAs (of which glycolic and lactic acids are the most common) are great exfoliants when you want to really rev up skin-cell turnover. AHAs help with the sloughing off of dead skin cells and are especially useful if you have sun-damaged skin. Most over-the-counter glycolic-acid products have too low a percentage of AHAs (under 10 percent) to be truly effective. Instead, doctor-strength AHA is your best bet. BHA (also known as salicylic acid) is better able to penetrate the pores where sebum and dead skin cells lurk, making it ideal for women who are still experiencing breakouts and clogged pores. Both AHA and BHA can increase your sun sensitivity, so make sure to use an effective sunscreen in conjunction with these products.

Oculus LactiCleanse is a great multitasking cleanser for women in their 40s and 50s because it kills two birds with one stone. It contains lactic acid, which is very hydrating to the skin, as well as a mild exfoliant to speed skin-cell turnover.

In the chemical-peel department, the prescription-strength SkinMedica Vitalize Peel uses retinoic acid. It delivers measurable results after just one use and significantly improves skin after several treatments. I also like the Rejuvenize Peel, which uses BHA to treat sun damage, pigment changes, and acne scarring, delivering visible results.

THE OLD NIP/TUCK

The old nip and tuck ain't what it used to be. With advancements in fillers and Botox, as well as other methods to camouflage the signs of aging, has come a reevaluation of what surgery can and should do.

The old-fashioned methods of plastic surgery called for stretching and cutting but did nothing to counter gravity — and gravity always won. Like stretching a tent or a drumhead over a frame, the old method essentially just pulled the skin taut over muscle and bone. As we intuitively know, things that are stretched too tight eventually become slack again. Gravity can only be addressed at the structural level, by putting things back where they used to be, rather than artificially tightening them to some imagined better place.

For example, everyone's midface tends to move downward and inward as they age. When I perform a cheek-lift procedure, it's imperative that I place the cheek pad back where it belongs, on the cheekbone, so the patient looks the way she used to look. Only now are we counteracting gravity. But if the cheek is left where it is, and it's merely filled or stretched, gravity wins. The "tent" approach disregards the essential scaffolding of flesh and bone beneath. It's the difference between temporary camouflage and long-term correction.

It comes down to your doctor's approach and philosophy. If you were my patient, I would stress that the look you want is an improved version of yourself — not a stranger looking back at you from the mirror. For too many surgeons too often, transformation doesn't necessarily mean improvement.

THE EYES HAVE IT

Surprisingly, the eyes — an area of the face that can show dramatic signs of aging — are often neglected. Crepiness and discoloration can occur as skin loses elasticity and begins to show veins. Since the skin around the eyes is the thinnest on the body, the underlying anatomy there is the first to reveal itself. As the cheek pads descend, the orbital rim of bone is revealed, accentuating the fatty tissue beneath the eyes. The subtracted volume around the eyes reveals irregularities and hollows, while the fatty pads of the descending cheek shift downward and inward, making the nasolabial fold thicker and deeper.

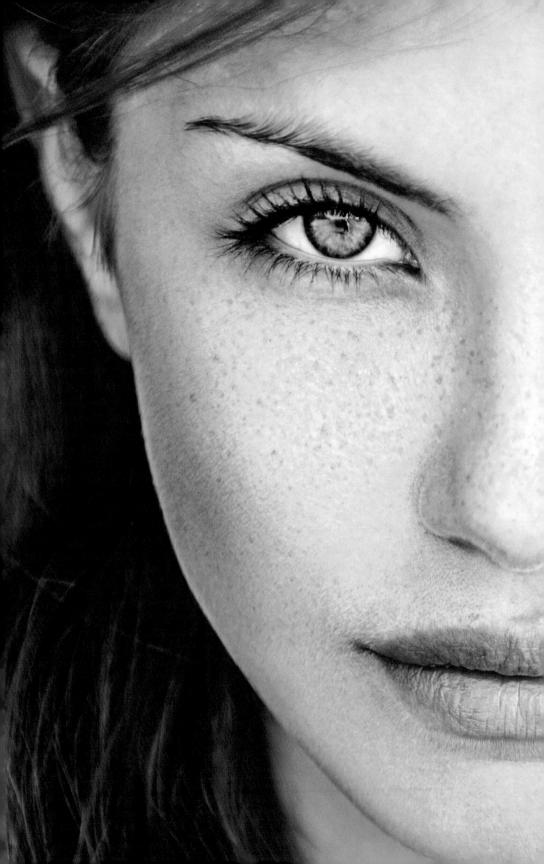

My patients often express concern over how they think they look, but also how others say they look. Comments such as "You look so tired," "You look sad all the time" or "Why are you so angry?" drive patients into my office. They ask what I can do about the puffy bags under their eyes, about the excess fat that has accumulated there, about the hooded upper eyelids that hinder proper vision and make them look so tired.

Over the past decade, I've seen many patients who had "eyelid tucks" by other physicians and did not see the improvement they expected. What these patients require is a multilayered rejuvenation approach that takes into consideration not just the upper eyelid skin, but the area around the eyes. Crow's feet, bags or hollows, angry brows, and hanging skin are all areas to be considered — not just the eyelid skin. When the brows are low and unstable, it's crucial to approach the brow and eyes in tandem, rather than treating the eyes in isolation from the brow, as is done all too often.

My response to the inevitable effect of aging is a patented Eyelight Blepharoplasty technique, which I developed to remedy this midfacial slackness. The procedure employs a laser and endoscope to rejuvenate both the upper and lower eyelids, as well as the brow and cheek area. The laser helps repair and restore the facial tissue to its original position and a more youthful texture, while the endoscope helps restore the proper distance between the brow and lashes. There are no visible incisions and no stitches to remove. This is an ultra-precise procedure that achieves wonderful, natural-looking results.

Stabilizing the brows endoscopically is very important at this point because they must be prevented from drooping. If the skin on the upper lid is tightened but the brow is not stabilized, the tightened skin will pull the brow down. Simply cutting away the extra eyelid skin removes the stimulus for the brow to stay elevated. It's like taking off sagging wallpaper and regluing it. The wallpaper isn't new, it's just been stabilized.

The Eyelight Blepharoplasty is a much less invasive procedure: instead of the usual cutting another doctor might do, my technique is to go behind the hairline and make a little access point in the temple area or through the mouth. The only time I make an exposed incision is in the crease of the upper eyelid, where it will be barely visible. The incision is thus hidden within the eye's natural fold. Most people without a microscopic surgical background aren't able to notice it. Most important, by using this method the brow is stabilized, then sutured, so no forehead skin is removed; the distance from hairline to brow does not change. The great thing about opting for a procedure like this in your 40s or 50s is that your skin has a far better ability to heal — and your collagen replacement is superior — than if you had waited until your 60s or 70s.

BEYOND THE CLINIC

A STYLE REFRESHER: SMALL CHANGES, BIG RESULTS

This is a time when people — men especially — can become set in their ways, and often need the wisdom of an outside perspective to help refresh their look. There are a lot of different approaches to staying beautiful as you age — beyond skin care, exercise, and anti-aging procedures — such as surgery, fillers, and Botox.

One of the biggest changes women can make at this age to help fuel their self-esteem is to begin a frank appraisal of their personal style. While women in their 40s and 50s are often hitting their stride (a good career, husband, home, children and friends), they can also get settled into a style that worked for them in their 20s, but maybe isn't so flattering in their 40s.

A good place to start in reevaluating your style might be a favorite department store or boutique, where a personal shopper can help you find clothes that fit your lifestyle and project the right image. Ask around, as small towns and big cities alike often have a wealth of style consultants, even outside of department stores, who can offer targeted wardrobe advice, as well as comprehensive tips on hairstyle, color analysis, diet, and the whole spectrum of appearance. Once found, this sort of style guru can become one of your golden allies in the battle to stay gorgeous and hip. If they work in a shop, this person can put aside outfits when they come in that will work with your taste and body type, and also help in giving you an honest, educated appraisal of what works and what doesn't — something your friends often won't do, and your poor husband can't.

A wardrobe or style consultant can help you transition from a stunted style that you are still clinging to (well into middle-age) into something more polished and appealing.

Men often use these services, too — especially men looking for a competitive edge in the business world but also younger men who might want to up their game in the dating realm, or transition from the style-impaired world of college to the more sophisticated demands of adult life. Out in the real world, the backward baseball caps and flip-flops that telegraphed "fun" in college can now register as immature in adulthood. A wardrobe or style consultant can help men transition from a stunted style that some men are still clinging to (well into middle-age) into something more polished and appealing.

Following are some things you may not have considered, and perhaps other things you have, that can dramatically affect your looks as you age. I don't profess to be an expert in fashion or grooming, but I have seen clear evidence that self-confidence can improve when surgical or nonsurgical changes are made in conjunction with a reappraisal of one's personal style. Over time I've observed that certain style choices made by both women and men can date them as much as wrinkles or age spots (more on that in Chapter 7). Even among men and women of the exact same age, some look effortlessly stylish while others have let time catch up with them. So just as important as taking care of your face is making sure you aren't adopting aging ways of dressing or applying makeup that counteract all that hard work.

LASHES AND EYEBROWS

You may notice your eyebrows and eyelashes becoming a bit more sparse as you inch toward middle-age. The lush lashes you once took for granted in your younger years can now show thinning or a lack of luster. A lifetime of plucking can also take a toll. Over time those poor tortured hair follicles just don't snap back as much with new hair growth, and you're left with the eyebrow shape you loved at 25 but now wish was just a bit more filled in. Luckily, we live in an age of beauty-restoring advances that can take most negatives and transform them into positives. To restore the full, lush look of your lashes there are a number of products you can use, including Latisse, an FDA-approved prescription treatment that restores the length and fullness of lashes. Latisse is not approved for use on the eyebrows, so patients are advised first to discuss potential side effects with their doctor before using the product in this off-label way. ("Off-label" is the term for an FDA-approved product used in a non-approved site; this accounts for 62 percent of all FDA-approved medications.)

Though you may not have needed it in the past, you might look into a brush-on brow powder or brow pencil for thinning brows. Either can subtly fill in gaps in brows and increase thickness in the brow, which can have a dramatic effect on your face. If the idea of filling in color with a brow pencil leaves you fearful, with visions of Joan Crawford's exclamatory super-brows dancing in your head, a tinted brow gel can do the work for you without looking artificial or forcing you to play Picasso each morning. A popular alternative we offer at Oculus Skin Care Centre is medical-grade permanent brow tattooing.

HAIR REMOVAL

As you age, you may notice an increase in the fine, downy white hairs on your face, or the darker hairs that can create the bane of women's existence, the dreaded lady mustache. There are a number of remedies — from home waxing to professional

Complaint: Slack skin on the face and neck; heaviness in her eyelids

An actor in the popular long-running stage comedy *Peachtree Battle,* about Atlanta's wealthy, eccentric residents, Deborah Childs was motivated to do something about the dramatic aging that had begun to claim her looks. She showed the classic signs of facial aging: the volume of her midface had started to shift, periorbital wrinkles were increasing, and her lower jawline was boxed off by jowling. She decided to take action after a conversation with a little girl.

"This adorable little girl with the innocence and honesty of a child asked me, 'Why are you so sad?'" Deborah recalls. *"I remember saying to her, 'Honey, I'm not sad, why do you ask?' She replied, 'Well, you sure do look sad.' Later, I went inside and took a long look in the mirror and I understood what she meant."*

Ah, the refreshing honesty of children.

Deborah recognized that in her business, it was time to make a change. Her career depended on it. *"God help you if you have the bad taste to become middle-aged in this business. All the celebrity magazines did big stories on Julia Roberts and Jennifer Aniston the nanosecond they turned 40. Those same magazines didn't give Brad Pitt or Tom Cruise the same treatment. Men just don't have to deal with the same things in our business."*

As they say, when men age they start looking like Robert Redford. When women age they start looking like Robert Redford.

Deborah wanted to avoid Botox because it would limit the facial movements a comedic actress needs to make to perform her role convincingly, especially onstage. *"As an actor, I have to keep my face very mobile. Trudy wouldn't get half the laughs she does if the audience couldn't read my expression from the 20th row."*

Outcome: Deborah underwent an endoscopic brow lift, periorbital laser resurfacing, endoscopic midface and cheek lift, and lower face lift with anterior platysmaplasty, which is the tightening of the neck bands and jawline. Deborah was so delighted with her results — and her surgery made such a powerful impact on her self-esteem — that she also lost weight, so her body would match her youthful face. With her new face came new roles.

With surgery, it's often necessary to begin a new beauty regimen to maintain your results, and for Deborah that meant no longer ignoring the crucial steps of moisturizing her skin and applying sunscreen every day. To maintain her results, Deborah has come in for small tweaks, including fillers, and has begun a therapeutic skin-care regimen.

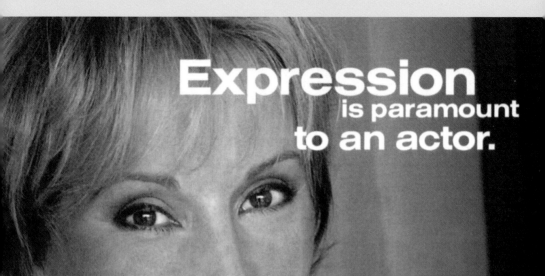
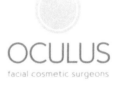

laser hair removal — to suit your particular needs and budget. But be vigilant if you're going to take the DIY route. For example, waxing of the delicate upper lip area can be painful (plucking is often best). And if you use Retin-A, be aware that your skin can be more delicate and easily irritated by waxing.

TEETH WHITENING

As we age, our teeth tend to yellow, and our daily coffee and tea habits certainly don't help. Few things can age you as quickly as yellow or gray teeth. Fortunately, everyone in this day and age can have white teeth. One quick and easy way to take years off of your appearance is with the array of bleaching options available, from whitening toothpastes to at-home bleaching and professional whitening procedures. With so many options, there is every reason to incorporate some bleaching into your beauty routine. If money is no object, porcelain veneers are the Cadillac of cosmetic dentistry, allowing patients to dramatically reshape their teeth and also add brightness to their smile.

WEIGHT TRAINING

If you don't exercise, this is probably not the first time you've heard that getting physical is an essential. That means increasing your heart rate for an hour at least four times a week. You may have been able to avoid exercise in your 20s and 30s and not gain weight. But what applied then does not necessarily apply now. Metabolism peaks in your 20s then begins to decline. The truth is, weight gain starts to be a serious concern as you get older, and if you don't find an aerobic exercise routine that you like and can stick with, then you may begin to see the slow creep of pounds. Exercise doesn't have to mean the drudgery of the treadmill, if that's not your thing. It can be a great opportunity for quality time with your children or husband, with a brisk nightly walk in the park or around your neighborhood. Set up a tennis date with a friend a few days a week. Take a Pilates or yoga class. The most important thing is to do *something*. Exercise early and exercise often. What often

> Along with dry-brushing, massage of both the face and body is a great way to stimulate the skin and the body's lymphatic system.

happens once you start making time for exercise is that it becomes easier and more rewarding to increase your activity as you begin to feel and look better.

If you do exercise you know the advantages are myriad: increased energy and longevity, glowing skin, better overall health, lowered cholesterol, fewer menopause symptoms, reduced cancer risk, less stress, and a sense of well-being. And freedom from that horrible feeling you get when the jeans you once effortlessly fit into can't be zipped up anymore. We've all been there, and it's not pretty. Even if you exercise with some frequency at the gym or running around your neighborhood, it's probably a good idea at this point to add some weights to your routine. Along with the incredible benefits of aerobic exercise — for the circulatory system and for burning calories and fat as we age — weight training helps to maintain muscle tone and definition, as well as bone density. If we're lucky and diligent, maybe by the time we're 70 we can all look as good as Jane Fonda. Feel the burn!

MASSAGE

Although it's generally thought of as a relaxing, stress-relieving pursuit (which can be beneficial too), massage can be also intensely therapeutic. Along with dry-brushing, massage of both the face and body is a great way to stimulate the skin and the body's lymphatic system. So the next time your husband asks, instead of saying you are going to get a massage, tell him you're off for some physical therapy. (Remember, you heard it here first.)

THE EMPRESS NEEDS NEW CLOTHES

Personal style is a tricky thing. What works for one person may not work for the next. I try to avoid rules or edicts, but as I have mentioned, as women age, certain adjustments to style can really take off the years. Dressing too young — especially after undergoing surgery — or too old and frumpy, because you feel self-conscious about your body, are two ways that you lose sight of your biological age and cling to some frozen-in-time vision of what you think looks good.

People change, trends change, life changes, and the best way to be prepared is to take an honest survey of how you're dressing, how you're applying makeup, and other elements of personal grooming. Small changes can have big impact, but a little ruthless honesty may be called for too. Spend a day with your daughter or a friend whose taste you trust — or with your new personal stylist — weeding through your closet and chucking anything you haven't worn in a year, or that's out of date or doesn't flatter you. It shouldn't matter how much you paid for it or how much you long to one day fit into it: if it doesn't look good, if it doesn't fit, get rid of it. And don't feel like you're being wasteful: We all make mistakes and we shouldn't have to wear them as penance, just to feel like we're getting our money's worth. You can donate the clothes to Goodwill, the Salvation Army or a women's shelter, and know that you're not only streamlining your personal style, you're helping someone in need.

EVALUATE (AND EMBRACE) YOUR BODY TYPE

First things first. Figure out what works for your figure and don't force looks that don't flatter. Think of how Sophia Loren would look in skinny jeans: maybe not so great. She's a gorgeous woman, but she knows what looks good on her curves. We could all learn a little from the style icons among us who retain their beauty because they don't cling to fads or some worn-out former identity of what was hip and cool. Just because everyone is wearing maxi dresses doesn't mean you have to, especially if your figure leans toward the zaftig. If you don't have the power arms to get away with a sleeveless look, work the three-quarter or cap sleeve. Know your strengths and your weaknesses and don't let a cute skirt (on the hanger) or the new Manolos everyone's wearing convince you otherwise. Many of us spend a lifetime striving for something we don't naturally possess. If we have straw-straight hair, we want it curly; if our hair is curly we spend hours taming it into sleek, straight strands. Same goes for our clothes. Fashion designer Michael Kors offered this wise advice in *Elle* magazine on working with your natural gifts, and I think these are words worth remembering. "Don't put a round peg in a square hole. Buy clothes based on your silhouette: 1950s — hourglass; 1960s — gamine; 1970s — small-chested." That's why you're more likely to see First Lady Michelle Obama wear a more forgiving A-line skirt that highlights her toned arms, rather than try to make a fashion statement in a fitted skirt.

> Many of us spend a lifetime striving for something that we don't naturally possess. Instead, figure out what works for your figure and don't force looks that don't flatter.

AVOID TRENDS

As you get older it's best to avoid the appearance of slavishly following every new thing, especially the cheap and transitory items you find in the chain stores. Teenagers and twentysomethings are supposed to try such things out because they don't know their own style. But women of a certain age should stick with the fashion cuts and the styles that suit them best. This is not to say that a dramatic new cut, color or accessory can't be incorporated into your look. The latest handbag or bangle can telegraph to the world that you still care about style, but that's not the same as wearing daisy dukes, tube tops or gladiator sandals, just because everyone else is. Aim to be a little more discriminating.

RETHINK COLOR IN YOUR CLOTHING

I know color analysis was a big fad in the '80s, but there's a lot to be said for the advantages of knowing what hues suit you. While it might seem like an outdated idea, I think it's one worth bringing back. Some people think that with age must come bright, cheery colors and no more "depressing" black and gray, but colorful doesn't always spell youth or energy. Often it's neutrals — like tan, white, black, navy and gray — that can provide a beautiful foundation to complement accessories such as a scarf, a purse, an amazing pair of shoes, or bold jewelry. Black and white can remain great go-to colors even as you age, because they're so versatile, and solids can often look more chic than prints and patterns, which soon can become dated and trendy looking. If you crave visual interest, try a neutral color but with great texture instead of a print. If a bold color really suits you, then remember to keep the shapes simple and don't overdo the accessories.

HAIR

Older hair often means thinner hair. Ask your hair stylist for a product that will bulk up the hair shaft during blow drying. Or try a volumizer, thickening shampoo or even dry shampoo, all of which can plump up thinning hair. Stick with a cut that works with your hair's texture, and don't over-tease (thinking that will hide thinning hair). If your hair is very thin, you might want to go a bit shorter. And don't overlook the importance of good nutrition in making your hair full and glossy. Make sure you're getting all your vitamin supplements, especially biotin, which has been shown to help with thinning hair.

Don't think that because you're over 40, you need to sport hair that's shoulder-length or shorter. If your hair looks great long, keep it that way, but be aware that longer aging hair may need more layering to lend body, depth, and movement.

Highlights of a slightly lighter hair color, with some variation in tones, can also make a huge difference in combating age — rather than a single flat color. Bright highlights concentrated around the face lighten and brighten the face. Of course, blonde doesn't look great on everyone and can, in fact, make skin look ashy and washed out with certain skin tones. Adjusting your natural hair color slightly (by one or two shades) can make a huge difference and rev up the luminosity of not just your hair but your face, too.

Also consider asking your stylist about a modified sweep of bangs, which can soften your face and hide forehead wrinkles at the same time.

PAY ATTENTION TO CUT

Before you buy a piece of clothing, check the silhouette in a full-length, three-way mirror to make sure it's as flattering behind as it is in front. And don't underestimate the effect of tailoring. Men will typically have a tailor hem pant legs or jacket sleeves to suit them, and women should do the same — not just for length but for fit. The cost is minimal and worth every penny. Best of all, tailoring adapts clothes to your particular body, making something off the rack uniquely flattering.

DON'T SHOW TOO MUCH SKIN

Trying too hard is for amateurs. If you have a great bust line, a clingy shirt can show it off as well as a shirt plunging down to your navel. Great gams will still look fabulous in a knee-length skirt, but wearing a miniskirt telegraphs an unappealing "look at me" bid for attention when you're over 40. Most of all, pick your winning battles. If you're going to show off your legs, then cut back on the cleavage, and vice versa.

By the same token, don't suddenly buy only A-line shapes, tunics, pajama-wide pants and voluminous square blouses. Very loose and boxy garments, too-long skirts and a covered-up look can actually suggest more pounds than the ones you're trying to hide. The best strategy is usually balance: If you're wearing an A-line skirt, you should wear something a bit more fitted on top. If you're crazy about tunics, go for some leggings or slim jeans underneath to keep from looking swallowed up by your clothes. And if you're wearing something black and want to brighten your face, never underestimate the power of a bright, shimmery or silky scarf tied at the neck or draped to add color and visual interest. Know the colors that work best for you and find a wardrobe of scarves in those hues.

MAKEUP

Most beauty editors will tell you that certain rules apply as you grow older. As with everything, keeping makeup minimal and subtle is key. The foundation that you once used to hide acne-prone or blotchy skin may begin to look too heavy and can make duller skin look even more ashy and lifeless. The better option is to use foundation sparingly, and in conjunction with a skin primer, tinted moisturizer (preferably with an SPF) or concealer. Face powder can also have a dramatic aging effect, so choose wisely. If shine is an issue, blotting papers or an oil-diminishing primer are effective remedies. A translucent or light-reflecting powder, very lightly applied and only on the T-zone, can be used if the thought of going powderless strikes terror in your heart. Many women find that using a cream rather than a powder blush gives their skin a much-needed luminosity, where powder blushes just dull. Avoiding dark, heavy lipsticks, which can accentuate lines around thin lips, is also important. Most experts agree that lighter, brighter, more translucent pinks and berries applied as a gloss or a balm are much better than lipsticks with a matte red, brown, or wine hue. Instead of purples, blues and other intense shades, neutral eye shadows often are more flattering and will last much longer if used along with an eye primer.

NAILS

Generally speaking, simpler is better. Nails that are too dark, too bright, too long and artificial looking (the "done" and fussy look) can become an inadvertent homage to Imelda Marcos. An elegant natural hue like white, beige or pink works best, unless you really have the schedule and the inclination to keep your long or bright nails meticulously chip-free and perfect. And who has that kind of time?

ACCESSORIES

TAKE A SECOND LOOK AT YOUR EYEWEAR
This is the age when many women begin to get glasses as their eyesight worsens. And what applies to teenagers applies to 40- and 50-somethings, too: embrace the fashion potential of glasses with light, colorful frames. Stay away from heavy,

dark-colored frames, which can age you. Like a great bag, glasses are with you every day, so invest in a few really great pairs. Head to a store with a wide range of European and designer brands — this is one place where you should not skimp on budget, whether you want glasses that fade into the background à la Sarah Palin's clear, frameless Kazuo Kawasaki glasses or something more fashion forward, like Tina Fey's darker librarian-chic tortoise-shell frames.

With sunglasses, make sure you're choosing pairs with 100 percent UV protection to protect the delicate skin around the eyes from sun damage. Also consider larger (or perhaps wraparound) sunglasses, or ones with wide arms to shield crow's feet. You may end up looking like an incognito movie star to boot.

HOSIERY

Opinion is divided on this one. Fashion-forward types say you should never, ever consider wearing panty hose and always go with bare legs. But women who live in cold climates, have less than perfect legs, or don't want to commit to constant self-tanner sessions, may beg to differ. Some women can't live without panty hose, especially because of their tendency to offer support and a sleek look to the hips and thighs. But be aware that they can have an aging effect. Aim for sheer instead of heavy and colored. And by all means, don't wear stockings with open-toe sandals. A more modern approach — if having a smooth silhouette under your clothes is important — is to look for Spanx products, which offer support without the necessity of stockings. There are few women today who don't understand the value of this Atlanta creation, after having tried them. Spanx have no panty lines, yielding a smooth transition. Not to mention that founder Sara Blakely does a tremendous amount for local, national, and global charities.

BAGS

A beautifully made leather bag with luxurious details is more glamorous and stylish than a million trendy or cheap bags. Do like the French and invest in quality when you can.

BOTTOM LINE

You've done everything you can to integrate proper skin care into your daily routine. You shield your face from the sun. You don't smoke. You eat a healthy diet. But looking older can also extend from a number of subtler aspects of our appearance that can change over time. In my opinion, the best strategies for combating the effects of age are subtle ones that allow you to put your best self forward. Start with gratitude for who you are and everything you can be.

A successful salesperson for a major media company, Bethany is a beautiful woman who has the genetic advantages of great bone structure. For Bethany, daily attention to diet, exercise, and her appearance has been a priority since high school. She takes great care of herself through a healthy Mediterranean diet high in fruits, vegetables, Omega 3–rich fish, and whole grains. Bethany also makes regular exercise a part of her routine, especially Pilates and cardio sessions at L.A. Fitness.

But like all of us, she felt she could use a little help. When she first visited Oculus, Bethany treated herself to facials; but over time she has ramped up her beauty maintenance. When she began to notice the first tiny lines around her eyes and mouth, she advanced to other nonsurgical treatments, including Botox, microdermabrasion, and dermal fillers. She was dealing with some volume loss around her eyes and some very early midface and cheek descent. She also had minimal thinning of her lip region and wanted some augmentation to complement her facial features.

Outcome: My recommendations to Bethany for restoration have primarily been maintenance procedures: fillers, Botox, laser treatments, microdermabrasion, chemical peels, vitamin supplements, and prescription skin-care products. She plans to undergo an endoscopic brow lift and cheek lift in the near future to counteract early descent of the brow and midfacial region. This is one of the most sensitive early signs of facial aging. When Bethany recently noticed small brown spots on the bridge of her nose, she inquired about the Oculus IPL photofacial treatment, where a pulsed light is used to treat damaged skin and reduce pigmentation as it promotes the production of collagen.

Currently, she is considering a more aggressive mid-dermal laser-resurfacing procedure. But again, since she's on top of her game, she's considering such a procedure now, while this shift in volume is in its earliest stages. As Bethany says, *"Skin care needs to be a daily ritual, like diet and exercise. If you pay attention to it every day, you're never going to look into the mirror and see a person 10 years older than you want to be. When I posted some vacation pictures of us on Facebook recently, my husband asked me, 'Why is it that I keep looking older and you look exactly the way you did when we got married?' I just smiled at him and said, 'A woman never reveals* all *her secrets.'"*

Bethany recently brought home a testament to her well-maintained good looks when she was awarded the "Best Catch" and "Least Changed Since High School" awards from her 20-year high-school reunion. I had to smile when Bethany said she felt like she should share the awards with me.

"I got to the point where if the clothes were clean, that's what I threw on. I had multiple pairs of Mom jeans. I figured, 'What's the point? With all the sags and bags and flapping skin, who cares what I'm wearing?' I went from being extremely meticulous about my appearance to leaving home and caring more about whether I had my coffee commuter cup than taking the time to look in the mirror."

When Rachel put a stop to her "one last look in the mirror" morning ritual, she realized there was a problem. *"All my life, looking good was a priority,"* she recalls. *"But over time, with a husband and two growing kids, how I looked became less and less important. My days revolved around my family and my career. I was more concerned about the kids forgetting their homework, what to do about dinner, and my husband leaving his ever-buzzing BlackBerry on the kitchen table."*

When she was younger, one of her favorite morning routines was standing in front of her closet doors, surveying her wardrobe options. But no longer. When she did take the time to look in the mirror, Rachel wasn't thrilled with what she saw. *"I had genetically inherited the turkey neck, the bags and sags under the eyes, and the jowls below my jawline,"* she remembers.

In the back of her mind, Rachel had been considering a face lift for 10 years, but her busy life hadn't always left time for her to consider her own needs. She was the classic giver in her family. *"My dentist recommended Dr. Cole to me,"* she recalls. *"Because I was considering having extensive work done, there was a fear factor there for me. My college-age son told me: 'Don't do it, mom. You'll look plastic.' I remember thinking: 'I'm beautiful on the inside. I'll let Dr. Cole take care of the outside.' I put my trust in Dr. Cole, and it turned out beautifully."*

Following my advice, Rachel asked her sister and best friend to come for a visit following her procedure, to help take care of her. They stayed in a hotel together and pampered themselves.

Just four days after surgery, under a scarf and sunglasses, Rachel treated herself to a brief shopping spree. *"For the first two weeks following surgery, makeup hid things,"* she says. *"After six weeks, friends were in awe of how I looked. Within three months, all the swelling was gone. I had no scars whatsoever. I look 15 years younger. It was worth every penny."*

These days, Rachel spends a fraction of her morning applying makeup and the rest of the time in front of the closet; she's back to selecting an outfit to suit her heightened mood. *"I actually care about styles and fashion again!"* she says, laughing. *"I'm dressing in brighter colors, not just beiges, blacks, or whatever is still in a dry-cleaner's bag. I want my clothes to complement the rest of me again."*

Rachel **Laser Light Treatment**

Prior to surgery, Rachel looked tired and her eyes looked heavy. After surgery, she had facial harmony and looked refreshed. Her eyes were rested and she appeared happy and energetic.

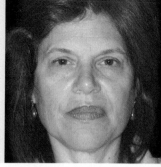

AFTER ▼   ▲ BEFORE

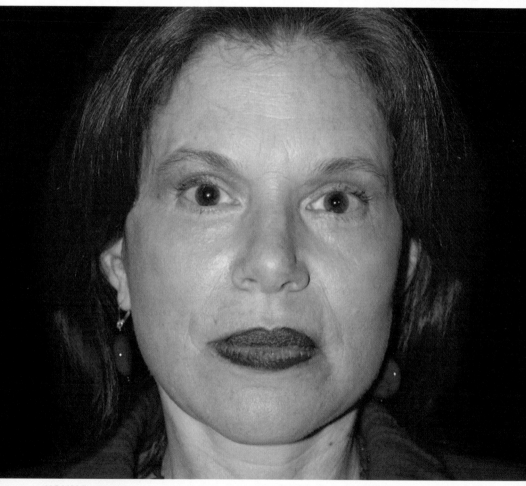

YOUNG▼

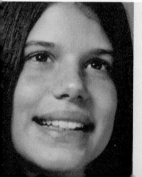

Rachel **Her Younger Years**

Rachel's younger picture is 35 years earlier for comparison. Great plastic surgery is defined by making a person look like a younger, refreshed version of themselves. Rachel was very happy, and thus, so was I.

When she meets girlfriends for lunch now, she's back to swapping style trends and fashion forecasts. *"I'm back in the game,"* says Rachel. *"I no longer feel like life's passed me by in favor of the younger, fresh-faced generation."*

One unanticipated side effect of Rachel's surgery was her renewed self-esteem. *"I realized that I'm more than just somebody's mother, wife, or nurse. I forgot there was a me in there buried under all my responsibilities to others. When I take care of myself, though, I'm better at taking care of everyone else I care about. I love that I have my old confidence back and that I can get up in the morning and not need all that heavy makeup. One thing that never gets old for me is hearing from others that I look good. Now, I'm saving for that touch-up in 10 years!"*

Outcome: On Rachel's first visit, I noted that she had a prominent frown line, which was creating a fold between her eyebrows; she also had laugh lines that were evident even when she wasn't laughing. I shared with her that she would be a good candidate for laser resurfacing, to give her a freshened appearance around her eyes and also help with some of the brownish pigmentation she was experiencing. Her upper lids were in a good position, and she only needed to undergo laser resurfacing to freshen up the fabric and overall skin quality. Her brows were sagging below her orbital bone rim, adding to her tired look. The midfacial descent of her cheek pad, which was causing an under-eye hollow appearance, made her a good candidate for an endoscopic cheek or midface lift. The jowling of her lower face, with the loss of jawline definition and banding of anterior neck lines, made her an ideal candidate for a lower face lift and platysmaplasty.

She selected as her restorative procedures an endoscopic brow lift, laser resurfacing of the eyes, an endoscopic cheek lift, and a lower face lift with platys-maplasty. Rachel's results were excellent, and she experienced normal, uncomplicated healing. She had some stiffness in the upper eyelids, which is normal following laser resurfacing, but she responded to lubricant therapy over a two-week postoperative period. She felt emotionally tense during her healing time, so I prescribed a muscle relaxer.

In my practice, it's pretty typical to treat mothers who take care of their family and spouse every day. They find it a stressful event to undergo normal recovery. They're not used to sitting around and healing, and having someone else wait on them. Rachel definitely fit this pattern, but several of her friends supported her during this process and she did remarkably well. I still see Rachel from time to time when she comes into the office for Botox treatments. She's considering a filler treatment for her perioral region (around her mouth) in the coming years, because this is an area that doesn't respond with a face lift as well as it does with a filler. I explained to her that if you perform a face lift tight enough to distort the mouth region, it doesn't look natural, so fillers offer a good supplemental option.

CHIP'S TIPS

1   If you're going to spend money on skin-care products, skip the fancy (but often ineffective) department-store brands. Instead, spend it on products that contain human growth factors and retinols, which are available through your doctor's office. They change the cell architecture, not just the surface.

2   A regimen of minor procedures over the years delivers more beautiful, subtle results. Start early. Start now. You'll be amazed at your body's ability to correct, restore, and heal.

3   Age is just a number, not a jail sentence. Don't overcompensate with youthful styles that are too trendy and send the wrong message. Don't. Try. Too. Hard.

4   Fillers can address a number of specific complaints for women of this age, though you should remember that fillers are just camouflage. Surgery is the only lasting solution.

5   For those in a long-term, committed relationship, discuss the idea with your significant other. You might be surprised by how many men respond viscerally and angrily to a change in their wife's or girlfriend's appearance.

6   Permanent fillers in the face are not recommended; you should keep your options open.

7   Now is the time to mount a three-pronged attack: human growth factor, antioxidants, and retinol. These three "best friends" are the key ingredients in the "fountain of youth."

8   Remember the forgotten benefits of dry brushing and microdermabrasion: increased penetration and, therefore, added effectiveness of topical prescription-strength products.

9   Lasers have the distinct advantage of sealing the vasculature as an incision is made, thus less bleeding and resultant bruising and swelling. This means you look better faster.

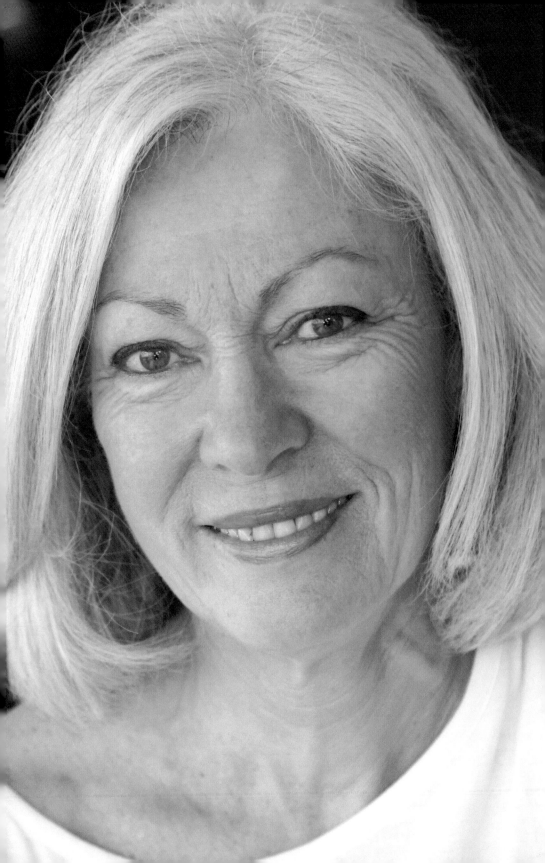

CHAPTER 6

* * *

MAINTAINING THE REAL YOU,
INTO THE GOLDEN YEARS

"Don't make me look like Joan Rivers. I don't want to be a joke."
— *Peggy* (see case study, page 137)

I have some radical news for you, which may be especially shocking to hear from a cosmetic surgeon: we are all going to grow old. Maybe not what you wanted to be reminded of. But in our youth-obsessed culture, seemingly fixated somewhere between 16 and 23, it's worth a friendly reminder that clinging to some media-defined ideal age is not healthy. And it's certainly not realistic. The best way to cope is not to deny your age but to find realistic ways to deal with it while striving to look your absolute best.

And the way to look your best at a certain age will most likely entail surgery, so the features that gravity conspires to drag down can be returned to their original position. The Restylane, Juvéderm, Perlane, Sculptra, and Radiesse that worked wonders in previous decades may not pay off now, because they can only plump what's there, not lift what's migrated. Those fillers and that Botox will no longer camouflage the truth that surgery is now a better choice for achieving the rejuvenating results you seek.

The key to looking fantastic as you age is to realize that you can never stop maintaining your looks through the regimens of consistent skin care and a healthy diet and lifestyle. Combine those with strategic surgical procedures and you'll get real results.

With surgery comes one important caveat. It can indeed work miracles, but it won't permanently keep you from aging. Have a face lift at 40 or 50 and you will most likely look 10, even 20, years younger than your friends. But time will eventually catch up. People often ask me how long a surgical procedure lasts, and usually I explain that after about a decade, you may begin to see changes that will make you want to consider supplementing an earlier procedure. You can turn back the clock, but you can't stop it. However, with effective skin care, you can slow it down going forward.

Think of it like a haircut. People usually will say a haircut lasts about six weeks. In fact a haircut lasts forever (in some ethereal sense). But after six weeks your hair grows out, changes shape, and makes you want to go in for a fresh cut to maintain that look and feel. The haircut analogy helps people understand that things continue to change, but the improvement is always with you. You're going to need maintenance every 10 years or so to continue looking your best.

REVISITING MATH: USE + INSTEAD OF −

The key to both looking natural and getting long-term results is to reposition and restore rather than make your skin so tight you could bounce a coin on it. One example is surgery to correct a drooping cheek pad. As we age, our cheek pads — which once sat high on our cheekbones — begin to fall, resulting in deeper nasolabial folds, jowls, and other indicators of age. Some doctors use the quick-fix remedy of slipping in a cheek implant, which fills in that fallen cheek-pad volume but doesn't really correct the underlying problem. I don't believe in camouflaging the problem; I'd rather correct it. My solution is to lift the descended cheek (your natural cheek pad) to its previous position and perhaps work with fillers, where appropriate, to create fullness. Returning a patient's anatomy to its natural position, as opposed to just inserting an implant, most often yields a more natural look.

Too many patients seek out stretching, tightening, and skin removal. Instead of cutting away, as with the removal of eye bags or saggy skin, I often choose to recondition the skin with a laser so that you don't have to remove the skin. The same thing holds true with fat: if it is out of position, it needs to be put back into position. It needs to be replaced, not removed, to avoid that hollowed-out, cadaverous look. Many times I'll take a dermis fat graft and place it in the eye area to refill lost volume; or I'll choose a filler to mimic the fuller face of a younger man or woman.

If you look at women like Michelle Pfeiffer, Christie Brinkley, and Madonna, who have maintained a youthful look well into their 50s, the first thing that becomes apparent is that their doctors understand the crucial new math of addition. Their faces are full, lush, and glowing with health. And the reason is that, instead of the too-tight face lift procedures of yore, their doctors are performing cheek lifts to replace lost volume or, more likely, very subtle face lifts to prevent that drawn, gaunt look that is a sure sign of aging. Fillers are then used for minimal maintenance and enhanced longevity after the correction is established.

Lasers are an amazing tool for subtly altering the quality of the skin without surgical cutting or tightening. Just be sure you have a doctor who has the very latest laser technology in his office and who performs laser procedures with great frequency. You certainly don't want a doctor who's still using first-generation lasers, which were associated with minor pigmentation problems and various other complications. Lasers have since been refined with advances in technology since 2010. I personally refuse to use a second-generation CO2 laser for facial resurfacing, because even after just three years, that technology has become outmoded. Right now the latest technology is Fractional CO2, which sends heat deep into the skin to ablate old skin cells and stimulate new collagen production. This is the type of thing you should discuss with your doctor to make sure he's keeping up with industry advances.

SKINCARE + LIFESTYLE CHANGES = DRAMATIC RESULTS

As you get older, a variety of lifestyle changes and topical treatments, in conjunction with surgical and nonsurgical upkeep, can help you feel fantastic. Mercifully, medicine teaches us that you're never too old to change your life, and if you're determined to do so, you can. I've listed a variety of solutions — most of them fairly easy to work into your routine — that can put you on the path toward better-looking skin, enhanced well-being, and renewed confidence. Growing older doesn't have to mean feeling old.

PULLED TIGHT ≠ LONG LASTING

Some doctors merely look at a patient's chronological age and decide it's time to take a cookie-cutter approach: they lift, tighten, and call it a day. While the results from that type of approach can be dramatic and quite noticeable, they won't last long. And I don't think patients should be viewed this way. The truth is people age differently — their lifestyles are different, their skin quality is individual to them. All of these things need to be taken into account before jumping into surgery. It's not a one-size-fits-all process.

Most people have a chronological age and an anatomical age. The chronological age is the number of candles on top of your birthday cake; it tells you how much energy you'll need to muster to blow them all out. But as we all know, one woman's 65 can look dramatically different from another woman's 65. That's where anatomical age comes into play. Our anatomical age is the age we actually look, which is related to a whole host of factors. By far the most important factor is to pick the right parents! Seventy percent of how you look is genetics, and the other 30 percent is negotiable. Our anatomical age extends from the effects of stress, sun, suds (alcohol), and climate (finally, a reason to be grateful for the humidity).

The amount of difficulty we've had over our lifetimes — whether we've smoked, had health problems, experienced significant weight gain or loss, suffered trauma — affects our anatomical age. It explains why, in some families, the sister who's been through several divorces; has worked at low-paying, stressful jobs; eats poorly and doesn't exercise can look 10 years older than her older sister who watches her diet, loves her work, has a happy marriage, and deals with minimal stress in her life. But small, seemingly insignificant things add up in positive ways, too. The woman who routinely takes the stairs instead of the elevator, enjoys long walks after dinner, and finds daily reasons to be active, is the one whose anatomical age is lower — who has better skin, better circulation, more energy, and more spring in her step.

Your lifestyle habits determine more than just how old you look. They can also contribute to your overall health. A 2008 study published in the Archives of Internal Medicine found a correlation between a sedentary lifestyle and anatomically advanced aging. As the study's author, Lynn F. Cherkas of King's College London, notes: "A sedentary lifestyle increases the propensity to aging-related diseases and premature death. Inactivity may diminish life expectancy not only by predisposing to aging-related diseases, but also because it may influence the aging process itself."

Cosmetic surgeons need to understand that people are complicated. That's why I don't recommend boilerplate, quick-fix, budget-conscious procedures. Your face is not the place where you should be pinching pennies, because the results are going to show. The rise in quick-fix procedures has led to some very unsavory practices that I am often in the position of having to correct. Those slapdash procedures range from permanent fillers badly injected (which I must perform surgery to remove), and "Lifestyle Lifts," which temporarily give the impression of tightened skin. The results with those procedures don't last and can even cause permanent damage.

Some people opt for cosmetic surgery because they believe it's the end-all. They think it will eliminate the need for regular maintenance and that their surgery won't need to be refreshed and tweaked over time. They falsely believe that if they have one dramatic face lift, the results will last longer. Not only is this not the case, but with drastic, too-tight face lifts come obvious, artificial-looking results. The gold standard now is subtlety, the kind of invisible procedures you see on Hollywood royalty like Madonna and Raquel Welch — not the trampoline-tight faces of wanna-be socialites. One super-tight face lift now does not mean you won't need another

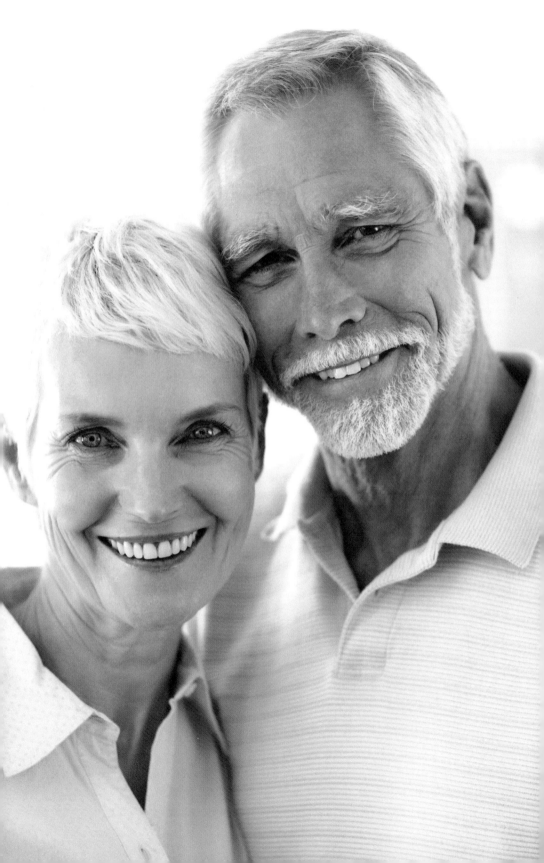

for 20 or 30 years. In truth, a too-tight face lift looks strained and artificial; it proclaims to the world that you've had a procedure. My approach is far more natural, because I restore your natural anatomy to its original position. You still look like you.

SEGMENTAL VERSUS COMPREHENSIVE

There are two different approaches to surgery — segmental or comprehensive — and they can yield very different results. A good surgeon will discuss the benefits of both approaches and offer a realistic assessment of what each can achieve.

Depending on the issue being treated, your plastic surgeon may elect to take a segmental approach and only target one part of your face for improvement. Or perhaps you are hesitant to do too much and prefer to ease into surgery with smaller, incremental procedures before tackling a more involved surgery. With a segmental approach, when a patient may find that one portion of her face is aging more quickly than others, targeting that trouble spot makes sense. This is often the case with the skin around the eyes, which can often age more quickly than other parts of the face. Blepharoplasty, for instance, which targets excess skin or excess fatty tissue on the upper or lower eyelid, can create a rejuvenated appearance by focusing on this one area — or segment — of the face.

Eyelid surgery is the third most common plastic surgery performed in the United States but is considered the highest yielding improvement for a single procedure. It can make a remarkable difference in diminishing signs of aging by removing excess skin and lifting a descending eyelid. Simply put, the eyes have it.

But some plastic surgeons find it difficult to correct problems in isolation. Certain doctors perform a blepharoplasty without taking into account how interconnected the eyelids and the eyebrows are, and how they work in tandem. Too many doctors make the mistake of correcting drooping eyelids without paying attention to stabilizing or lifting the brow. In many cases, if both eyelid and brow surgery are performed at the same time, the effects will look better and last longer. You could be happy with those results for a decade or more, rather than just five or six years.

I call this comprehensive surgery, because a more harmonious and natural result is achieved by tackling the face as a whole. Comprehensive surgery looks at the face as a totality. Rather than merely tackling one portion of the face, which can create an unnatural, unbalanced look, a comprehensive procedure — like a face lift performed in conjunction with a brow lift, cheek lift, and liposuction around the jawline — will create balance and a more congruent appearance.

In most cases, I recommend the comprehensive approach, because the pro-cedures work in harmony and can even disguise the fact that a procedure has been done at all. The comprehensive approach is the foundation of a procedure like the Eyelight Blepharoplasty, an Oculus-patented procedure, which creates a more youthful appearance by performing several procedures together, rather than simply focusing on altering aging eyes with a traditional blepharoplasty. With the Eyelight Blepharoplasty, an endoscope and laser are used in a customized procedure to stabilize the brow, and to tighten and restore the eyes and cheek region. Performed together, these procedures restore the harmonious, natural youthfulness to the midface region, with minimal scarring and only monitored anesthesia required.

A common misunderstanding is that comprehensive surgery takes longer to heal and results in more complications or risks. The stages of wound healing are exactly the same whether it's a one-inch incision or a ten-inch incision. No extra time is needed to heal.

COSMETIC VERSUS RECONSTRUCTIVE

The distinction between cosmetic surgery and reconstructive surgery is one with potential health and safety implications for my older patients. Reconstructive surgery incorporates functional work that can repair damage or offset debilitating conditions, while cosmetic surgery centers on aesthetic improvements that are not medically necessary. Cosmetic surgery is not covered by insurance, but recon-structive surgery usually is.

As you get older, you may encounter problems that can — and should — be corrected through reconstructive surgery and will therefore be covered by your health insurance. A good doctor will be able to help a patient determine when a condition merits a health-insurance claim. For example, while blepharoplasty addresses some of the aesthetic issues involved in facial aging, there are other medical conditions treated by plastic surgery that are not simply aesthetic. Ptosis, for instance, is a condition that also affects the eyelid, but it's the result of an internal muscle problem and not just natural aging. It occurs when the muscles that raise the eyelid are not strong enough to function properly, or have lost their previous attachment point. This condition — whether caused by aging, injury, a congenital condition, or disease — can cause the height of your eyelid to droop down in relation to your pupil.

In more advanced cases, ptosis can interfere with a patient's vision. If you feel that your field of vision is impaired and putting you in harm's way, you might be a good candidate for reconstructive surgery. While surgery to correct ptosis might improve your cosmetic appearance, the improvement to your vision justifies health-insurance coverage.

To simplify, if it's broken and we fix it, that's reconstructive surgery. If it ain't broke but we make it prettier, that's cosmetic. Oftentimes when a procedure is performed for reconstructive reasons, you still get the cosmetic improvement. In New Orleans, we call that a lagniappe.

FACE SHAPE AND AGING

If you're contemplating comprehensive surgical correction to maintain your youth, consider the geometry of beauty. As we age, our face shape fundamentally changes. A face shape that once resembled a heart or a base-up triangle or an oval begins to descend; the symmetry of high cheekbones and a narrow jaw becomes more square and boxy, less defined. The soft fullness we associate with youth is replaced with a heavier rectangular or square-shaped face. The cheek pad, once located close to the eyes, begins to slacken even as the contours of the chin become more indistinct, softer, less articulated. The purpose of surgery as you enter your 60s is to restore that triangle shape, to take what gravity has pulled down and return it to its optimal position. We are aiming for a pillowy lushness, rather than a masculine, squared-off look. One of the primary goals is to restore facial harmony, and that's the hallmark of superior plastic surgery.

> To simplify, if it's broken and we fix it, that's reconstructive surgery. If it ain't broke but we make it prettier, that's cosmetic. Oftentimes when a procedure is performed for reconstructive reasons, you will still get the cosmetic improvement.

SURGERY TATTLETALES

So you've had a face lift, or a combination of surgeries — maybe a blepharoplasty and a brow lift. You can see the difference, and you look great. But if you haven't paid attention to two crucial areas of your face when having surgery, your true biological age can be given away without your realizing it. It's an issue I see more and more as I treat CNN and Fox anchors who must deal with the unforgiving effects of high-definition TV, which glaringly reveal such flaws on camera.

Those tattletales? The neck, ears, and hands. If you ignore these areas and only improve your face, you will see what I call the lollipop effect: a smooth, uncreased face bobbing on a wrinkled, loose-skinned neck. The hands are another talebearer. I routinely use chemical peels, fillers, microdermabrasion, or lasers to treat the hands so they correspond to facial improvements. The overall goal is the visual harmony of the face, ears, neck, décolleté, and hands.

Fortunately, there are opportunities to make sure your youthful appearance is the total package and not just a collection of unrelated procedures. Incorporating a laser treatment to tighten and condition the skin of the ear, for example, will make your ears match your new appearance. And a complementary chemical peel on the neck can ensure that the skin there looks as refreshed and natural as the skin on your face.

FACIAL HAIR

Joan Rivers jokes that as we age we lose hair in the places we want it and grow it where we don't. I'm reminded of the Italian spokeswoman for upper-lip hair bleach: "Shhh, nobody has to know…you're Italian."

A number of options are available to women who are unhappy with fine (or not so fine) hair growth — especially on the face — that seems to accompany age. A number of options are available to the modern hirsute woman. Laser hair-removal treatments or a prescription for Vaniqa — or better yet, the two used in tandem at your cosmetic surgeon's — can provide longer-lasting results.

Another option is face shaving, a practice widely used in Eastern cultures. Many women have found that shaving their face not only gets rid of that downy, delicate hair that often begins to sprout on the cheeks and jawline with age, but has other beneficial effects. It's also a form of daily exfoliation that removes dead skin cells, reduces pore size, removes blackheads, and allows makeup to go on smoother. There's a reason husbands sometimes look younger than their wives, and the reason is the daily exfoliation they undergo with shaving. (Of course hair appears to grow back more thickly when it's shaved, because it's all even, but let's not split hairs.)

HUMAN GROWTH FACTORS

I can't recommend strongly enough that women start using a topical human growth factor — which stimulates collagen production and gets rid of fine lines, brown spots, and wrinkles — in their 40s. If this recent advancement in skin-care science isn't yet a part of your routine, hightail it to Oculus to make human growth factors part of your daily skin maintenance. The earlier the better, too, because it's always better to maintain what you have rather than scramble to replenish what you've lost.

MENOPAUSE

Hormone replacement therapy, with natural or bioidentical hormones, is crucial as you age. It truly is the future, and for that reason, it's a cutting-edge division of Oculus. Bioidentical pharmaceutical hormones (FDA-approved, plant-based hormone products) are superior to the synthetic hormones peddled by drug companies. The marketing behind synthetic hormones can be deceptive, stressing that they're just like natural hormones. It's like marketers saying, "It's just like Coke." My response would be, "then why not drink Coke?" If I were a woman, I would want the real thing — not a facsimile.

PAY ATTENTION TO YOUR HEALTH

Take care of yourself and you will not only feel and look better but you'll be a better candidate for surgery. Upping your intake of vegetables, salmon, nuts and seeds, fruits, chia, and flaxseed will improve your sense of well-being while increasing luminosity and improving skin tone. Exercise is also vital. I've said it before and I'll say it again: whether you're 10 or 90, some form of exercise is essential for looking and feeling great. With the advent of your 60s, exercise will help you fight osteoporosis and maintain that absolute essential for a happy life: a positive outlook. To me, 60 is the new middle-age.

DRESSING THE PART

With surgery comes the need to adjust your wardrobe and makeup. A change in dress and makeup, combined with cosmetic surgery, can result in a dramatically refreshed and youthful appearance. And following the advice of Joan Rivers, a woman who knows what she's talking about when it comes to plastic surgery, "I don't believe makeup should be optional after age thirty-five." I think Joan is right on that one. The natural look starts to look less breezy and carefree come 60 or 70. Here's what matters at this age: polish, sophistication, and attention to detail.

A LITTLE HELP FROM YOUR FRIENDS

You need a fantastic support network as you age, and especially when you undergo surgery. You'll want your close friends and family nearby to help you through the recovery period and to provide emotional support. Let them know you're doing the procedure for yourself, and that the best thing they can do is to not try to talk you out of it — that is, tell you that you're too old to bother, or that you're already beautiful. Ask them just to be supportive as you begin your journey. If this doesn't seem possible, we'll recommend a host of medical assistants and nurses who are available to perform any service — from a few hours of help to weekly monitoring to 24/7 assistance, including travel.

GOT BOTOX?

For years that was the headline of a popular Oculus ad in Atlanta magazines. It featured a trio of adorable shar-pei puppies, with the tagline, "Not everyone looks this cute with wrinkles." It was my lighthearted take on the very serious and stressful situation of aging. I've found that the best approach when it comes to wrinkles, lines, and jowls is to laugh in times of stress — but then get down to the brass tacks of fixing the problem.

PRENATAL VITAMINS

Most ladies who lunch know that avoiding the dreaded effects of osteoporosis means getting enough calcium in their diet. If they don't eat cheese or drink milk, for instance, they faithfully take a calcium supplement to fight bone-density loss. According to the National Institutes of Health recommendations, women should take a thousand milligrams of calcium each day starting at age 30. In women over 50, the recommended amount increases to at least 1,200 mg. To prevent the calcification of arteries and associated risk of heart attack that can come with taking calcium alone, take a calcium supplement containing magnesium and vitamin D. I advise women to check with their doctors to adjust their calcium needs to their individual circumstance. For a serious dose of skin-improving vitamins, I advise my older patients to significantly rev up their nutrients with a daily dose of the same prenatal vitamins that enhance the health of expectant mothers and their unborn children.

END RESULTS

I really enjoy the final consultation following surgery, because I get the opportunity to see what kind of impact the procedure has had on my patient's life and relationships. You can feel the enthusiasm in the room. Perhaps due to increased self-confidence, her business life has improved because her presentations are better. Maybe she feels freer to take risks in the workplace. She might be confident enough to join her friends for girls' night out again or to take a chance on love following divorce or widowhood. I love it when patients tell me, "I haven't felt this confident in 10 years. I feel like I've stepped back in time."

One of the greatest compliments in this job is when a patient comes back a decade or more after surgery; she has a high-school reunion or a 60th birthday party coming up, and she comes back in for a tune-up. We can do a little enhancement to get her look back to where it was. When scheduling a tune-up before one of those milestone events, I recommend patients come in at least three months prior, and even earlier if possible.

When a daughter or son gets engaged, for instance, that's the time to start thinking about how they want to look at the wedding — not a few weeks before the event itself. People often don't realize how much activity there is a month or two before a wedding. Patients certainly don't want to schedule an appointment in the midst of planning for a big event, or be recovering from a procedure on that special day.

Often, I'll recommend some bridge procedures, like Botox or fillers, to get someone looking good through the wedding. Just remember, the focus should be on the bride. Naturally, everyone wants to put their best face forward, but let's not make you a distraction. I always ask the mother of the groom if she knows what her role is at the wedding. She usually says no. My advice is to wear beige and blend into the background. But remember: It's OK to look damn good while you're doing it!

And as we discussed above, zero birthdays are a huge deal. We use them to gauge where we are in life. Did we meet our goals? Are we the people we set out to be at this stage in our lives? We all want to look our best for those milestone birthdays.

And let's not forget divorces. Suddenly, you have a shot at a new life, a clean slate. Here's your opportunity to lasso that Mr. or Ms. Wonderful you wish you'd wrangled the first time around. You want to look your best when you're putting yourself back out there in the social scene.

However, when it comes to such milestone occasions, I will try to see a patient two or three times before scheduling a procedure. I want to ensure that they're not just making an impulsive decision — that they're psychologically ready for it.

It shouldn't be about "Oh my God, I'm going to change my life and my looks and I'm going to go to court, and he's going to regret ever divorcing me." I've had patients use those very terms to tell me why they need to look good by their divorce-court date. They'll literally sell stock or valuables to do it, too! It becomes a personal vendetta to them. Believe it or not, patients have had their attorneys seek a postponement or file a continuance on their behalf because they're still recovering from a procedure.

And then there are the couples who are still very much together. Do you want to know one of the biggest fringe benefits of this job? When a patient tells me, "My husband and I are having date nights again. We haven't done that in years." When you amp up that attraction again, things can reach a new plateau. As a plastic surgeon, it's never been my goal to save a marriage, but sometimes that's been an unintended consequence.

I know we've accomplished our mutual goals when a patient's inner beauty finally merges with a more youthful-looking exterior. We're ready to say hasta la vista, baby, when she looks in the mirror and what she sees matches how she feels. But at Oculus Plastic Surgery, we never say good-bye.

"Never say good-bye because
saying good-bye means going away,
and going away means forgetting."
— Peter Pan

Peggy, *homemaker* **Age:** 67 **Complaint:** Crisis of confidence due to grandchildren who teased her for looking unusually older and tired.

Peggy was a 63-year-old wife (and the sweetest lady you'll ever meet) when I first met her. She had been caring for her sick husband, enduring many difficult months of long-term illness. In our first meeting, I discovered that she had family who had attended Vanderbilt University — where I had done my oculofacial plastic-surgery training — and was a huge Vanderbilt fan. This got us off to a good start.

In our initial consult, I noted that Peggy had classical facial aging changes, with a descending brow and midface; periorbital skin changes; and laxity of cheek, lower face and jaw region. Her main interest was to freshen up. She felt like her aging had accelerated because of what she'd been through with her husband — family stress is one of those factors I mentioned earlier that can increase anatomical age.

I told her what I tell a lot of my patients: Aging comes in bursts; it's not consistent all the time. It's not unusual for your looks to age a decade during a few stress-filled years (just look at pictures of U.S. presidents at the beginning and end of their terms).

In Peggy's case, she had experienced hypermetabolic aging due to the stress and strain of everything she had been through with her loved ones.

I think her story is worth telling.

Peggy stared at herself in the mirror, under the unforgiving fluorescent light of the ladies' room at St. Joseph's Hospital. She thought, *"I look like death warmed over."* In the months following her husband's aortic aneurysm and his subsequent coma, this had become her home away from home. Supporting him in his extended illness, she hadn't taken the time to consider her appearance at all.

And then the unthinkable happened. William did not survive.

Having married at the age of 20, Peggy was now alone. After grieving and acclimating to the realities of widowhood, she began to think about dating for the first time in 45 years. *"I was devastated and at a very low point in my life,"* she reflects. *"Having your husband die really brings it all home. You only have so much time on this earth. But I was in good health and still relatively young."*

Then Peggy remembered that William had told her to do whatever she could to be happy. So she did.

Outcome: After consulting with me and listening to my recommendations, Peggy opted to have a brow lift, a mid and lower face lift, laser resurfacing on her eyes, and a neck lift. Before proceeding with Peggy's work, I advised her to undergo a complete physical to ensure her overall health, a necessity for anyone considering comprehensive cosmetic surgery at this age.

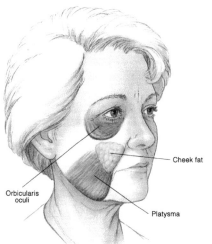

Cheek fat

Orbicularis
oculi

Platysma

Internal anatomy (what I see)

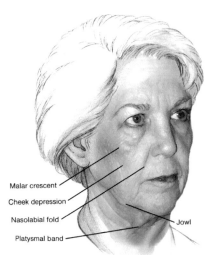

Malar crescent

Cheek depression

Nasolabial fold

Platysmal band

Jowl

External anatomy (what you see)

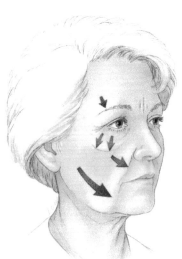

Force vectors of aging

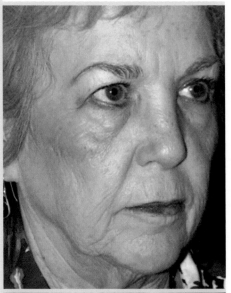

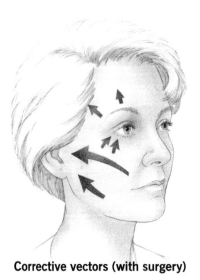

Corrective vectors (with surgery)

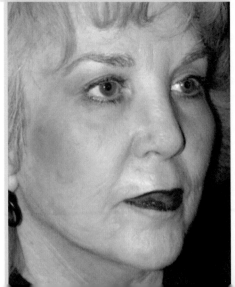

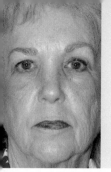

Peggy Facelift Procedure

Peggy is a 67-year-young widow who felt depressed and tired of "looking tired." Basically, her inside feelings and spirit did not match her outside presentation. She wanted comprehensive facial harmony. She felt she had "found herself" after her outpatient surgical procedure.

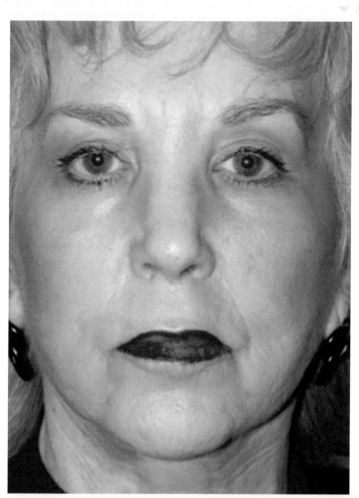

Improving on the Past

Peggy's younger picture is 40 years earlier for comparison. Notice how her facial shape, jawline, and eyes have recaptured an earlier, more rested appearance. She was a huge hit at her 50-year high-school reunion, receiving the "Least Changed Award."

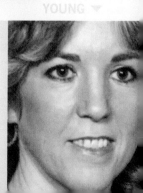

Peggy just had one request for me, one that made me laugh: *"Don't make me look like Joan Rivers. I don't want to look like a cartoon character."* I assured Peggy her new self would look completely natural.

"The beauty of Dr. Cole's work is that he doesn't pull the eyes the way other surgeons do," she explains. *"If I'd gone to a doctor who just yanked tight the skin around my eyes, I would have looked younger, but ridiculous!"*

During her three-week recovery at home, Peggy decided she would be completely up front with her friends and family about getting work done, and she's happy she did.

"I recommend being transparent with people about it," she says. *"Secrets have a way of coming out. Be honest. I would much rather people talk to me about it than talk about me behind my back. Besides, having plastic surgery isn't exactly an immoral act!"*

Peggy was quite pleased with her results. She told me how she had transformed before her own eyes during the healing process. We noticed a change when she came to the office, too. She had become a lot more talkative; she dressed nicely, changed her hair, and would bring in homemade baked goods for the office. She became a true advocate of my entire practice and has referred several people to us.

A few months later, a recent widower walked into Peggy's Sunday-school class. Stephen had recently lost his wife of 50 years. He and Peggy ended up going to the same support-group meetings. Afterward, over a glass of wine, they would discuss how to move past the pain. Hours were spent chatting on the phone. A friendship blossomed into romance, and Peggy and Stephen were married in 2009. Today, with the blessing of their six adult children, the couple vacations in the Canadian Rockies, goes on family ski trips to Big Sky, and takes Disney cruises together.

I joke with Peggy that we've watched her transform from a depressed widow to a hot globe-trotting grandma with a new life. To me, Peggy is the epitome of the modern woman: beautiful, spirited, and not one to let age hold her back.

"I'm not going to say that looking years younger resulted in Stephen proposing to me," Peggy quips, *"but it certainly didn't hurt! Aside from my looking rested and more youthful, it restored my confidence. You feel like a new person, and people notice that."*

Peggy still checks in with me for regular Botox appointments and filler to keep her looking fresh. Most recently, she was in to have a Sculptra treatment, which is a stimulatory filler for the cheeks and perioral region that helps keep aging at bay. It's always a pleasure to see her whenever she visits. (And the homemade treats are a bonus.)

"Having my work done with Dr. Cole was the best thing I ever did for myself, next to marrying two wonderful men," says Peggy.

Who am I to disagree?

CHIP'S TIPS

1 Regarding spur-of-the-moment facelifts: In a nutshell, don't go there.

2 Any facelift procedure done quickly with local anesthesia should come with a warning: penny-pinch on surgery and you may find yourself regretting the results.

3 If you undergo lower priced and often lower quality body surgery, you can always camouflage a less than desired result under clothing. Your eyes and mouth are seen by everyone you talk to. Don't cut corners on quality, proven surgical skills.

4 Quality of skin is *never* improved by surgery with a scalpel. A laser surgical procedure will improve both the quantity and quality of your skin.

5 Protect your investment in your facial rejuvenation by not smoking, eating healthy and getting adequate rest.

6 Remember to address the two "tattletale areas" when undergoing facial rejuvenation: the neck and ears. Not only are most phone cameras HD, but your "attentive" girlfriends are, too.

7 When you want to look your best for that important upcoming event (wedding, birthday, or reunion), plan ahead, because life is full of surprises and an unexpected party or unscheduled event may present itself.

8 Your plastic surgeon is your quarterback, but you get to be the coach. Discuss all of your concerns and do not keep any secrets. The goal is to take the best care of you possible and give you an outstanding result. Your surgeon can only do his best work if he encounters no surprises.

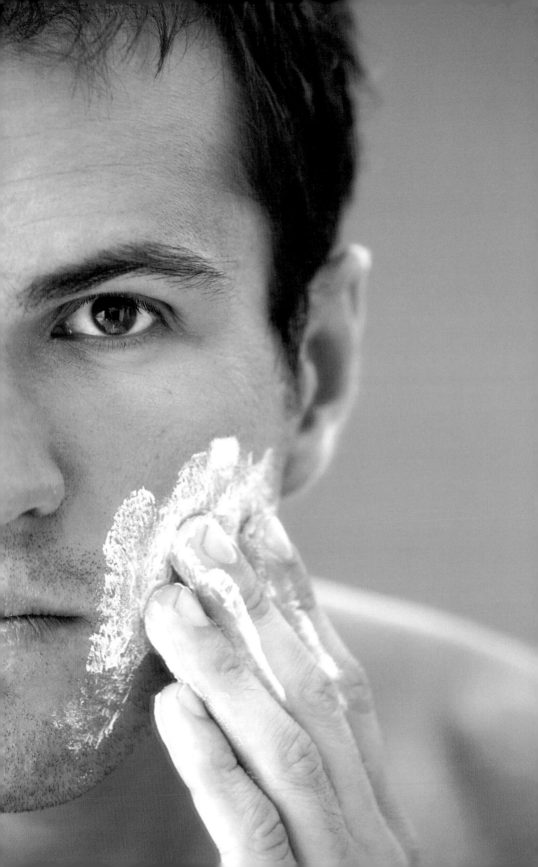

CHAPTER 7

∗ ∗ ∗

REAL MEN GET BOTOX:
HOW MEN CAN PROLONG THEIR PLASTIC-SURGERY RESULTS AND PROTECT THEIR INVESTMENT

"It's not something you're ever going to catch guys talking about. You'll never hear a group of guys shift the conversation from stock tips and how the Falcons did on Sunday to 'Hey Tripp, how did you eliminate those unsightly heavy eyelids, buddy?' It's just not going to happen. But that's not to say that men aren't having plastic surgery." — *Tripp*

While not every man who seeks plastic surgery would describe himself as a metrosexual, more and more men are exhibiting a distinct interest in the details of their face, body, and dress. It's a fact that we live in a more visual age, and a more democratic one. Men today feel as able to seek out physical improvements as women do — or almost, anyway. Where manicures and man jewelry once seemed the province of the Rat Pack and Jersey mafiosi, such maintenance and accessorizing are now commonplace, even expected.

If you think it's only women seeking surgical and nonsurgical approaches to looking good, think again. Figures released in 2012 by the American Society of Plastic Surgeons (ASPS) make it abundantly clear that men are as concerned with their looks as women are. Plastic surgery for men saw a 5 percent jump in 2012 over 2011, with more than 1.5 million cosmetic procedures (at an expense that tops billions) performed on men each year. The number of cosmetic procedures for men increased more than 121 percent from 1997.

The six most popular surgical procedures for 2012 were:

- Liposuction
- Eyelid surgery
- Face lifts
- Rhinoplasty
- Breast reduction surgery
- Tummy tucks

As this list indicates, procedures we might think of as more for women, such as fillers and Botox, are popular with men, too. But just as I tell my female patients, men need to be aware that while fillers and Botox can go a long way toward diminishing the signs of aging, they are just a temporary fix. To really reverse the aging clock and see truly significant improvement, you may need surgery to effectively lift and erase those sags and bags that bother you.

Where I advise caution, to avoid the overly feminized Bruce Jenner look (for more on instructive celebrity plastic-surgery mistakes, see Chapter 11), is in using a very accomplished plastic surgeon. A great surgeon will not take your face to a place it never was. An experienced and skilled surgeon will not make the mistake of thinking that extreme tightening — treating your face like a piece of clay to shift and mold at will — is a remedy to facial aging. Jenner's surgery took an unfortunate detour when his face lift was accompanied by a nose job that was far too small and pert for his face. If that weren't enough, he chose a doctor who seemed not to appreciate the difference between male and female facial anatomy, giving Jenner a far too radical eye lift.

I feel for men like Bruce, who grapple with the same neuroses about aging that women do, and I feel even worse when they choose an unskilled cosmetic surgeon in their effort to correct an aging issue. The techniques and procedures that work well on women's faces cannot be applied to men. Plastic surgery isn't a one-size-fits-all overhaul; it needs to take into consideration every person's unique physiognomy as well as the significant gender differences.

One example of how the wrong procedure can lead to a strangely feminized appearance is the upper eyelids, illustrating the need for a conservative and artful approach when it comes to plastic surgery for men. Some men want an eyelid crease, like women naturally have. I strongly advise against this procedure. When you take away that fullness of a man's upper lids and give him a lid platform he doesn't naturally have, it looks unnatural and — to be blunt — feminine.

Make sure you find a cosmetic surgeon who can show you in words and pictures that he understands that difference, whether you are seeking fillers or a face lift. Your doctor should know, for instance, that men tend to need more Botox than women, to correct the deeper, harsher lines that typically affect them.

Men are increasingly being evaluated based on their appearances, especially in high-profile professional arenas. For instance, lawyers are increasingly turning to Oculus for the Botox injections that keep them from looking harsh, tough, and angry. Instead, they need to sway juries by looking rested, down to earth, and — perhaps for the first time — *nice,* instead of looking like they're itching for a fight. They want to look friendlier and more relaxed, and cosmetic improvements are a great way to achieve those results. Botox for men has become huge at the corporate level. It is now just as much of a required accessory as having the latest handheld mobile device or the newest BMW or Porsche.

More men choose cosmetic "bridge" procedures like fillers, neck liposuction, and laser procedures, because they require less downtime. They want a quick freshening up — one they can recover from over the weekend. In the current economy, I'm doing 300 percent more filler and Botox work for men than I was just a couple of years ago.

Men's needs differ when it comes to lifestyle, too. More men are taking care of themselves in the extreme. They compete in triathlons and marathons, and they cycle and hike on the weekends. On one hand, nothing is better than regular exercise for a man's self-esteem (as well as his looks). But there can be some unwanted side effects too. They're out in the sun for long periods of time, testing their bodies — and skin. As a result, many more men are coming to see me about aging issues associated with this intense approach to mega-fitness. These men tend to seek out weekend procedures — like Botox, facials, and fillers — where the effects are subtle, and no one has to know they've visited a cosmetic surgeon.

Fillers are especially popular for camouflaging some of the hollowness that comes with too much exercise. A filler like Sculptra, which generates and builds your own collagen gradually, is a great choice for my fitness-obsessed guy patients.

Men think very differently about surgery as well. Typically men treat a youth-enhancing procedure in much the same way they would handle a stock transfer: as a transaction free of emotional investment. For women, an elective facial procedure is psychologically a more complex undertaking. Perhaps it's because they feel so much hinges on their looks. Female patients have told me they carried around one of my *Atlanta* magazine advertisements in their purse for a *decade* before making the final decision to have a procedure. Men don't seem to engage in that kind of prolonged deliberation. They are practical, they want the facts, and they want to see results. Because of this, I've had to adjust the way I think about my patients and do my best to make all of them, both men and women, feel comfortable.

I've learned a lot from the men who come into my office. I've discovered that you can communicate with them most effectively by using a business vocabulary and sports analogies. Men feel more comfortable when you use that vernacular, perhaps because some still fear plastic surgery carries a feminine "stigma." I'll say to the guys: "This is your investment. Let's take care of it. How do you want to look in the boardroom? Are you going to look as rested and relaxed to your client as your main competitor does?"

THE COVER UP

If you just can't admit to others that you're taking steps to improve your appearance, you're not alone. People make up some pretty creative excuses for why they look red, puffy, or bruised after a cosmetic procedure.

If you're worried that people will notice *your* procedure, just give one explanation — but don't feel like you need to explain everything. People just want to understand why you look different, or why your skin is red or bruised. You don't have to give them TMI.

Here are some of the most creative excuses I've heard; use whichever one best fits your healing process:

- Allergies
- Sinus surgery
- Wisdom-tooth removal
- Laser treatments for sun damage (this is one of the better excuses, since saying you've had a procedure done for health reasons can distract from the fact that you've had a more extensive procedure done for cosmetic reasons)
- Sports injury (not always successful since tennis balls don't tend to give you two black eyes, though Senator John Kerry proved a hockey stick to the face can do the trick)
- Waterskiing or snow skiing injury (a serious spill here can result in the kind of dramatic allover bruising and trauma that would also accompany, say, a face lift)

If you'd rather not make up an excuse about why your face looks different, try some of the following strategies for disguising it.

- Alter your facial hair (either growing or removing it).
- Change your style of dress.
- Get a new haircut to deflect attention from your face.
- Wear glasses or try a different style to replace the old ones.

Lasers, Botox, and fillers fit right into the modern male lifestyle. Social stigmas about men having a little work done have receded in our culture just as things have become hyper-competitive in the current corporate climate. And in some ways, gender distinctions are even becoming blurred.

A lot of advertising has now shifted to a more unisex theme. Look at an ad for Guess Jeans. You can't really tell *who* the garment is made for now. In fact, it's often hard even to identify the gender of the model. Much of that attitude and approach has crossed over into the mainstream. It's now quite common for men to be aware of their skin-care needs. Gone is the embarrassment of having "product" on your bathroom counter. Men are even coming in and asking for Latisse to grow their eyelashes. The culture is really changing.

While younger patients embrace the need to look their best, my older patients can be a tough sell. The biggest obstacle I've had to overcome with older male patients is letting them know that it's OK to do something for *themselves.* And that plastic surgery isn't going to take away from their masculinity, as long as it's done by a skillful surgeon.

One thing I've learned in dealing with men is that you've got to break through that old-school John Wayne mentality and educate them on the benefits of some of the products and services available. If you can properly explain the functionality of a specific surgery, it legitimizes the procedure for them. A useful metaphor is the automobile. No man I know would leave a classic Mustang convertible to molder in the garage. It's not only accepted but expected that he'll restore it when needed and, in the meantime, maintain it with regular washing, waxing, and lube jobs. If an older man comes in and has heavy eyelids, jowling, and a heavy beard/jaw line, it helps to "tighten the hammock." Over time, a hammock can still function well but it can get stretched out. Tighten it by a link or two on the tree and it works better. It's like an entirely new hammock.

If a man can relate that analogy to his lower eyelid and we tighten it a little, it's going to hug up against his eye better. He might also experience a little less tearing when he's out in the wind on the tennis court or on the boat. It gives him a functional way to look at the procedure. It's not just vanity.

At Oculus I have definitely seen an upward trend in the number of men seeking cosmetic surgery and other procedures to look their best. At this point nearly 20 percent of my patients are men, and I expect that figure to be even greater as cosmetic surgery and skin-care regimens increase in acceptability. In our culture, with so much emphasis on youth and good looks, I have found men responding to that pressure much more readily than in the past.

WORKING IT

There's a reason James Bond has remained a pop-culture icon for decades. I see author Ian Fleming's super-spy creation as the earliest form of the modern male. No matter what variety of mission he was on, 007 *always* looked great. That pulled-together look is what guys strive for these days.

Of course, there's another reason James Bond has endured.

Every time an actor got a little too old for the role, the film studio hired a younger one to keep the franchise going. But unlike Bond, we can't recast ourselves. Thankfully, men are discovering that skin rejuvenation isn't just for the ladies anymore, and they also have the option of slowing the progress of aging with attentive skin care and a variety of surgical and nonsurgical cosmetic procedures.

There is also a practical explanation for why cosmetic surgery is becoming increasingly popular among men in American culture. Competition means men worry about their careers. We all know someone who's lost his job. Guys who are currently between jobs are getting procedures that will give them that edge in a job interview. It's not enough just to have a hot résumé, good references, and solid work experience anymore. You've got to have the whole package. To stay competitive in the workplace, men are coming in for regular facials and requesting nonsurgical procedures — simple things they can do to spruce up their appearance. They want to stay competitive longer. Often a fresher look yields that extra measure of competitiveness.

University of Texas economist Daniel S. Hamermesh is an expert on the correlation between looks and earning potential. In *Beauty Pays: Why Attractive People Are More Successful*, the first book to quantify the economic advantages of looking good, Hamermesh determined that looks come into play on the job for men more often than they do for women. Being good looking can mean 15 percent higher earnings for men says Hamermesh, and he's not the only one to reach that conclusion. A study published in the 2004 issue of *Aesthetic Plastic Surgery* found that cosmetic surgery could yield significant rewards for patients, including better relationships, financial success, and the appearance of being more intelligent and better educated.

Studies show that taller men traditionally do better and make more money in business. A more attractive man does better too. But while you can't change your height (at least by any reasonable means), you *can* do something to improve your appearance. Women have always had to fight ageism in the workplace. But until the economy worsened in 2008, men had largely escaped this corporate trap.

Now, the playing field is becoming more level. Older men used to be regarded as authoritative. The last couple of economic downturns have had a curious effect

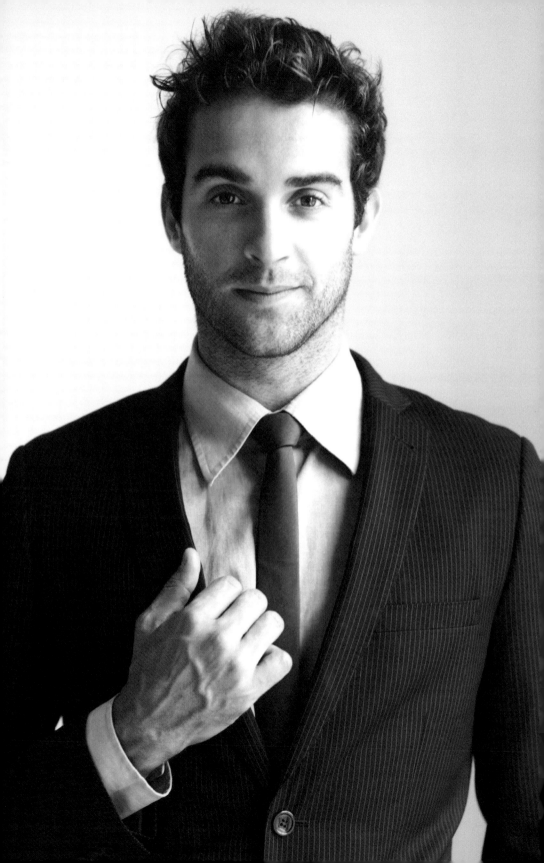

on men in the workplace. Suddenly, the cushy corner office was up for grabs. As profits plunged, younger, cheaper, more tech-savvy guys began pushing out the veterans. Younger men are often more comfortable with the technological advances so prevalent today, and they don't demand the salaries and benefits that the older generation once expected. Unlike so many men of my generation, they have a natural comfort level with the social media employed by so many businesses now. They're able to adapt more quickly. If you're perceived as an older man in the work-place, you're more likely to be labeled a dinosaur and seen as someone who isn't up for learning new skills as readily.

In my practice, I've seen an increase in the number of middle-aged men who are dealing with the profound effects of what I call "age-sizing." The situation has led to some very dramatic, often quite sad consultations in my exam rooms. Men will now sometimes break down in tears. Stress is high. Jobs are on the line or have already evaporated. I feel for these guys. Our culture still clings to the residual tenets of the '50s, which state that the man is the breadwinner and his social standing is defined by the work he does. Women have made enormous gains in the workplace and are frequently able to dip in and out of their careers when they have children. But men still have their identities defined by being well-employed. When they suffer a job loss, it can be a devastating blow to their sense of self and their masculinity.

> The techniques and procedures that work well on women's faces cannot be applied to men. Plastic surgery isn't a one-size-fits-all overhaul; it needs to take into consideration every person's unique physiognomy as well as the significant gender differences.

"Everyone has felt the shift," says one of my patients, Tripp. An engineer, Tripp explains, *"With today's economy and workplace challenges, I totally understand why cosmetic procedures for men are such a growth market for plastic surgeons. For some guys, this may be the first time in their careers to feel this vulnerable."*

I hope I can help my male patients feel better about themselves and more empowered by learning the things they can do to improve their appearance. Because while there are still significant differences between men's and women's cosmetic-surgery needs, those differences disappear when it comes to matters of self-esteem. Improve your outward appearance, whether through surgery or better skin care, and more than likely you will feel better physically and psychologically.

SKIN CARE

Recently, I met with a returning patient who is a very successful businessman. He owns houses, a yacht, a plane — everything you can think of that exemplifies a satisfying, financially secure life. This man has also had some facial cosmetic surgery, and he looks great. He came back in to consult with me about a series of skin-pigment changes that are occurring on his face.

We ended up having a lengthy conversation about lifestyle factors that were contributing to those changes in the color of his skin. For years, he has been a heavy smoker. A few months back, he was finally able to quit.

However, he's now chewing a considerable amount of nicotine gum to compensate for those cigarettes. Even though he's a very bright, successful businessman, he didn't understand that the nicotine, whether in gum or cigarette form, was still a drug coursing through his blood stream and affecting his blood vessels. While making the switch from smoking to the gum was an important step in his overall health, he couldn't stay on the gum forever. The nicotine was still having an adverse affect on his skin tone, metabolism, and overall health. I gave him this advice: "In order for us to protect this cosmetic-surgery investment you've made in yourself, you've got to protect your skin health as well."

Many of the patients I see in my practice don't understand that skin health and skin care are interconnected with every other lifestyle choice they make. I refer to it as your "skin fitness." That is the primary reason we opened Oculus Skin Care Centre, to complement the surgery practice. We have skin-care professionals here to assist you in the daily skin maintenance that's important for each of us to practice. That's also why I urge each of my patients to take advantage of our computerized VISIA skin-health analysis as well, which can show you how the sun and bad habits have affected your skin. After the analysis, you'll be more motivated to take steps to correct that damage.

How you maintain your skin health can mean the difference between the positive effects of a surgical treatment lasting five years or 15. Taking a multivitamin every day; using sunscreen; maintaining a healthy diet, including plenty of leafy green vegetables, fruits, and whole grains; and minimizing the intake of dairy and sugar are crucial for good health and great skin tone.

A lot of patients, especially men, think they can have a surgical procedure then go straight back to the patterns of behavior that led to their needing surgery. But ultimately, it's all up to you and what you do after you leave my office. After I've explained the benefits of good skin care, most patients get it — it's all about maintenance, it's about protecting your investment.

In some ways, men are lucky. As previously mentioned, the shaving they've been doing since they were teenagers regularly removes a layer of surface skin — an exfoliation process that helps speed cell turnover and keeps wrinkles at bay. They also aren't as prone as women — who have been enticed their whole lives to seek out miracles in fancy potions — to fall for every new skin-care product. Not that men don't have their own buttons pushed by savvy Madison Avenue ad men. You only have to read the back-page ads for Viagra, hair-loss treatments, and libido enhancers in *Esquire* or *Men's Health* to realize that men can be just as susceptible to appeals to their vanity.

At the drug store or department store, you are on your own, surrounded by confusing and exaggerated claims about what certain products can do for you. That's why a doctor-supervised skin-care regimen is so important.

Another advantage for male patients is that they are very loyal and dedicated in carrying out treatment plans. Women are more likely to stray from a skin-care regimen by trying new products, which can counteract the benefits of their prescribed skin-care plan. Once I give my male patients a list of recommended products to address their skin-care issues, I've found that they tend to stick with them. The aestheticians at Oculus certainly appreciate that.

In general, men benefit from some of the same skin-treatment approaches women use: that holy trinity of cleanse, exfoliate, and moisturize. As they grow older, a serum can be added to greatly enhance that troika of essential skin care.

THREE AND OUT: CLEANSE, EXFOLIATE, MOISTURIZE

Keeping your skin healthy and clean — it's not rocket science, just a matter of habit. For women, standing in front of the mirror and cleaning and treating are second nature. An endless assortment of tonics, lotions, and unguents work themselves into the female grooming regimen. But men are generally less willing to spend their time experimenting with new products. With guys, it can be a harder sell. So I like to keep things simple. In general, a creamy cleanser is best for dry skin and a gel cleanser is best for oily skin. If you're lucky enough to have normal skin, find a cleanser that makes your skin feel clean but not tight and dry.

Seek out a recommendation from a doctor or aesthetician, since they will be able to suggest a product that can multitask to combat signs of aging, acne, or whatever your concern, *while* cleaning your skin. And once you've found some-thing you like that works, stick with it. Don't revert to that cheap bar of Ivory soap that once comprised your total skin-care routine.

A moisturizer — oil absorbing, if shine is a problem — with an SPF is essential, especially considering the drying effects of shaving. A good moisturizer will protect your skin from the sun, keep your skin smooth, and help stave off signs of aging. **Men can also benefit from weekly use of a skin mask and from an exfoliator two or three times a week to more aggressively rid the skin of dead skin cells and to keep breakouts at bay.**

I often recommend Illuminize Peel from SkinMedica to my male clients; it offers a superficial chemical peel without the downtime involved in a traditional peel. For my executive clients, the lack of peeling involved means they can use the product without the irritation that signals "procedure." The product is great at tightening the skin and improving skin color, clarity, and texture.

Another great product available exclusively in our office is the multi-functional Oculus TeaDerma Pad. These are especially appreciated by our male patients since they're so easy to use: just a quick swipe over your skin. They contain epigallo-catechin gallate (EGCG), which is associated with a variety of biological effects including free-radical scavenging, inflammation reduction, and UVA/UVB photo protection. And when you're feeling lazy, that quick, refreshing swipe of the pad can count as your cleansing regimen too!

If wrinkles and fine lines are an issue, there's no reason for men not to consid-er Retin-A or another retinol product. But there are non-prescription moisturizers and serums that offer anti-aging benefits as well. Look for the active ingredients coenzyme Q10, which repairs skin cell damage; alpha hydroxy acids, which shed skin cells and clarify skin; and polyphenols, which diminish inflammation. At the drug store or department store, you are on your own, surrounded by confusing hyperbole and exaggerated claims about what certain products can do for you. That's why a doctor-supervised skin-care regimen is so important. Your medically trained aesthetician can be invaluable in guiding you to the products that work best for your skin.

GROOMING: BROWS, BOOZE, AND B.O.

If you've made it to manhood without incident and managed to offend no one with your haphazard self-maintenance, your grooming habits may already be topnotch. But even the most immaculately pulled-together men could often use a bit of a refresher course in grooming basics. The following are some of the small but key details that complement a round of Botox or a face lift, giving you far more bang for your buck.

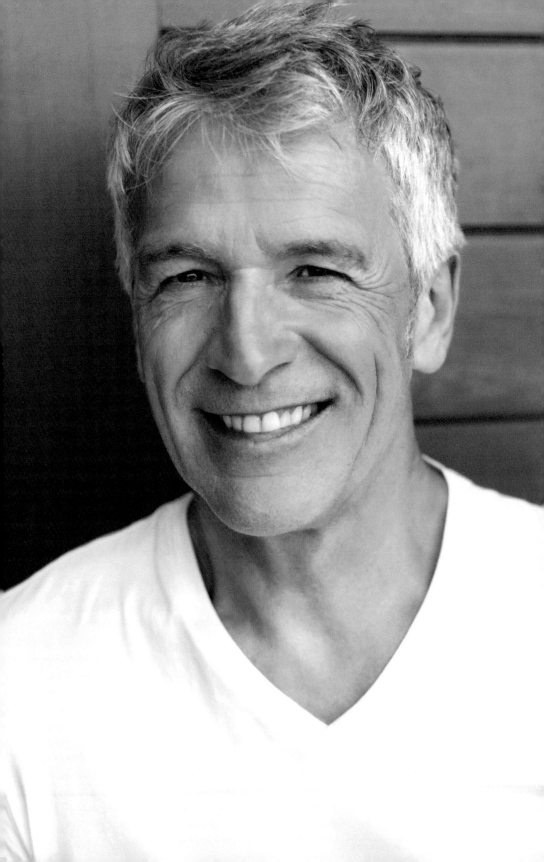

BROWS

In a nutshell, if you have a unibrow, seek out professional help at a high-end salon (ask your wife, girlfriend, or chic female office mate for a recommendation). If your unibrow embarrasses you, tell them you need a really great haircut. An experienced aesthetician will shape and prune your unruly brows to help you in your "manscaping" quest.

BOOZE

The older you get, the more careful you need to be about drinking to excess or too frequently, which can have a definite aging effect. Not only does alcohol translate to dreaded belly fat, but too much imbibing can mean broken blood vessels in your face, as blood vessels become dilated or in some cases burst, increasing the tendency toward facial redness.

B.O.

It's unfortunately a result of the high-stress, very active lives many men lead that body odor can at times be an issue. Beyond the obvious fixes of showering at least once a day, wearing deodorant, and keeping a spare shirt at the office to slip into à la "Mad Men," there are several solutions for both excessive body odor and excessive sweating.

One crucial step is to always make sure your body (especially your feet) is scrupulously dry before dressing. Wear cotton garments, especially cotton socks, and try an antibacterial soap. If pungent feet are an issue, wash your feet before going to bed each night and use a foot powder or even a spray antiperspirant on your feet in the morning.

If excessive sweating (or hyperhidrosis) is an issue, there are prescription-strength deodorants available from your doctor. Or look for clinical-strength over-the-counter antiperspirants that contain aluminum chloride, a very effective perspiration inhibitor. Injections of Botox in the underarm area, which temporarily block the chemical signals from the nerves that stimulate the sweat glands, are also very effective for up to six months. There are also some surgical options available for both excessive underarm, foot, and palm sweating, but they should only be used as a last resort, once all other methods have been tried and exhausted.

NAILS

Manicures and pedicures often aren't necessary, but by all means, pay attention to the look of your nails. Keep your fingernails short and scrupulously clean. And nothing can put a chill on a romantic evening as quickly as claw-like toenails, so don't think that because such things are out of sight they're out of mind. Remember, those toenails are attached to your feet, which are often on display in summer sandals, at the pool, or with your significant other. If your skin becomes too dry, it can crack — especially around the heels. The best way to treat and prevent the condition, short of getting regular pedicures, is to use a pumice stone to file away the hard, dry skin. Once the softer skin is exposed, apply therapeutic ointments or creams, purchased at any drugstore.

YOUR PEARLY WHITES

Teeth can be one of the most obvious places to begin showing one's age. Whether you seek a dentist's help or use a home-bleaching method, keep your teeth bright and white to avoid the yellowed look of aged teeth. If uneven, small, or discolored teeth are an issue, consider veneers, which can take decades off your age.

HAIR LOSS

The American Academy of Dermatology estimates that 80 million men and women in the United States suffer with hair thinning or hair loss. For most men, hair loss (or a dramatically receding hairline) can be a devastating blow to their self-esteem. Hair is associated with virility, and its retreat is too often a visible reminder of aging. Rest assured, though, that if your hairline is retreating, you're in very good company. Iconic men, from Jack Nicholson to Prince William to Bruce Willis, suffer from balding, but clearly they appeal to some of the most beautiful women in the world. And if it's any consolation, male-pattern baldness is associated with higher testosterone levels, meaning the men most likely to experience it are generally the most masculine among us.

And chances are that what is devastating to you is not even registering to the rest of the world. Maybe you're overthinking it. Like most things in life, how you handle balding, whether by trying to deny it or by strategically coping with it and getting on with your life, will define the type of person you are.

Men can exercise various options to combat thinning hair or balding heads. The easiest is to just shave it all off. Even men with a full head of hair shave their heads to look more masculine. If your head has a good shape and extreme hair loss can't be denied any longer, this is a remarkably easy and often very flattering option. With so many young, stylish urban men taking this course, shaving your head can often look like a fashion statement. It's also remarkably cool in the summer (just don't forget the sunscreen for your newly chromed dome), though you may find yourself needing a knit cap or other headgear to stave off winter chills.

A radically shorter cut is another option. The merest whiff of a buzz cut can hide the fact that your hair is beginning to retreat.

The thing to avoid, though, is trying to hide the balding; it won't fool anyone. You know what I'm talking about: laughable, you're-not-kidding-anyone Donald Trump comb-overs, bad hair plugs, and old-man toupees. Better to shave your dome than signal to the world your anxiety about your retreating locks. Women will like you better for your honesty and self-confidence.

There are also a number of hair-growth stimulators, such as the nonprescription drug Minoxidil, applied topically, and the oral prescription drug Finasteride, both of which have helped some men maintain the amount of hair they have and in some cases regrow new hair. Especially with Finasteride, the earlier you begin using the medication the better, because it seems most effective when hair loss is just beginning. Generally, once you begin these treatments you must stay on them, or your hair will go back to its previous rate of shedding.

If it's any consolation, male-pattern baldness is associated with higher testosterone levels, meaning the men most likely to experience it are generally the most masculine among us.

HAIR DYE

First of all, there is no shame in going gray. Gray hair connotes experience and sophistication. On the right man it can be attractive and distinguished. You will probably find as many women turned on by gray hair, if not more, as there are women who find it unappealing. Look at Giorgio Armani or Richard Gere, and you will observe men who are at ease in their own skin (and hair), who have embraced the masculine appeal of age and experience. If you do go gray, or white, all the more reason to put a little color in your face to offset it. Self-tanner is a great way to achieve the perfect contrast between fair hair and a face that advertises healthy virility.

But if gray is not your thing — if you think it sends the wrong message for your particular office, where experience and maturity are undervalued — then there is no shame in dying your hair. Getting rid of gray is becoming more and more popular as men hold on to their sex appeal and keep their competitive edge, especially on the job.

You have two options on this front. There is the salon option, where a skilled colorist will help you choose a color as close to your natural, pre-gray shade as possible. Keep it real by not going too far astray from your natural hair color.

If you are the do-it-yourself type, there are drugstore products that will mask the gray, such as Clairol Natural Instincts for Men or Redken's Color Camo; but again, the key is to keep the color as close to your natural shade as possible to avoid looking like you are trying too hard or have entered the witness-protection program. I can't stress enough that you need to be extremely cautious when you take this approach. Find a color that suits your skin tone, one that isn't too light and brassy or so dark and monochrome that it obviously comes out of a bottle.

A third option is to find a hairdresser who is willing to help you achieve a balance of at-home and salon color. Maybe you go in every three to six months for color, but the colorist helps you find a kit and a shade for touch-ups between visits.

BEWARE THE HAIR

There are two schools of thought on this. On one hand, with the proliferation of Grizzly Adams beards has come the tendency to let things get a little too out of control hair-wise. Keep it clean, fellas, which means if you're going to sport a mountain-man look, make sure your beard is free of crumbs, sauces, vermin, and any other surprises. On the other hand, if you go for a more curated facial-hair look, it's possible to take things too far.

Once upon a time, men had a choice: mustache or no mustache, beard or no beard. Now, the opportunities for facial hair have exploded. There are mutton chops and Elvis sideburns, soul patches and handlebar mustaches, and the two-day shadow that's supposed to look sexy. The danger is in taking things to such a grooming extreme that you begin to treat your face like a garden and your hair as some exquisite topiary to groom and weed. Too much facial-hair fastidiousness can border on the creepy and indicate control issues. There is such a thing as looking too groomed... indicating to the world that you have just spent the previous two hours in front of the mirror shaping your Van Dyke with needlepoint scissors. That definitely qualifies.

HAIR REMOVAL

Back hair, chest hair, ear hair, excessive nose hair. There are a host of places that require a little pruning. Laser hair removal is one typically painless option, generally requiring five or more sessions to significantly diminish the texture and prevalence of hair, though the procedure will not get rid of hair altogether. A good nose-hair trimmer or a judicious barber is another option. While how much to shave or pluck is a matter of personal opinion, the fact is: too much hair sprouting from your neck, nose, or ears can telegraph a disinterest in personal grooming that could have repercussions on the job or in your love life.

SELF-TANNER

What women already know, men can stand to learn, too. Self-tanner is makeup without makeup, giving your skin a consistent tone and the glow of good health without dangerous exposure to the sun. The more we learn about the sun's dam-aging effects, the more appealing self-tanners look. Just make sure you exfoliate before using to remove dead skin cells, and moisturize before application to help the tanner apply more smoothly and stick to the skin. Also be sure to wash off your hands following application to avoid telltale tanned palms. Don't overdo it, though; you wouldn't want to be called out as an obvious self-tanner, like House Rep. John Boehner, whose orange face is a dead giveaway.

STYLE NOTES

So what does a cosmetic surgeon know about men's style? Working in the field of aesthetics, one's eye becomes adjusted to what works and what doesn't, both in surgery and in personal style. In my case, I work in an office with a staff of smart, opinionated women who are not afraid to let me know about my own style infractions. You could say that over time I've picked up a tip or two from my female co-workers, but also from my equally observant wife and daughter. They're always more than happy to share with me some of the mistakes men (like me) make — and they have suggestions for the best way to correct them. I am, in the spirit of brotherhood, passing along their advice to you.

Just like most women, every guy could use a style overhaul at some point in his life. Everyone needs a refresher course on what works and what doesn't. There are several approaches you can take. If you have a wife or girlfriend whose style advice you trust, she would most likely be more than happy to help you update your wardrobe, cast off some of the relics, and assess your style strengths and weaknesses. A close female friend or stylish co-worker might also be more than happy to spend a Saturday with you at the mall, helping you figure out what styles and cuts suit you.

Or you can do as the ladies do and take it to the professionals. Hire someone to come work with your existing wardrobe, while bringing in some new pieces; or

Tripp is an old friend who first began discussing a procedure with me when he was 54. An engineer, his main concerns were the aging changes to his eyebrow and eye region. Like many middle-aged men, Tripp was beginning to notice some wrinkles around his eyes and some puffiness underneath, along with the dreaded dark circles. He always looked tired and was receiving negative comments from friends and co-workers. He also noticed that he had some decreased side vision while driving and was concerned that it could become a safety issue for him in traffic.

"Most guys aren't going to schedule a session with Dr. Phil to discuss their feelings on the subject, but aging can be a real blow to the ego," says Tripp. *"You always think of yourself as a young guy. It can be quite a reality check when the guy looking back at you in the mirror looks more like your dad than you. Since Dr. Cole is a friend, I listened when he suggested surgery for my eyelids,"* Tripp recalls. *"He also advised laser resurfacing to eliminate some wrinkles around my eyes and to get rid of the puffiness and dark circles below. To be honest, if I didn't know Chip personally, I probably wouldn't have had the work done. But the trust factor was there for me. I have a lot of close friends, but there aren't many I'd allow near me with a laser."*

Outcome: Tripp underwent laser resurfacing to tighten things up from a skin standpoint and also had an upper-lid blepharoplasty. Some skin was removed and his eyebrow tissue was tightened.

"Following surgery, I couldn't believe the difference," Tripp reflects.

His healing took a little longer than normal. He went on a ski trip five or six days after surgery, and the elevated altitude and lower oxygen level prolonged some of the natural swelling. I had told him that after a week he'd be about 85 percent healed. He may have been a bit overly optimistic, thinking he would be more like 99 percent back to normal. So he opted to tell friends and co-workers that his lingering puffiness was the result of allergies.

In a lot of respects, Tripp is like many of my male patients. He chose to keep his procedures a secret from those he does business with.

But whenever I see Tripp — who, despite keeping pace in a very competitive industry, looks rested and relaxed — that's thanks enough for me.

Tripp Laser Resurfacing, Upper-Lid Blepharoplasty

Prior to surgery, he appeared stern and overworked. After surgery, he looked relaxed and rested. His hooding over his upper eyelids was reduced while maintaining his masculinity.

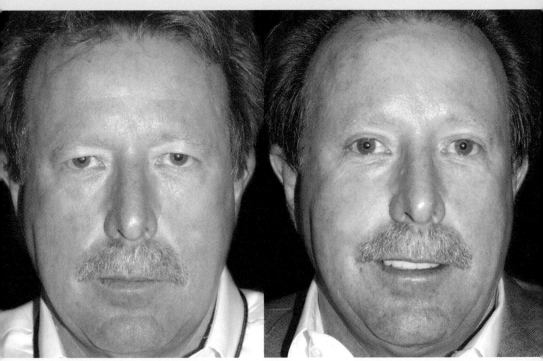

BEFORE ▲   ▲ AFTER

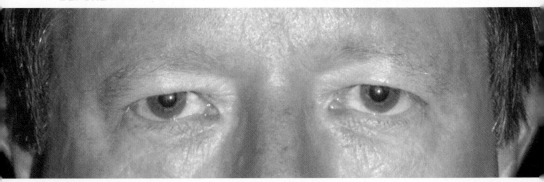

BEFORE ▲   ▼ AFTER

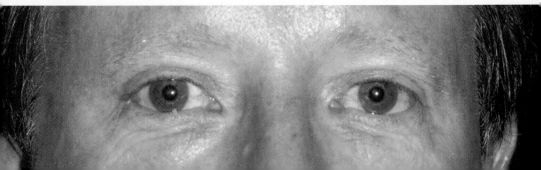

shop at a higher-end store that suits your style, like Brooks Brothers or Nordstrom, then find a personal shopper you click with. A general rule of thumb, which works for men as well as women, is that if you haven't worn it in a year, get rid of it. And don't get stuck in a rut. Embrace the positive changes that can come when you let go of old habits and let someone with a fresh vision help lead you to the light! I think you'll find that a style refresher, combined with a cosmetic procedure that takes years off of your looks, can be a pretty potent combination.

MAN UP

Look at a man and woman in their 20s or 30s going out on a date, and you may notice something radically wrong. The woman is dressed to the nines in a sexy dress and sky-high heels. And the man? He's in cargo shorts, jumbo sneakers, and a T-shirt stating "Will Work For Beer." Do you see anything wrong with this picture? The woman is dressed as if the occasion is important. She has made preparations for it in grooming and probably also logged some shopping miles to pick out a great outfit for the occasion. But the man is saying, "I could be going out for Italian with a beautiful lady, or I could be lying on my sofa eating corn chips and watching football. Same diff." In other words, he's not bothering to make the effort. This is, to me, a major problem. Grown men (I'm talking about anyone over 20 who should know better) who are unable to distinguish between occasions, who cannot adjust their wardrobe for different events, who refuse to budge from a chronic casual mode signal to me that they have some growing up to do in other departments as well.

We have obviously lost some serious ground from the days of Sean Connery and Steve McQueen, when men had different outfits for different occasions and put some time and money into their "look." Back in the day, becoming a man was something boys looked forward to. Now they seem to be kicking and screaming to return to the womb. In our present age of perpetual adolescence, everyone wants to act as though they're 12. But I have news for you: just because you dress like you're 12 doesn't mean you're going to magically transform. If you are one of these Peter Pan men, it's probably time to consider ditching the short pants and running with the big boys. Dignity can be a powerful thing.

THERE'S ALWAYS A GAME ON SOMEWHERE

Save the tribal gear for game day. When you are *at* the actual game or watching it along with similarly outfitted men and women in your living room, it's OK to rock those Bulldog and Gator colors and insignia. By the same token, don't let your super-casual weekend wear fool you into thinking you have an endorsement deal with Nike, Adidas, or New Balance. Head-to-toe logos on your shorts, shoes, shirt, and hat make you look like your soul is owned by Sports Authority.

NOSTALGIA DRESSING

Your high-school and college years may have been the best times in your life, but while you can hold onto the memories, don't hold onto the clothes. Just because a look worked for you in the '60s, '70s, or '80s doesn't mean you have to keep rocking it today. So stow the acid-washed jeans, the Member's Only jackets, the Hawaiian shirts, and all the other looks that indicate you're due for a style overhaul. They don't signal to the world that you're ever-young, just that you're stuck in a style time warp. More often, hanging onto the style fixations of the past can date you, making it clear you're a fashion dinosaur.

THE 24-7 BASEBALL CAP

I recognize that sometimes this phenomenon is related to balding. When I was hard pressed for several years to find a photo of Ron Howard without a baseball cap on his head, I knew something was up. And that *something* was self-consciousness about his receding hairline. But sometimes this phenomenon is related to the perpetually-up-for-fun, always-on-vacation, don't-want-to-bother-washing-my-hair litany of bad grooming habits. When women spend as much time as they do to make themselves presentable just to go to the grocery store on a Saturday, don't you think it's only fair that you wash and comb your hair every day? C'mon.

KEEP THE THEME-DRESSING IN CHECK

Say you're one of those weekend bikers who loves to head up into the mountains with a group of other lawyers and doctors harboring *Easy Rider* fantasies. Nothing wrong with that. A guy needs an outlet. But try not to look like the five-year-old who prepares for a rain shower by donning his Big Bird slicker, boots, umbrella, and rain hat. Don't dress in top-to-toe leather; some leather pants will probably do it and advertise just fine to the locals on your hog-ride into the mountains that you are one tough hombre and mean business when you order your mesclun salad with dressing on the side. As I like to say, nothing exceeds like excess.

By the same token, avoid fashion accessories that scream "costume." It's a short list, but one worth committing to memory:

- Themed ties or bolo ties
- Bow ties (unless you're over 65)
- Cowboy hats (unless you're a cowboy)
- Holiday-themed attire
- Denim-on-denim (denim shirts or jean jackets with jeans)
- Fanny packs (unacceptable under any circumstance)
- Cell-phone belt holsters
- Jackets with epaulets, unless you work as a doorman
- Leather blazers
- Patterned sweaters (do you belong on "The Cosby Show"?)
- Shirts unbuttoned to your navel
- Tank tops (they're underwear, plain and simple; no self-respecting guy, unless he's headlining in a rockabilly band or pumping iron, should be caught dead in public wearing a tank top)
- Crocs, unless you are in the operating room
- Flip-flops — save 'em for the pool

SHOES AND WATCHES

Nothing indicates to the world the kind of man you are more quickly than these two items. Invest in good ones and/or classic styles and you can wear the most pared-down, basic outfit and still look pulled together. The watch doesn't have to be a Rolex — a classic Timex can be cool, too. Just whatever you do, don't be the guy with the digital watch whose entire shoe wardrobe consists of various incarnations of the sneaker.

OCCASIONS

Some guys wear their clothes like a uniform, and they're terrified to appear in public without being suited up. That uniform can include jeans and a t-shirt or Carharts and a work shirt. My advice is, don't be afraid. You can sport different attire based on the occasion. Wear what is appropriate and don't think that the rules exist for everyone but you. If the occasion is black tie, a tux is in order. If someone is getting married, you need to wear a suit. The same goes for funerals. It shows respect for your hosts (as well as the dead), and it shows that you know the difference between any other day and this day. It's the mark of a gentleman.

CLASSIC TRUMPS TRENDY EVERY TIME

Something about a man who only wears "the latest" suggests that they're slaves to the dictates of fashion, that they don't know what suits them, and that their clothes are wearing them. There's nothing wrong with looking stylish, but beware of fads, like ripped jeans or detective-novel fedoras, that can make you look like you're trying too hard.

Instead, model your look on a man who is considered an exemplar of style — James Dean, Cary Grant, Leonardo DiCaprio — and you'll always look great. All of these men prove a point: before the present proliferation of clothing styles and endless misguided trends (parachute pants, anyone?), the classics were a foundation that allowed the man wearing them to shine. Follow their lead and stick with the tried-and-true basics.

THE SUIT

Most men know that a suit is a power move, a mode of dress that instantly confers style, sophistication, and a certain world-wise savoir faire. One great suit is better than five mediocre, cheap suits. In a word, *quality matters*. Buy the best you can afford and make sure the fit is perfect — especially behind the collar, where a gap is the mark of a bad fit. The shoulders also need to fit straight off the rack while allowing for range of movement, because a tailor can fix almost everything *except* the shoulders on a suit.

Comfort is key. If the suit you put on doesn't make you look better, more handsome, more dignified, it's time to start over. Cuffs or no cuffs, two or three buttons, single- or double-breasted are all matters of personal taste, but if you get the fit and quality right, you're 99 percent of the way there. The remaining 1 percent is up to you.

PAY ATTENTION TO FIT

Some men make the mistake of thinking that because they're in non-work, casual mode, fit doesn't matter. But shirts that are too tight, pants that are too baggy — in general, clothes that make you look like you don't know your size — are never flattering. One of the benefits of being a man is that when you purchase clothing from a reputable store, tailoring is complimentary. Use it.

BE A GENTLEMAN

Reality TV, boorish behavior, and the eroding boundary between private and public behavior means that sometimes what seems obvious needs to be restated. Thank people for kindnesses proffered, from your hosts at a dinner party to the valet who opens your car door for you. Real men don't make distinctions according to social station, and are polite to everyone they encounter. Hold doors for women — not just the young, attractive ones you want to impress, but the Rubenesque women and the cleaning ladies and those of a certain age. A gentleman doesn't extend good manners only to the women he thinks might date him. It doesn't matter how rich you are, how handsome, how well-dressed or how smart: if you have bad manners all of that crumbles away, revealing your true colors.

"Men want the same thing
from their underwear
that they want from women:
a little bit of support,
and a little bit of freedom."
— Jerry Seinfeld

CHIP'S TIPS

1 Skin-care products aren't just for women anymore. Regardless of gender, as we age our skin requires more moisturizing and maintenance. Don't have a John Wayne mentality about freshening procedures being unmanly. Chances are, your top competitors are having them regularly.

2 Keep a water bottle handy for the gym or the golf course. Your body requires more water than what you get from melting ice cubes in that glass of scotch after a long day. You'll see a real difference in your sense of well-being — and your mental acuity — with increased water intake.

3 Smoking, alcohol consumption, and diet all play a role in how your skin looks. Remember: everything (except smoking) in moderation.

4 James Bond has endured for decades. His secret is that he is well-dressed, beautifully groomed, and takes great care of his skin. Is it any wonder he's surrounded by gorgeous women?

5 Plastic surgery isn't a one-size-fits-all overhaul; it needs to take into consideration every person's unique physiognomy as well as the significant gender differences.

6 Fitness is an important concept in many areas, including physical, mental and spiritual. Skin fitness is key.

7 Real men eat quiche, wear pink, *and* take care of their faces.

8 Women like to be pampered and respected. Be a gentleman.

9 Just give in and put down the toilet seat. Each flush spreads airborne germs that impact your environment. The ladies will think you're their hero!

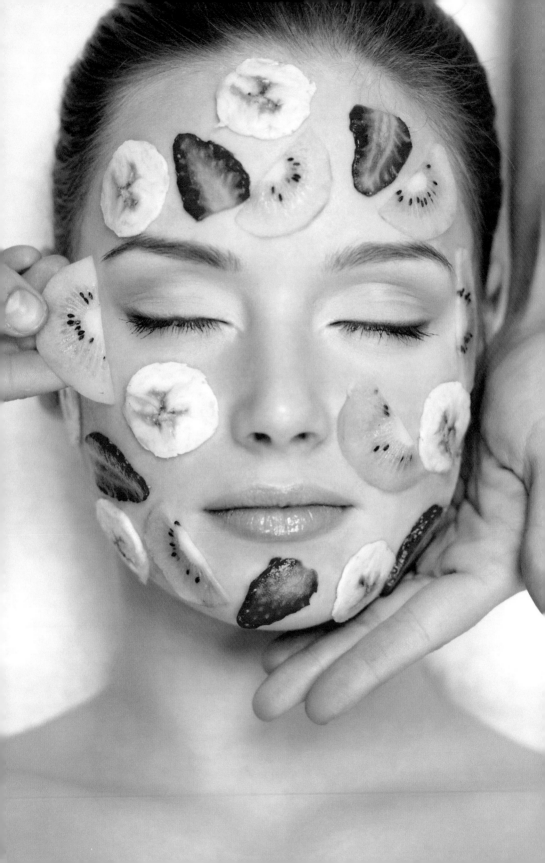

CHAPTER 8

* * *

FEED YOUR SKIN:
REVITALIZING FOODS AND VITAMINS

It's a simple fact: your skin is an indicator of your overall health. Lost amid the latest fad diets, expensive designer face creams, and quick-fix cosmetic surgeries is a fundamental truth: what you put into your body reveals itself on the outside. If you feel lethargic and your skin is breaking out, before heading for that energy drink or a trip to the dermatologist for an antibiotic, think about what you have been ingesting lately.

As citizens of the 21st century, we all should have drunk the Kool-Aid of good health. Thanks to the Atkins diet, we know that carbohydrates pack on pounds. Thanks to Michael Pollan's *The Omnivore's Dilemma,* we've learned that processed foods and factory-farmed meat is bad for us and bad for the planet. Thanks to Mireille Guiliano's *French Women Don't Get Fat*, the chic-mystique–busting best seller, we know that walking, small portions, and plenty of yogurt and leeks — as well as a certain amount of dark chocolate — can keep the pounds and yo-yo dieting at bay. And thanks to our moms telling us to eat our vegetables, we know that a diet rich in fruits and vegetables is better than one that's heavy on fatty meats and white flour. Thanks, Mom.

As someone who works in the beauty industry, I have a certain amount of wisdom to share regarding healthy eating. After all, expensive skin-care products may make us feel like we're pampering our skin; but the best way is to indulge in a great diet loaded with fruits and vegetables to fuel the health of our entire body. Believe me, that health will show up on the outside, too.

Some people think cosmetic surgery is just about surface beauty. But as I often tell my patients, the look of your skin, the brightness of your eyes, the sheen of your hair — all the things that lend the appearance of beauty and good health — reflect what's going on deep below the surface. Being in this business gives me a unique pulpit from which to preach the sermon of diet and vitamins. Because while a patient will often humor her family doctor when he gives her the same advice, she tends to take it to heart when it comes from her plastic surgeon. People might not eat right to stave off high cholesterol and sluggishness, but tell them tomatoes and vitamin C will make their skin glow and fight wrinkles, and they start changing their diet — STAT.

If you're going to invest in the expense and healing time of surgery, why not prolong your results? Better yet, delay that surgery in the first place by sticking to a healthy diet and abandoning the kind of yo-yo dieting that robs your skin of vital nutrients and upsets your metabolism.

The best ways to keep your skin, hair, and body healthy and vibrant are for the most part found in the things you eat. While supplements are great, it is the foods themselves, with their natural vitamins and minerals, that give you the most glow for your greenback. That being said, I also recommend some additional vitamin supplements to enhance your good looks (notice how I use the word "supplement," which means an addition to, not a substitution for, healthy eating).

As a doctor, I can tell a lot about people's health just by looking at their skin, hair, and nails (although the latter proves a little harder with all the acrylic nails out there). If your skin is sallow and dull, if your skin exhibits bad turgor (the ability to snap back when pinched), then you may be dehydrated and not getting the proper nutrients. Your collagen and elastic fibers are enormously affected by the foods you eat and the things you drink, which translates to wrinkled, less-vibrant, slack skin. I see a lot of fad dieters in my practice who pay much more attention to calories than to nutrients; the evidence is a sallow complexion and increased levels of fatigue. Nails also reveal a lot about diet. If yours are yellow, streaked, brittle, and easily broken, or if your cuticles are unhealthy, these are all indications of a poor diet.

How can eating affect your hair? Thin and dull hair can result from crash dieting, but foods high in cysteine, an amino acid found in keratin (which forms the basis of hair and nails) can make your hair lustrous and strong. Keratin is found in such readily available foods as broccoli, Brussels sprouts, chicken, garlic, onions, oats, red pepper, and egg yolks.

Amazingly, most medical-school curriculums do not cover diet or even consider holistic health. To me it's a scandalous oversight, when you think how much we've learned about the link between food and overall health. It's up to doctors to educate themselves about these matters. The reason places like Whole Foods and juice bars are booming is because people see the benefits of fruits and vegetables. The fact is, we know that limiting animal fats in our diet, which includes dairy, decreases our cancer risk — and especially the risk of skin cancer. And we know that leafy greens and fish are vital to maintaining good health.

So here's your chance to catch up, and even get ahead of the game...but you'll have to put in the work. Changing your diet means changing your lifestyle, and that's not easy to do. Eating is a social and communal activity. It unites us as family and friends and fellow diners at the table of life. My simple rule is, don't deprive yourself or make a drag out of occasions where food is the centerpiece. Instead, gravitate toward the things you know are good for you, and live fully in the moment. It's something that Europeans — a notoriously fit lot — have known all along. Slow down, enjoy time with friends and family, leave the bun off your hamburger, or better yet, choose a salad instead. Don't make a spectacle of avoidance and denial, because it makes everyone feel bad. The bigger deal you make about your diet, the harder it will be to maintain it in the long run.

Those of us who live in the South are, unfortunately, surrounded by the all-you-can-eat, super-size, more-is-more philosophy. We've learned the hard way that food is linked to weight. But what some of us haven't digested is that food is also linked to the quality of our skin, the brightness of our eyes, and the luster of our hair, not to mention truly transformative qualities like energy, outlook, and zest for life. We're all familiar with that sluggish feeling that accompanies a midday meal that's heavy on the meat and carbs. If it's doing that to our attention span and our energy level, it must be doing it to our skin, too.

Here's my simple list of things you can do right now, starting today, to make your skin look better and your overall health improve — the CliffsNotes version of what to what to avoid and what to embrace. Nothing about this list should intimidate or scare you. Slowly implement these changes, and I'm certain that your great-looking skin and hair, along with an increased sense of well-being, will encourage you to make more changes.

FOOD

LIMIT SUGAR
Harder than it sounds, I know. Sugar is a wily substance that likes to hide in a range of common foods, including ketchup, salad dressing and cereals. Ingredients like corn syrup, honey, molasses and maple syrup are also sugar rich, as are foods that contain dextrin, maltodextrin, sucrose and fructose. If you really do crave something

sweet occasionally, go with honey, which at least is a pure and unprocessed sugar. When blood sugar is elevated, the body reacts with increased insulin production, which has definitive hormonal effects — such as increasing androgen levels — resulting in excess oil and increased skin-cell production. Translation: pimples. The way your body reacts to the ingestion of sugar is to create enzymes that can destroy healthy tissue and interfere with your body's ability to make collagen and elastin; so your skin is less elastic, which makes it thinner and weaker. Limit your intake and you'll start seeing a difference in the quality of your skin.

LIMIT DAIRY

If you've been feeling listless or tired, or you want to improve the health of your skin, abstain from dairy for a week and see how you feel. You may be so motivated by the improvement that you'll naturally want to cut back on your dairy intake. You don't have to be lactose intolerant to have a sensitivity to dairy products. If cutting it out for a week makes you feel and look better, you might even consider living without it.

Why is dairy problematic? For one thing it's full of animal hormones. It's well known that dairy products boost the levels of sex hormones (testosterone and androgens), which increases insulin levels, in a way that's similar to sugar and starchy carbs, in turn giving a rapid rise to blood-sugar levels. Elevated blood sugar has a direct impact on the look of our skin. As I often tell my patients, the cure to acne is at the end of their fork, not in a prescription pad.

Many cows are also injected with the artificially engineered hormone rBGH (recombinant bovine growth hormone) to make them grow faster and produce more milk. Many experts believe that these trace hormones, which we ingest with our beef and each glass of milk, carry significant health risks. The intake of hormone residue in beef has been linked to early onset puberty in girls, and could upset the human hormone balance, leading to the development of cancer of the colon, prostate, and breast. Though there is some debate about how these hormones affect human health, the European Union does not allow the use of rBGH in cattle production and has for decades banned the import of American beef. To me, this is a red flag that should force us to look carefully at what kind of beef we consume, and especially the hormones they contain. Limiting dairy or choosing hormone-free organic beef and milk is your best option for dairy consumption.

Sustainabletable.org has a handy state-by-state list of dairies and farms that do not use rBGH; but most of the big organic brands, like Stonyfield and Horizon, advertise their products' absence of rBGH.

If you love milk and can't live without it, consider using almond milk or coconut milk, which offer a comparably creamy addition to coffee or cereal (some even like it better). In addition, soy contains isoflavone, which improves fine lines and elasticity. Be advised, though, that soy's plant estrogens may have negative side effects for women prone to breast cancer, and can interfere with testosterone production. So, men and women alike should check with their doctor before considering a soy diet.

LIMIT GLUTEN

You can't open a magazine or newspaper without hearing about gluten intolerance and bakeries opening to serve this apparently booming segment of the population. You may not be allergic to gluten, but you could be intolerant. If this is the case, you may find that just cutting back on this protein — found in wheat, barley, oats, and rye — dramatically impacts your overall well-being. Gluten is also hidden in pizza, pasta, buns, bread, wraps, rolls, and most processed foods — all staples of the American diet. There are a lot of places now where you can find gluten-free products, and most of the better restaurants now offer a gluten-free menu, so just ask. Often, the chef can prepare a gluten-free version of any dish, and it will taste just as good.

AVOID ARTIFICIAL SWEETENERS

Regular ingestion of chemicals disguised as diet aids is a bad idea. According to the Centers for Disease Control and Prevention, the side effects of aspartame (the key ingredient in NutraSweet) read like a Who's Who of maladies: headaches, dizziness, mood alterations, and gastrointestinal and dermatologic symptoms. Try Pure Via or Truvia instead, natural sweeteners that are derived from the stevia plant.

DON'T DRINK YOUR CALORIES

Why would you consume beverages like sodas and diet sodas, with their laundry list of ingredients made in a lab, when you could drink something natural instead? Drinking soda is like consuming pure sugar. Because it's a liquid, you tend not to consider the high-calorie factor, but ultimately you're taking in the caloric equivalent of 15 teaspoons of sugar for each 20-ounce can you consume. It's like drinking a candy bar or a slice of German-chocolate cake through a straw. Soda (both diet and regular) is the epitome of useless calories, filled with ingredients that provide no benefit to your body and may contribute to adverse health conditions, from osteoporosis to obesity. If you want something fizzy, mix your own cocktail free of corn syrup and chemicals by adding a splash of fruit juice or lemon to carbonated water. Or try Perrier or Pellegrino with a twist of lemon or a squeeze of lime.

MAKE OMEGA-3 FATTY ACIDS YOUR NEW FRIENDS

These "good fats" will do just about everything but wash your car and put your children through college: They aid in joint health, brain health, and cell function. They keep the skin plump, moist, and elastic, and prevent elements of skin aging.

You can find these friendly fats in salmon, tuna, sardines, fresh basil, flax seed, chia seed, walnuts, and almonds. And the linoleic acid found in olive oil, safflower oil, and walnut oil is an essential fatty acid that also keeps your skin resilient.

DRINK WATER LIKE YOU'D CRASHED ON A DESERT ISLAND
Whatever the amount of water you're drinking now, you can stand to drink more. Work toward 8 to 10 glasses a day as a goal. Your body is 60 percent water, your brain is 70 percent water, your lungs are 90 percent water. And our blood — which helps digest food, transport waste, and control body temperature — is 83 percent water. In other words, your body craves hydration.

Your skin will show immediate results in suppleness if you increase your water intake. Every day, we need to replace 2.4 liters of water through food and drink. To deny ourselves this natural elixir is like denying breast milk to a baby. Start every meal, the moment you sit down at the table, by drinking a full glass of water. Make that your rule. If you want to have a glass of wine or a cup of coffee later, that's fine; but always counterbalance these diuretics with water. You need to compensate for each glass of wine with two glasses of water.

People make the mistake of thinking that they're hitting the eight 8-ounce glasses of water requirement if they're consuming something with water *in* it. Sure, there's water in Coca-Cola, and folks drink it like it's going out of style. But the harmful ingredients in soft drinks negate any benefit of that water.

DINE AT FARM-TO-TABLE RESTAURANTS
Why? Because chef-driven restaurants like these favor quality over quantity. The portions may be smaller than at the big chains, but the cuisine packs a punch: it's more flavorful, with higher-quality ingredients and more interesting preparations. And chances are, the waiters at these restaurants will be more informed and have a greater sense of pride in the food they serve than at the homogeneous chains. Try asking a waiter at one of the formula restaurants whether the salmon is farm-raised, or where they source their asparagus, and he'll look at you as if you were speaking Mandarin.

By the way, if you ever get to Atlanta, treat yourself (and your palate) to an indulgence at Brooklyn Café — ask for Jeff, the owner. He has assembled knowledgeable staff who serve a healthy, delicious menu, including gluten-free options.

CONTROL YOUR PORTIONS
That means one helping. Only. Don't be guilt-tripped by waiters in restaurants into ordering an appetizer, salad, or soup before your meal. These first courses — appetizers especially — are where the high-fat, deep-fried options hide, tantalizing you with the notion that because they're junior-sized and can be shared they aren't as

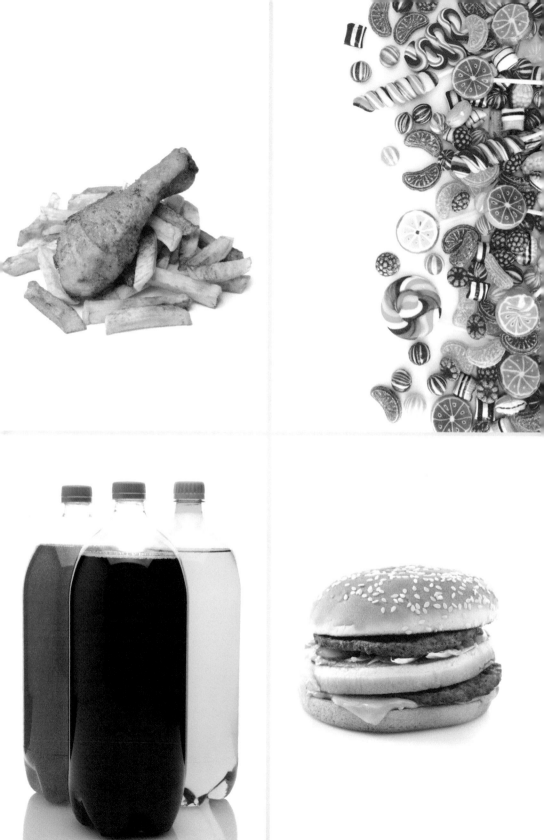

bad. Oh, and steer clear of any restaurant with buffet, factory, or trough in the name. 'Nuff said.

DRINK GREEN TEA

The suggestion to drink green tea has been floating around the popular consciousness for some time. Green tea (and dark chocolate, too) is so good because it contains flavonoids, which protect your skin from cancer and inflammation. A 2008 research study at the Harvard School of Public Health even determined that those who eat chocolate and sweets up to three times each month live almost a year longer than those who abstain. Sounds like a good argument for all things in moderation!

RECONFIGURE YOUR STARBUCKS ORDER

It's the adult version of a pacifier: sometimes you just need something creamy and warm to get you through the day. Don't avoid the little treat we all occasionally crave, but be sure to make smart choices. Skip anything with a pumped-in flavor option, like chai. No whipped cream (sorry). And choose skim milk or, better yet, soy. Think about a green tea option. And don't even *look* at that pastry case (trust me on this: banana chocolate-chip pound cake is sinfully delicious, but addictive).

DIVERSIFY YOUR FOOD PORTFOLIO

It's a smart approach for investing, and it's smart for eating, too. A diet rich in a diverse mix of fruits and vegetables (have fun with it!) will fight off the free radicals that damage collagen and can lead to skin cancer. Gravitate toward fruits with lower fructose — such as strawberries, oranges, blackberries, lemons, and blueberries — rather than high-fructose options like grapes and apples.

WHEN IN DOUBT, EAT A TOMATO

You know the expression, "an apple a day keeps the doctor away"? Well, here's one you may not have heard: a tomato a day is even better. This is my shout-out for tomatoes, in many ways the perfect food. They help protect the skin from sun damage and antioxidants, which in turn improves skin elasticity and radiance. And they're so easy to incorporate into your diet, between the great sauces, salsas, and sun-drieds out there. Reduced tomato products like tomato paste boast the beneficial substance lycopene, a carotenoid in human skin, that protects your skin. Many studies have found that people who eat lots of lycopene-rich foods have a reduced incidence of cardiovascular disease, cancer, and macular degeneration. Yet another reason to order Italian (with a glass of red)!

ADD FOODS RICH IN HYALURONIC ACID

This primary ingredient in cosmetic fillers (as well as your skin, connective tissue, and neural tissue) is found in many foods that are incredibly beneficial to the skin. Without enough hyaluronic acid, you're more likely to see wrinkles and irregular scar formation. The best foods for hyaluronic acid are those rich in magnesium: almonds, peanuts, kidney beans, black-eyed peas, lentils, pinto beans, asparagus, avocados, broccoli, carrots, cauliflower, green beans, green lettuce, soy, tomatoes, apples, bananas, melons, oranges, papayas, pears, pineapple. Also beef, chicken, lamb and veal. Foods containing zinc (lamb, beef, pork, chicken, beans, brown rice, potatoes, pumpkin seeds, whole grains), also help in the synthesis of hyaluronic acid in the body.

This is my shout-out to tomatoes, in many ways the perfect food. They help protect the skin from sun damage and antioxidants, which in turn improves skin elasticity and radiance.

NO CRASH DIETING!

You're generally not getting the nutrients your body needs when you make radical changes to your diet, and you adversely affect your skin and collagen levels, which means accelerated aging. If you skip meals, you slow down your metabolism, which means your body starts holding onto fat. To avoid blood-sugar fluctuations (which can also affect your skin), eat regular, healthy meals and choose occasional snacks of good foods like nuts and fresh fruits to maintain steady blood sugar.

THINK HIGH-QUALITY PROTEINS

Collagen is a naturally occurring protein found in the skin and connective tissue; it's responsible for skin strength and elasticity, which diminish as we age. The reason I recommend that my patients increase their consumption of high-quality proteins, such as fish, poultry, eggs, nuts and seeds, soy (like tofu), and some lean meats before surgery is that it helps build tissues and speed the healing process. The amino acids found in collagen — glycine and proline — are also found in beef, lamb, lobster, scallops, shrimp, and cabbage. Bison is another good, lean protein; and thanks to Atlanta's own Ted Turner, it's now easy to find in supermarkets — and at Ted's Montana Grill. Choose extra-lean ground beef and lean cuts like flank steak, sirloin, top loin, shoulder steak, and tenderloin. (Say, this is sounding better all the time.)

LIMIT SATURATED FATS

Saturated fats are plentiful in margarine, fatty beef, cheese, milk, cream, butter, and sour cream, which all contain high levels of saturated fat, as do cocoa butter, coconut oil and palm oil. The American Heart Association recommends moderating intake of these saturated fats. Healthier fats for cooking, like olive oil and canola oil, are an easy choice. And if you eat meat, choose the leanest cuts.

AVOID PROCESSED FOODS

Foods we find in bags, microwave packages, and plastic bowls — the ones that last for months or even years on your pantry shelves — should be limited. Remember that fresh is best. If it's hard to make frequent trips to the grocery store, or you're too busy to stay on top of all that shopping, frozen is better than processed.

Also consider a CSA membership. Community-supported agriculture programs allow you to order weekly supplies of fresh, often organic, fruits and vegetables you can either pick up at a designated spot each week or even have delivered to you. CSAs encourage you to try new vegetables (with some groups you have some choice over which fruits and vegetables you receive; with others, you get whatever's recently been harvested). It's like getting a present of good health every week! Some groups, especially in big cities, are even beginning to offer organic meats and farm-fresh eggs this way.

Farmers markets are also great, because they're generally held in the same location once or twice a week and are easy to integrate into your schedule. This rising phenomenon gets you out of your normal comfort zone of the local grocery store, encouraging you to break away from routine habits and familiar products. In many cases, surrounding yourself with farmers and other shoppers who are interested in health, and where their food is sourced, allows you to keep it regional, seasonal and sustainable (and pick up some healthy recipe ideas along the way). My wife Susan and I attended a free guided tour of our local Whole Foods Market; it was most informative and loaded with perks, like savings tips and food samples.

ESCHEW WHITES, CHEW GREENS

White bread, white sugar, white rice — all are simple carbohydrates and high-glycemic foods to avoid, many of which represent processed food that is no longer in its natural form. So instead of reaching for the white, go green, as in green juices. I am a big fan. A great Whole Foods or Arden's Garden habit involves a mix of kale, spinach, carrots, celery, and wheatgrass with a shot of ginger (calming to your intestinal system). It's my go-to breakfast. I know it sounds like a seven-year-old's nightmare food, but you'll be amazed at the increased focus and energy that result from this combination of pure foods. Plus, it's an amazing vitamin kick in natural form. Especially when you're busy with career and life, this works wonders. It's the kind of habit — like picking up a latte at Starbucks — that we as human beings seem to need each day, but this one's actually healthy. For green variety in your diet, try collards, dandelion greens or Swiss chard sautéed in a little olive oil and garlic.

Doing the occasional detox can be very healthy, as long as it's not being used just for weight control. Detoxing with healthy liquids should be used more to rest your system and get away from some of the bulk, like chicken and meat products, and the processed foods that are hard to digest and really put your body through its paces. Without a doctor's supervision, I don't recommend a detox program longer than 10 days. If you're interested in something beyond that, by all means, speak with your doctor first so you can both monitor your health status.

GO WHOLE GRAIN

...Because it tastes better, it's more satisfying, and it has a depth of flavor that you'll love after all the gummy white breads you've grown accustomed to. With all the great options out there in whole-grain pastas, breads, muffins, and other low-glycemic options, there's no reason to still be eating foods made from refined grain. Just remember that multigrain isn't the same as whole grain; it can be a mixture of various refined grains that isn't any better for you.

LIMIT ALCOHOL

The benefits of red wine have been widely demonstrated, and a glass every now and then could be advantageous to your health. But avoid alcohol on a daily basis if you can, since it's not only dehydrating and a source of empty calories, but can also cause you to lose your focus in following a healthy eating plan. It's amazing how a martini or three can somehow lead to a thick, fatty T-bone, a baked potato with everything on it, and a slice of cheesecake. Don't ask me how it happens, it just does. A patient once told me that he limits himself to one highball. "Just one highball *glass*," he says. "Of course, I refill it all night."

VITAMINS

As I've already said, you should get the majority of your nutrients from food. But vitamins are crucial to good health and for covering our bases and making sure we're consistently armed to fight disease and aging every day of our lives. Everyone should take a multivitamin/multimineral every day. That's the foundation of good health.

There are other vitamin supplements you should strongly consider putting into heavy rotation in your diet. But since capsulation is a problem (because nutri-

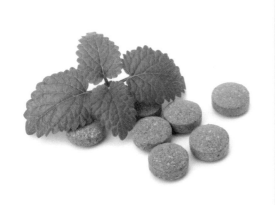

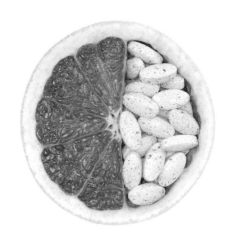

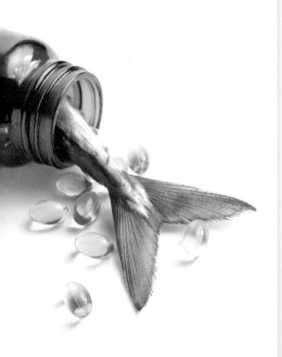

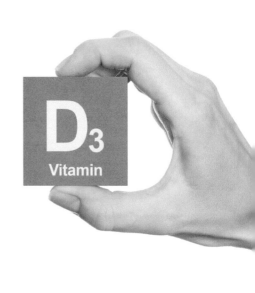

ents never make it out of their capsule containers to reach your digestive system), liquid and powder vitamins may be your best bet. And a liquid vitamin or a vitamin powder can easily be stirred into your smoothie or your child's soup. It beats swallowing the horse pills that most of us know from the vitamins of years past. I'm a huge believer in the power of vitamins. I always recommend to my surgical patients a course of vitamins that help in healing. There are also various homeopathic treatments, like arnica montana and bromelain (found in pineapple), that help reduce swelling and bruising.

VITAMIN C

Vitamin C is essential in the synthesis of collagen, which we all know has a dramatic effect on skin and muscle health — not to mention its benefits for good bone health. Every doctor has an opinion about the right dosage of this key vitamin. If you talk to ten doctors, you'll probably get ten different opinions. The Christopher Columbus of vitamin C, Linus Pauling, argued for megadoses of 10,000 International Units (IUs) a day, but that is probably overkill. I recommend 3,000 IUs a day (I break this down to 1,000 three times a day), and when I'm getting sick or feeling bad, I'll double that. But I only get sick once every three or four years, so I'm inclined to think that a regimen of healthy eating and supplements does work.

IRON AND ZINC

For glossier, thicker hair, foods rich in these minerals can help: beef, lamb, lentils, spinach, turkey, kidney beans, pork. Think about adding 8 to 11 mg of zinc each day if your dietary intake isn't covering it, as well as 8 mg a day of iron for men and 18 mg a day for women 19 to 50 years old. Both men and women can taper back to 8 mg a day at age 51 and over.

VITAMIN E

One of the best-known antioxidants found in the human body, vitamin E protects lipids — the building blocks of cell membranes — from free-radical damage. This antioxidant ramps up the skin's natural repair process and has even been found to help treat wrinkles and discoloration caused by aging and the sun. Taken orally, 400 IUs of vitamin E is a good daily dose. For topical use, 2 to 5 percent of vitamin E moisturizing cream, typically 25,000 IUs per four-ounce jar, is the best. For healing incisions only, read the label to make sure it's 100 percent vitamin E and not diluted with other ingredients. You can also break open capsules of vitamin E and apply it directly to your incision, which can also help diminish the appearance of scars.

SELENIUM
The trace mineral selenium has antioxidant properties that help prevent cell damage that can be caused by free radicals. Brazil nuts, beef, chicken, turkey, cod and tuna are good sources of this mineral.

VITAMIN D
With more people avoiding the sun because of skin-cancer concerns, a supplement of this essential vitamin can also protect against cancer of the breast, colon, and prostate. Most milk is also fortified with vitamin D, so if you're trying to cut back on dairy, as I recommend you do, a supplement is a good idea. Since it's difficult to find foods that contain vitamin D — beyond fatty fish such as mackerel, tuna, and salmon — the National Institutes of Health recommend that people age 19 to 70 take 600 IUs a day, and women and men over 70 increase it to 800 IUs.

GREEN LIVING, INSIDE AND OUT

Equally as important as your daily intake of food and drink is what you ingest in terms of chemicals and substances that have a detrimental effect on your health. There has been a movement toward green and sustainable consciousness, vis-à-vis preserving the planet. Humans recycle, compost, grow vegetable gardens, conserve energy, and (those who can afford it) drive hybrids. In other words, we fret over ways to reduce our carbon footprint. But what about applying those green principles to Planet You?

It's not hippy-dippy to pay attention to the many potentially toxic substances that surround us — it's just good common sense for 21st-century citizens living in an increasingly hazardous world. Many of these substances have not been conclusively proven to increase cancer rates, even as scientists continue to study their health effects; but many can be found in large quantities in human urine, which means they are being absorbed on a wide scale even if their long-term health effects are not conclusive. And with many countries already banning such substances as genetically modified food, certain hair dyes, pesticides, and irradiated meat, to name a few, I choose to err on the side of caution. Following are my tips for going green:

DON'T SMOKE
Smoking is the single worst thing you can do — not only for your health, but also for your looks. It steals oxygen from your body (and we kind of need that for essential things like breathing) and it produces free radicals that rob your skin of collagen and elastin, which means weak, thin, aged skin. **People who have**

cosmetic surgery and who smoke take twice as long to heal. And their results last half as long. It's a sad fact that people who subject themselves to the carcinogens in smoking take other risks with their health as well. Consider giving up smoking and enjoy the enormous benefits to your health and lifestyle.

AVOID EXCESSIVE SUN EXPOSURE

Believe it or not, consistent sun exposure is better than the weekend-warrior blast, because it's sunburns that cause the most skin damage. And regular low-dose exposure can help your body absorb vitamin D more effectively. Someone who golfs four or five times a week, for instance, often has healthier skin than someone who lays out a few times a month and gets burned almost every time. Sunscreen can protect your skin against both UVA and UVB rays, and SPF 30 is the minimum amount you should apply to your skin each day. But just as important is the frequency of application. Even when the label says the sunscreen is waterproof, it needs to be reapplied every two hours.

AVOID BPA

Bisphenol A is used to manufacture polycarbonate plastics and is most often found in canned goods, pizza-box linings, plastic dinnerware, and plastic containers. For your own health, as well as that of the environment, I advise staying away from plastic water bottles, which have been linked to liver problems, thyroid dysfunction, and even obesity. These plastics have even been called "obesogens," because of their link to increased weight gain. You can avoid BPAs by never heating plastic containers in the microwave, by avoiding the most toxic of plastics (PVC 3, PS 6, and number 7 plastics), and by limiting your consumption of canned foods. Fresh or frozen is tastier and more nutritious anyway. Eighty percent of water bottles end up languishing in landfills or floating in ocean garbage patches. When these water bottles are heated, they can release toxic chemicals such as phthalates. (More info in Cosmetic Alert below.)

AVOID NITRATES

These preservatives, used in foods to prevent botulism, can be found in preserved and cured meats, including bacon, salami, hot dogs, lunch meats, rotisserie chicken, and smoked salmon. Nitrates are known carcinogens. Children who eat more than 12 hot dogs a month have an elevated risk of childhood leukemia — scary when you think of how many children subsist on this quick, easy-to-eat food. There are bountiful and delicious no-nitrate options for bacon, hot dogs, lunch meats, and other meats available at Trader Joe's, Whole Foods, Publix and Kroger. Even Hormel puts out a gluten- and nitrate-free Natural Choice line, containing no preservatives. With all the alternatives, why eat nitrates?

Another reason to avoid the above processed meats: they can contain other cancer-causing agents such as HCAs (heterocyclic amines), created when meat is cooked at a high temperature (which is a good reason to avoid charring your meat on the grill). Other carcinogenic compounds formed in the cooking process are polycyclic aromatic hydrocarbons (PAHs), formed when meat is smoked, which are prevalent in processed meats; and advanced glycation end products (AGEs), which have been implicated in diabetic kidney disease, peripheral nerve damage, and Alzheimer's disease. AGEs are formed when high-protein foods are cooked with sugars in the absence of water. Try to eat your vegetables and fruits either raw or steamed. Avoid processed carbs and browned foods, because the caramelization and browning processes directly increase the levels of AGEs in those foods.

> Nitrates are known carcinogens. Children who eat more than 12 hot dogs a month have an elevated risk of childhood leukemia — scary when you think of how many children subsist on this quick, easy-to-eat food.

AVOID SULFATES
Used as a foaming agent and emulsifier, principally in toothpaste but also in shampoos and body washes, this suspected carcinogen (often called sodium lauryl sulfate) is already banned in Europe. It can increase skin inflammation and irritate the eyes, so those with sensitive skin or allergies may wish to carefully read the labels of everyday products to avoid these substances. If you are susceptible to cold sores, this is definitely an ingredient that can trigger them. You can find certain toothpaste brands without sulfates, such as Burt's Bees. If you buy Sensodyne, check the label: not all Sensodyne toothpastes are free of sodium lauryl sulfate, which is generally listed as an "inactive ingredient." There are also a number of companies that offer shampoos without sulfates, including L'Oréal's EverStrong line. This is a fairly easy change to make, too: just find the brand you like without sodium lauryl sulfate and make it your go-to brand. Sometimes, in our world overloaded with endless decisions, it's nice to streamline.

WATCH YOUR MERCURY LEVELS
People scoffed at "Entourage" star Jeremy Piven when he complained of mercury poisoning from a sushi-heavy diet (some thought is was just a ruse to back out of his Broadway contract). But if you're eating a lot of sushi or sashimi with ahi, yel-

lowtail, or king mackerel, your body is absorbing the high mercury levels in those fish, too. And mercury can be toxic if ingested in too high a concentration. I advise limiting your consumption of those fish to once a week or switching to low-mercury seafood, like scallops, eel, squid, octopus, wild salmon, and clams.

COSMETIC ALERT

A number of ingredients to avoid are commonly found in a whole array of skin creams, sunscreens, nail polish, body lotions, and cosmetics — many of which have already been banned in Europe (and yet, somehow Italian and French women manage to still look great. Maybe we need to follow their lead). Some suspect these substances are linked to nerve damage, certain cancers, and developmental delays. Limit your exposure or seek out product lines (many of them available at Target and Walmart) like Burt's Bees, Weleda, or Dr. Hauschka, which avoid the ingredients listed below.

If you must have a fancy department-store foundation or lipstick that contains one of these ingredients, strike a balance by lessening your exposure in another area. No one has the time to go around scanning lists of cosmetic ingredients, but an awareness of certain potentially unhealthy substances should be in the back of your mind, so you can ask your manicurist for formaldyhyde-free nail polish, for example, or make sure you're lessening risk where you can. Be especially aware of the following dangerous ingredients:

PHTHALATES

This substance, used to make plastics more flexible, enters the body through food or drinks housed in containers containing phthalates. Rates of this chemical have been found to be higher in women, most likely because they use more of the personal-care items like shampoo, moisturizers, and body washes that contain them.

PARABENS

Common parabens include methylparaben, ethylparaben, propylparaben, and butylparaben, which enter the body when they are ingested or absorbed into the skin. This preservative is found in cosmetics, moisturizers, hair-care products, and shaving creams.

HYDROQUINONE

This skin-lightening agent has been banned in many developed countries, but not in the United States, and it has been suspected of containing carcinogenic properties. If you are interested in skin lightening, try niacin instead, which lightens your skin naturally. Our office offers EpiQuin Micro, which contains tretinoin and hydroquinone, but this is closely monitored under a doctor's supervision and not available without a prescription. Don't risk using hydroquinone on your own.

TOLUENE
Found in hair dyes and nail polish, toluene has been discussed as potentially having an adverse effect on the nervous system.

The best six doctors anywhere
And no one can deny it
Are sunshine, water, rest, and air
Exercise and diet.
These six will gladly you attend
If only you are willing
Your mind they'll ease
Your will they'll mend
And charge you not a shilling.

—A nursery rhyme quoted by Wayne Fields in
What the River Knows *(1990)*

CHIP'S TIPS

1 Your rule of thumb should be five servings of fruits and vegetables a day, plus a multivitamin. These are the basics of good health.

2 Limit your consumption of milk. It is nature's perfect food — but only if you are a calf.

3 Get an oil change. Ditch the saturated fats and vegetable oils. Fish oil is best, because it's high in anti-inflammatory omega-3 fats.

4 Support your local farmers. Take a guided tour of your natural grocer, and discuss organic and hormone-free options.

5 Multigrain is not the same as whole grain. Always choose the latter.

6 Food is your best source of vitamins. Watch for organic or hormone-free options.

7 Take a multivitamin/multimineral every day; it's the foundation of good health.

8 Use sunscreen daily; reapply every two hours when in the sun — even if the label says it's waterproof.

9 Gluten-free and dairy-free are the best and fastest ways to improve your health and energy level. Even if you are not allergic.

10 Green is keen. Don't forget "Planet You"!

11 Don't forget what our skin nation is founded on — life, liberty, and the pursuit of happiness. Don't worry — be happy! Healthy skin is happy skin.

12 Remember: A tomato a day may keep the wrinkles away!

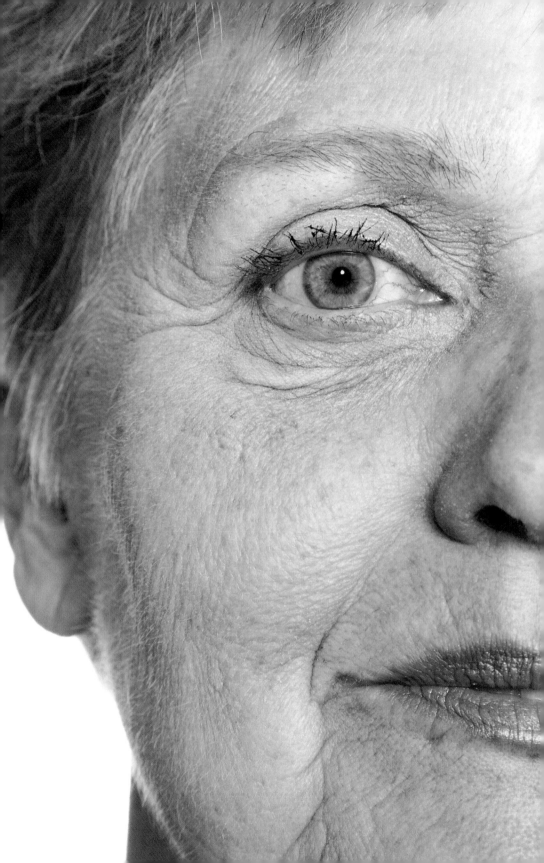

CHAPTER 9

* * *

SURGICAL SOLUTIONS:
WHEN IT'S TIME TO BRING
OUT THE BIG GUNS

At a certain point, all the filler, Botox, and serums in the world won't reverse the natural effects of gravity and facial aging. Inevitably, these factors will conspire to make a surgical solution necessary. Though there may be some reluctance to "go under the knife," I advise my patients that taking the leap will make them happier and more pleased with their appearance in the long run.

This chapter is designed for patients who have exhausted their presurgical options — whether Botox or fillers, Retin-A or human growth factor — some of which are temporary strategies rather than long-term corrective measures. Surgery is really the only way (outside of Ponce de Léon's fountain of youth) to reverse the ravages of time. When camouflage just isn't working or gets too expensive and time-consuming, it may be time for surgery.

Beyond improvements to your appearance, there are practical matters to consider (like your pocketbook). In many cases, surgery offers the best value. Case in point: I have several patients who have spent upwards of $50,000 on skin care, injectables, and Botox over the years. But the better strategy for some of these big spenders would have been to invest in face lifts, brow lifts, Eyelight Blepharoplasty,™ and cheek lifts — procedures that can really deliver impressive, noticeable results less expensively.

And there are additional practicalities to consider. While some patients opt for a conservative approach, dipping a foot in the pool with one isolated surgical procedure at a time, I remind my patients that combining procedures often gives them the most value for their investment.

For instance, suppose you're considering both a cheek lift and a brow lift. Tackling one at a time might *seem* more budget friendly. But the truth is, what applies in a restaurant also applies with surgery: when you order à la carte rather than selecting an entrée that includes salad and sides, you pay more. When you choose to stagger surgical procedures, you double your recovery periods. This requires more time away from work and more time recuperating in bed. You also duplicate certain surgical costs, such as that of an anesthesiologist. And most important, segmenting procedures can yield a more unnatural appearance than taking a holistic and comprehensive approach.

If a patient is already thinking he or she will come back for a supplementary surgery in a year or two, I almost always recommend that they combine surgeries and finance the amount they're unable to pay out of pocket. Beyond financial reasons, if the surgeries are completed together, on a single day, you'll be able to enjoy the results over the years you might otherwise have waited.

When it comes to creating facial harmony, a smart and sensitive plastic surgeon is going to explain the interrelationship between your features. For example, he may not recommend a rhinoplasty without also considering how a weak or undefined chin can also play a part in making the face appear unbalanced, especially when the nose becomes better sculpted. A good plastic surgeon is aware of facial balance and is therefore more likely to recommend an integrated approach for the sake of harmony.

To some patients who imagine that correcting their sagging eyelids will magically transform their entire face, such a recommendation might seem as if the surgeon were trying to upsell more procedures. But most realize there's a good reason for doctors to suggest several coinciding procedures. Such recommendations underscore the contrast between a trained professional and a patient who is new to the world of plastic surgery. When a patient is considering blepharoplasty to correct sagging eyelid skin, for example, a good plastic surgeon may also recommend an endoscopic brow lift, to diminish the descent of the features downward and refresh the entire face.

In the interest of saving you time, I have assembled a CliffsNotes-style breakdown of the most common surgical and nonsurgical procedures available at Oculus, with relevant information about the recovery time, cost, and results you can expect from each surgery. The arsenal of surgical options primarily includes seven major procedures and five complementary procedures, to achieve overall facial harmony. If you read no other chapter in this book, read this one. I hope it will familiarize you with the incredible array of treatments available to tackle everything from fine lines to wrinkles, from "turkey neck" to sagging brows. Surgery is central to my practice because of its dramatic ability to turn back the clock.

Before I proceed, let me offer an important disclaimer: we're all adults here, so let's understand that when we're talking surgery, we're also talking risk. With any surgery comes the possibility of infection, scarring, even death. Almost everything worth doing in life carries some degree of risk: sex, childbirth, swimming in the ocean, crossing the street, driving a car, and countless other activities all entail potential danger. Even the simple act of taking an aspirin has an attendant risk. There have been more deaths from aspirin than from any complications from Botox, whose proven safety profile is better than that of aspirin. But with all medications and with all surgeries, it's important to be aware of the potential hazards. Be sure to ask your doctor about the perils of your particular surgery.

People naturally want and expect their results to be positive. They also tend to believe that complications, many of which are uncommon, will not happen to them. This is not an accurate assumption. Despite the best care, complications *can* happen. Although the overall incidence of a given complication may be low, if it happens to you, the incidence is then 100 percent in your case. So as I have advised in previous chapters, choose your doctor wisely, know the risks of your particular surgery, and treat the surgery you are about to undergo with the respect it deserves. With laser surgery, to use one example, keeping the skin hydrated and lubricated minimizes the discomfort. But if it's allowed to become dry and crusty, it hurts, because nerve endings become irritated. So follow your surgeon's postoperative instructions to the letter. You will achieve better results and lower the chance of complications.

The arsenal of surgical options primarily includes seven major procedures and five complementary procedures to choose from, in order to achieve overall facial harmony.

Procedures are measured by factors including investment and recovery time.

INVESTMENT	RECOVERY TIME
$ = <$5k	R = 1 week
$$ = $5k-$10k	RR = 2 weeks
$$$ = $10k-$15k	RRR = 3 weeks
$$$$ = $15k-$20k	RRRR = 4 weeks

BLEPHAROPLASTY (AKA EYELID LIFT)

WHAT IT IS: In this procedure to tighten sagging eyelid skin, fat or skin is removed (or repositioned, ideally), using a laser.

WHAT IT TREATS: Sagging and/or puffy eyelids

COMMON SCENARIO: At age 52, Margaret had started to notice that when she was driving, cars seemed to sneak up on her a bit, because her side vision was not what it used to be. The skin of her upper lid, which had descended to partially obscure her vision, was to blame. After a simple eyelid lift, Margaret was able to regain her confidence behind the wheel, much to the relief of her family.

THE PROCEDURE: In the lower eyelids, if puffiness (not excess skin) is the problem, an incision can be made inside the lower eyelid to remove or reposition bulging fatty pads. This sidesteps traditional skin incision and is called "transconjunctival blepharoplasty" (using an internal incision). However, if there is significant excess skin, in addition to puffiness of the lower eyelid, a traditional incision just below the eyelashes (called *external blepharoplasty,* because of the visible external incision) allows for conservative removal of that excess skin.

By using the laser in blepharoplasty, rather than the conventional scalpel, the surgery is nearly bloodless, because the laser cauterizes the small blood vessels with each precision cut. Not only does this allow better visualization for the surgeon, but it markedly diminishes the amount of time necessary to perform surgery and, therefore, the amount of time the patient is in the operating room. The other significant advantage this provides is less bruising and swelling after surgery and a more rapid recovery.

INVESTMENT: $ **RECOVERY TIME:** RR

In the upper eyelids there is usually minimal to no bruising and only mild swelling. Tiny sutures are hidden in the natural eyelid crease, and dissolve in place over the course of a week. In the lower eyelids, the bruising varies from none to moderate. Moderate bruising may take a week or two to completely disappear. Makeup, however, can be used to cover any bruising once the sutures dissolve. Contact lenses are usually left out for one week.

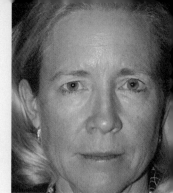

Margaret
Blepharoplasty

At age 52, Margaret appeared tired, and her upper eyelid makeup always smeared. After surgery, she had renewed confidence and enjoyed accentuating her eyes with makeup.

AFTER ▼   ▲ BEFORE

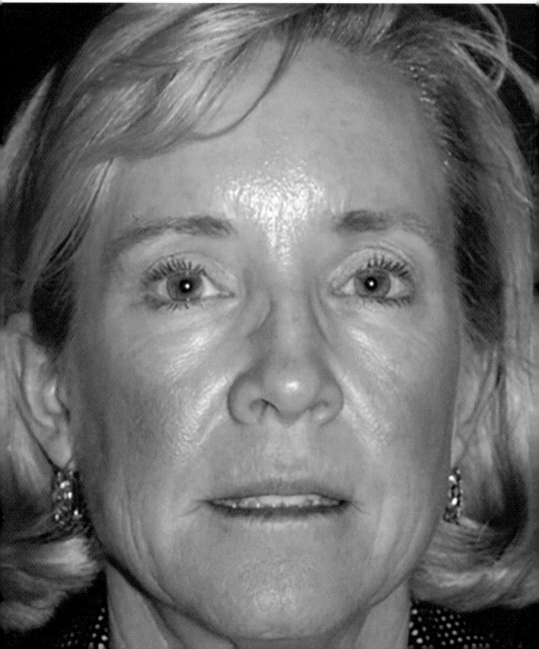

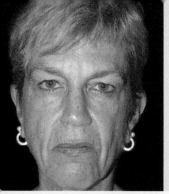

Katherine
Endoscopic Brow Lift

At age 49, Katherine had angled, stern-appearing eyebrows that made her appear angry or like she was frowning. After her endoscopic procedure, she appeared rested.

BEFORE ▲   ▼ AFTER

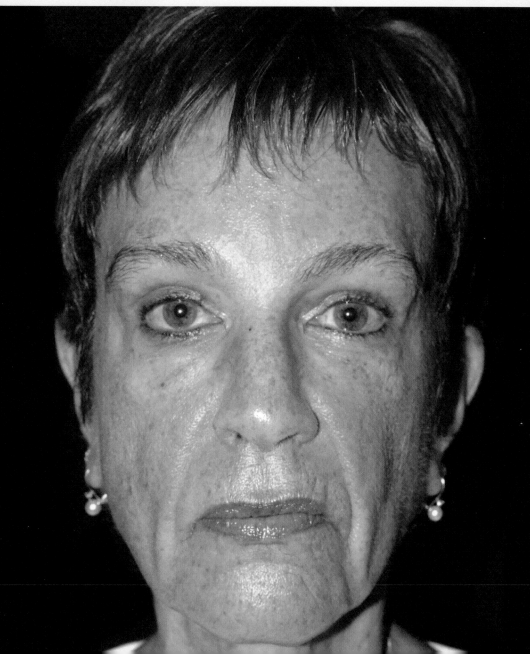

ENDOSCOPIC BROW LIFT

WHAT IT IS: The surgical lifting of the brow, using the far-less-invasive endoscope technique.

WHAT IT TREATS: Drooping eyebrows and worry lines. An endoscopic brow lift stabilizes the brows at their original, natural position. Additionally, wrinkles on the forehead and frown lines between the eyebrows can be reduced. Asymmetry of the brows can be corrected at the time of the surgery as well. The endoscopic brow lift is often performed in conjunction with upper-eyelid surgery to achieve optimal results. The procedures work in tandem with one another, much like a curtain rod (brow) and curtain (eyelid).

COMMON SCENARIO: Katherine's drooping eyebrows made her look old and tired, even at 49 (although she looks older because she is a smoker). She opted for a combination of an endoscopic brow lift and blepharoplasty, in which her brow was raised and stabilized, and drooping eyelid tissue was removed to give her a more rested, youthful expression.

THE PROCEDURE: A tiny fiber-optic lens called an endoscope is inserted into small incisions made behind the hairline. The lens is attached to a camera that is connected to a monitor screen, allowing for visualization of the surgery. Additional half-inch incisions are made for the insertion of tiny graspers, scissors and retractors. The surgeon performs the procedure while viewing the monitor and manipulating tiny instruments externally. Skin is not removed — muscles are lifted, tightened, and held in place with absorbable sutures.

INVESTMENT: $ **RECOVERY:** RR

The amount of discomfort following a brow lift is minimal. There may be swelling and bruising around the cheeks and eyelids. The doctor may recommend keeping the head elevated to reduce these effects. As the incisions heal, the patient may experience some itching and numbness (these symptoms will diminish over time), but the patient can return to a normal routine after two weeks. Strenuous physical activity should be avoided for two weeks until all healing is complete.

ENDOSCOPIC CHEEK LIFT (AKA MIDFACE LIFT)

What it is: A sagging cheek region is lifted for a more youthful appearance.

What it treats: Drooping cheeks, skin laxity, hollowness where the eyelid and the cheek meet.

Common scenario: A 60-year-old former fashion model, Elizabeth was still a remarkably good-looking woman. But with age and the effects of gravity her cheeks had begun to sag, giving her a drawn, tired look. After a simple cheek lift, Elizabeth regained that youthful glow that had graced the pages of many a magazine.

The procedure: Done as an outpatient procedure under general anesthesia, a cheek lift is best performed in conjunction with a lower eyelid blepharoplasty to give a smooth appearance from beneath the eyes to the cheeks. Small access incisions are made in the temple region above the ears (no hair is removed) and inside the mouth above each eye tooth. Using an endoscope for visualization, the surgeon lifts the cheek region and secures it back onto the cheekbone, using a fixation device called Endotine. Endotine is an absorbable material, about the size of a cotton-swab tip, that acts as a suture and usually dissolves within six to eight months of surgery.

Investment: $ **Recovery:** RR

Bruising, swelling, numbness, and rare cases of facial motor weakness can occur postoperatively. Numbness and facial motor weakness can last up to two years in some patients but typically resolves within six to eight months. Bruising and swelling usually resolve within two to three weeks. External sutures, completely hidden in the hair of the temple, are absorbable and will usually dissolve or fall out on their own after a week.

Elizabeth
Endoscopic Cheek Lift

As a former model, Elizabeth felt she had begun to sag and her eyes had a tired look. After her endoscopic cheek lift, her own cheek fatty cushion was placed back on her natural cheekbone, restoring her own youthful glow.

AFTER ▼   ▲ BEFORE

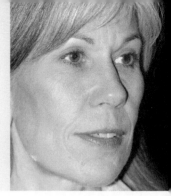

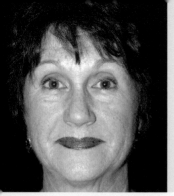

Mary
Laser Light Treatment

As an ex-smoker, Mary showed dull skin with many fine lines and crepey skin striations. After Active FX light laser, she felt and looked refreshed and was back to work, with the help of makeup, in one week.

BEFORE ▲   ▼ AFTER

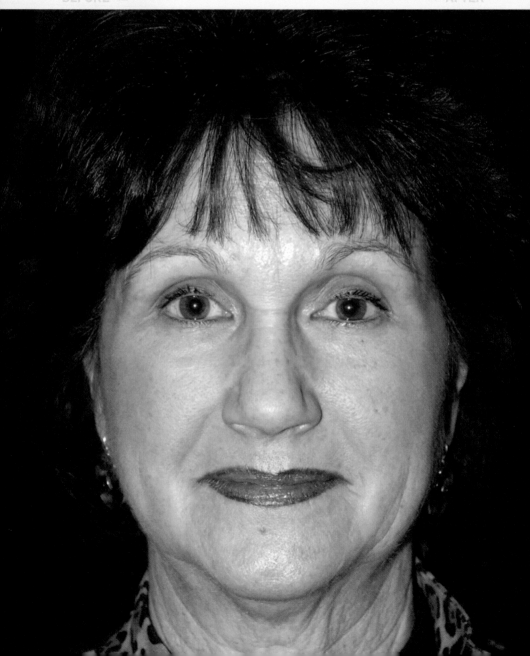

LASER LIGHT (ACTIVE FX) TREATMENT OF THE EYES

What it is: A high-energy beam of laser light is applied in a fractional pattern, leaving some areas of skin untreated, which yields a faster recovery time. New collagen formation plumps the skin. Most patients will see immediate results, and improvement will continue for up to six months after treatment.

What it treats: Fine lines, wrinkles, skin laxity, and dyschromia (irregular skin pigmentation, such as brown spots). Patients will feel a sunburn-like warmth during treatment. The Active FX (light) and the Deep FX (dermal) are both used to customize the best treatment for each facial area, depending on skin thickness, pigmentation, vascularity, and overall treatment goals.

Common scenario: A longtime smoker who had quit 10 years earlier, Mary still showed the residual signs of her habit: dull skin and fine lines around her lips and eyes. With Active FX treatment, her somewhat harsh appearance was softened considerably, and she was pleased to report more-positive interactions with her husband and coworkers.

Investment: $ **Recovery:** R

Healing from CO_2 light-laser resurfacing takes a minimum of two to three months. However, most people are able to wear camouflage makeup at seven days. After resurfacing, the skin is red or pink, resembling a sunburn. It is necessary during the first seven days to keep the skin protected with moisture coverage. The skin will continue to fade back to its natural color as healing progresses. However, patients will experience flushing of the skin for a few months when exerting themselves and can stay pink for two to three months. Healing from resurfacing is virtually pain free. Some people report itching, but this can be controlled with medication.

EYELIGHT BLEPHAROPLASTY™

What it is: This proprietary Oculus surgery is a combination of the four procedures listed above. It utilizes endoscopic and laser surgery to treat sagging eyelid skin, fine lines, and crepiness (crepe-paper skin) in the cheek area, which are all brought about by facial aging.

What it treats: Loose and baggy eyelid skin and eyelid hooding, in which the eyelid skin sags enough to occasionally interfere with vision and makeup application. Eyelight surgery is a precision procedure that repairs the upper and lower eyelids by reducing crepiness and skin laxity, or looseness. Utilizing a laser, the procedure surgically removes overhanging skin and either removes or repositions the fat that causes puffiness in the eyelids. Eyelight surgery can be combined with that of the midface, where cheeks are repositioned to restore a younger, healthier look to both the eye and cheek areas with minimal downtime.

Common scenario: Madeleine, 48, had good skin mostly free of lines, thanks to long-term Retin-A use. However, over time, bags of loose skin had begun to form beneath her eyes, and there was significant sagging of her midface region, including her cheek pads. Together, this slackening of her features made Madeleine appear doughy and exhausted. After surgery, Madeleine recaptured the bright, poised look that had defined much of her younger life.

The procedure: Eyelight Blepharoplasty™ is generally a series of procedures, depending on the patient's needs and goals, which are performed simultaneously for greater facial harmony. It achieves results that are far more lasting and dramatic than those of injectables.

Investment: $$$ **Recovery:** RR

Laser skin incisions leave scars, but they are minimal and well-concealed. The skin may remain pink for several months as it heals. Scars from the upper eyelid blepharoplasty are concealed by the natural crease of the eyelid, while scars from the lower eyelid blepharoplasty are either internal and completely concealed or hidden by the lower eyelashes. The incisions for the endoscopic cheek lift are hidden in the hairline and inside the mouth. Bruising, swelling, and mild discomfort are normal for a few days after the procedure. You may return to normal activity in seven to ten days after surgery. Patients should avoid strenuous activity for a week and sleep with their head elevated to minimize swelling after surgery. After two weeks, 50 percent of normal activity may be resumed, with a return to full activity after three weeks.

Madeleine
Eyelight™ Blepharoplasty

At age 48, Madeleine felt she appeared stern and exhausted. After undergoing a proprietary combination of the preceding four procedures, she now feels she has the rested and relaxed look that defined much of her younger life.

BEFORE ▼   ▼ AFTER

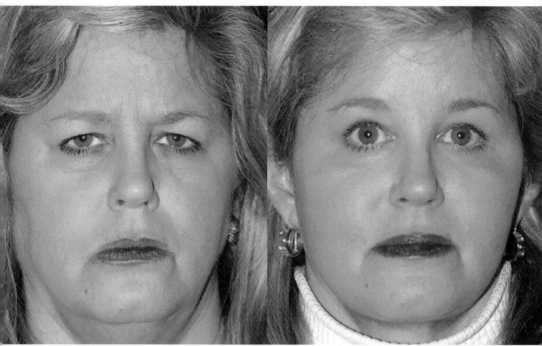

BEFORE ▼   ▼ AFTER

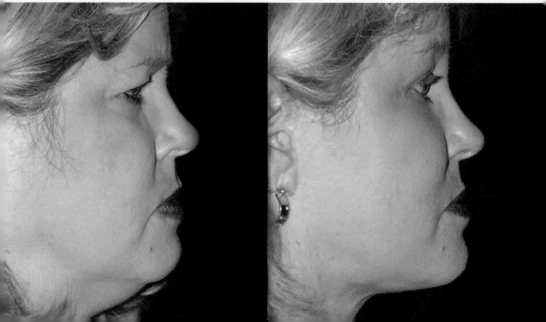

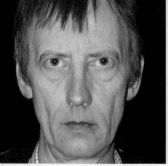

Frank Lower Face Lift

At age 54, Frank had an inherited tendency toward facial volume loss with jowling and a heavy neck. After surgery, he regained his youthful contour and his success in the courtroom was much improved.

BEFORE ▲   ▼ AFTER

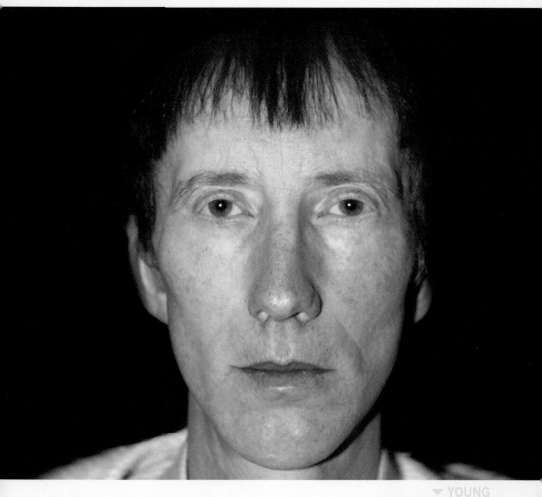

▼ YOUNG

Then and Now

Frank's younger picture is 35 years earlier for comparison. He felt like he had "found himself again" and was pleased to no longer resemble his father. Maybe a coincidence, but he was elected to full partner in his law firm six months after surgery.

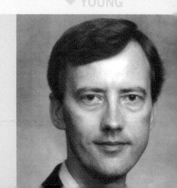

LOWER FACE LIFT

What it is: Performed while the patient is under general anesthesia, this procedure tightens loose skin and lifts descending facial features.

What it treats: Facial descent, jowling, excess skin, fat and muscle in the neck. The best results are achieved when the skin still has some elasticity and the facial bone structure is strong and well-defined. Most candidates who are considering a lower face lift have jowls that extend below the jaw line and into the neck area. There will often be excess skin, loose muscle, and fat in the neck, as well. A lower face lift can be performed safely in conjunction with other procedures, including eyelid surgery, endoscopic brow lift, and cheek lift.

Common scenario: Frank had inherited the heavy jowls that had appeared on his father's face in his mid-50s. But unlike his father, who retired at 60, Frank was determined to stay at work, going strong, well into his 70s. However, he felt his aged appearance made him look less fit and competitive than the junior partners in his law firm. But one outpatient procedure later, he was back in the courtroom and winning over juries with renewed gusto.

The procedure: Improvement of the visible signs of aging can be achieved by making an incision around and behind the ear. The deep tissues are then repositioned and tightened, excess fat and skin are excised, and the skin is re-draped while the patient is typically under general anesthesia. The incisions are then closed with absorbable (dissolving) sutures that fall out on their own after about a week.

Investment: $$ **Recovery:** RR

For the first week after surgery, patients wear an elastic neck support 24 hours a day. The following week, the wrap should be worn in a minimal capacity, during any eight hours of the day (in two-hour increments) or during eight hours of sleep. Patients may experience postoperative stiffness, numbness, and bruising of the neck, with only mild discomfort. The stiffness and numbness can last up to two years in some patients, but typically resolve within six to eight months.

NECK PLATYSMAPLASTY

What it is: Repair of the underlying neck muscle (platysma).

What it treats: "Turkey neck," sagging skin.

Common scenario: Sally, 67, had always dreaded the family turkey gobbler that she had laughed about at so many family reunions when she saw her older relatives. Now that she was the older one, it was not "very damn funny," as she sternly presented to me. We discussed the anatomy and strong genetics, then proceeded to allow her Southern charm and grace to once again shine through over her famed apple and pecan pies. Reunions were once again cherished, and she was thrilled. Oh how I love it when she brings me one of her pecan pies!

The procedure: Platysmaplasty is performed through a one-inch incision made under the chin. The platysma muscle is tightened and reattached along the neck-line. A platysmaplasty involves the neck area only. It does not include the jowls or areas above the jawline. In some cases, to achieve the best results, a lower face lift should be performed with the platysmaplasty to smooth the jowl area. Platysmaplasty is often done in conjunction with a neck lift.

Investment: $ **Recovery:** RR

During the first week after surgery you must wear an elastic neck support 24 hours a day. The following week, the wrap should be worn eight hours a day. You can choose any eight hours of the day to wear the wrap, and you are allowed to break up the time into smaller increments (i.e., wear the wrap for two hours then take it off for two hours until you have achieved a total of eight hours). The sutures are absorbable and will therefore fall out on their own after about one week. You may have stiffness, numbness, and bruising in your neck postoperatively. The numbness can last up to two years in some patients, but typically resolves within four to six months.

Sally
Platysmaplasty

At 67, Sally had the family neck that she had so dreaded when she was younger. This had come to make her feel very self-conscious. After her neck-muscle tightening, she had renewed confidence.

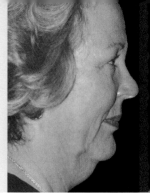

AFTER ▼   ▲ BEFORE

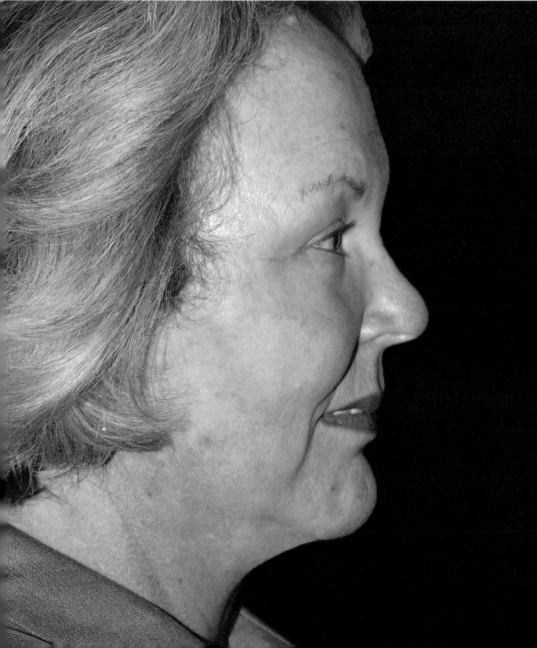

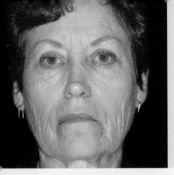

Kim Laser Light Treatment

At age 68, Kim had spent many years in the hot Alabama sun. Her grandkids told her she looked mean. After fractionated laser, she now appeared rested, and everyone called her "nice granny"!

BEFORE ▲   ▼ AFTER

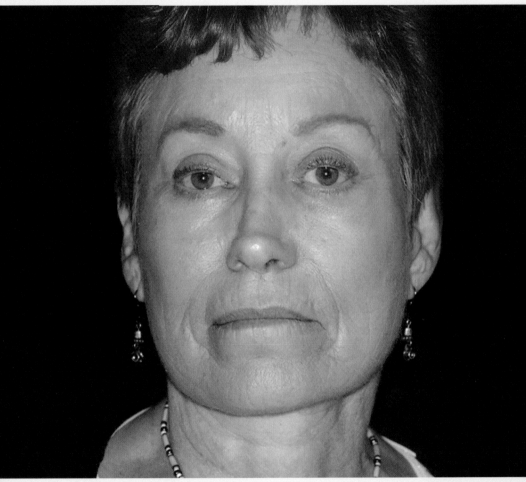

▼ YOUNG

The Wisdom of Youth

Kim's younger picture is 40 years earlier for comparison. She felt that she now looked like her picture's "older sister" instead of that younger lady's "mother." At age 68, she took great pleasure in "being carded" for her senior blue-plate specials at each diner.

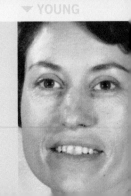

LASER (CO2) SKIN RESURFACING (DEEP FX) OF THE FACE

What it is: A fractional CO2 laser microbeam is used to target the deep dermal layers of the skin and vaporize the superficial layers of the skin. The resulting skin-repair responses lead to collagen formation and tissue regeneration.

What it treats: Scars, wrinkles, and uneven skin texture. Laser skin resurfacing is especially effective for aged, sun-damaged, or scarred skin.

Common scenario: Kim had spent every day of her high-school summers baking in the Alabama sun. Now that she was in her 60s, the results were beginning to show up in uneven skin tone and rough skin texture. After just one round of resurfacing, Kim's skin was noticeably smoother and more balanced in tone.

The procedure: The treatment generally lasts about 20 minutes. An anesthetic cream may be applied before treatment to numb the affected area, which will feel warm during the treatment. The patient's skin will appear sunburned after treatment and will peel, revealing improved skin.

Investment: $ **Recovery:** R

Healing from CO2 laser resurfacing takes a minimum of two to three months. However, most people are able to wear camouflage makeup at ten days, while protecting the skin with moisture coverage. The skin will continue to fade back to its natural color as healing progresses. However, patients may experience flushing of the skin for a few months when exerting themselves and can stay light pink for three to six months. Healing from resurfacing is virtually painless. Some people report itching, but this can be controlled with medication. Note: If you have used Accutane in the past 12 months, tend to heal poorly, have hyperpigmentation issues, or a history of keloid (scar) formation, avoid this procedure.

CHEEK IMPLANTS

What it is: Implantation of either a surgical-grade synthetic material or fat, transplanted from other areas of the patient's body, to counteract descent with lift, and to lend youthfulness to the midface region through added volume.

What it treats: With age, the fat pad and soft tissues in the cheek area begin to slip down and inward toward the mouth. Hollow depressions can form beneath the cheek, and deep folds can develop around the mouth. Cheek implants can also enhance facial harmony, mitigating a prominent nose or chin.

Common scenario: Forty-year-old Daphne suffered from the significant descent of her cheek pad, which gave her a gaunt, chronically tired look. Though she wanted to undergo a face lift, she needed more structure around her cheekbones to hold the soft tissue in place. Daphne opted for submalar augmentation, in which implants are placed below the cheekbones to lift and support sagging midface tissue, and she chose to combine that procedure with a face lift. The results have been deeply gratifying and have restored Daphne's youthfulness.

The procedure: Cheek implants are usually inserted through incisions made in the mouth between the upper gums and the cheek, which conceals any resulting scars. Supportive tissue will grow around the implant as the patient heals, integrating the implant with his or her facial contours.

Investment: $ **Recovery:** RR

Expect some swelling, which should diminish within seven to ten days. Patients should drink liquids and restrict themselves to soft foods, and avoid brushing their teeth until their incisions heal, which can take from seven to ten days.

Daphne
Cheek Implants

At age 40, Daphne had some descent of her cheek pads that had exposed her orbital bony rims. After her surgery, she had an improved facial proportion, softer eyes and a more feminine appearance.

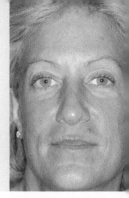

AFTER ▼   ▲ BEFORE

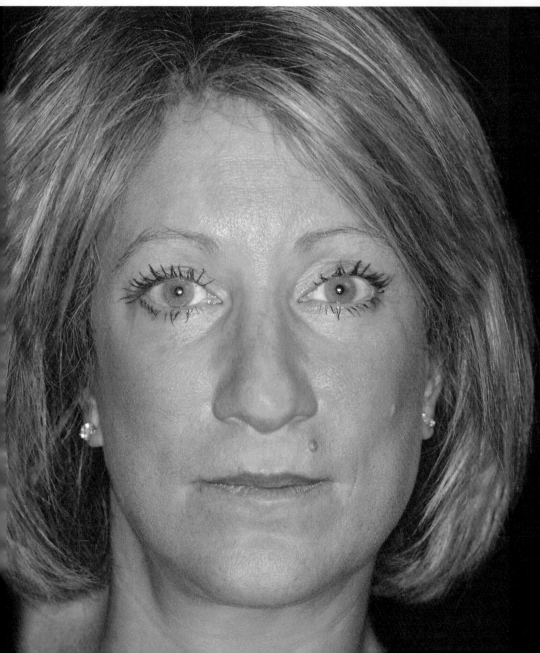

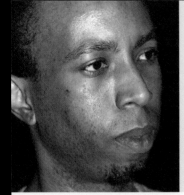

Daryl
Chin Implant

At age 34, Daryl was an extremely successful West Coast executive but felt that his recessed chin reflected poorly on his presentation and confidence. After surgery, he felt more physically balanced with his confident and authoritative nature.

BEFORE ▲   ▼ AFTER

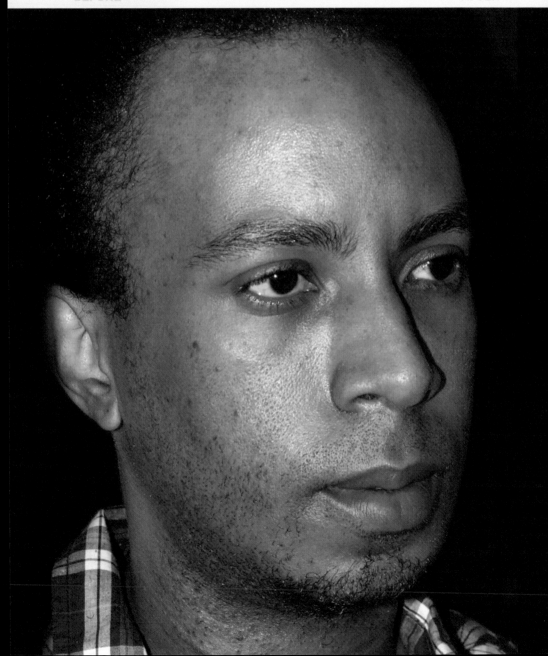

CHIN IMPLANTS

What it is: The insertion of a surgical-grade implant material, like silicone or the patient's own bone or fat, to correct a weak or receding chin.

What it treats: A less-pronounced chin that causes the nose to appear more prominent. It can also give balance to a less-defined face and is often done in conjunction with rhinoplasty.

Common scenario: Daryl was a high-powered executive who had always felt that, especially in men, a feeble chin suggests a weak will. He opted for a silicone implant, which immediately gave him the masculine, authoritative appearance that matched his personality.

The procedure: The implant is placed either through incisions in the mouth, or into a pocket beneath the chin to hide the scar. The implant is generally sutured to bone and adjacent connective tissue, or fixated with a titanium surgical microscrew.

Investment: $ **Recovery:** RR

Sutures will generally be removed within a week. You may be asked to sleep in a surgical brace after surgery to keep your implant in place, and to promote healing in the proper position. Swelling generally diminishes after a week.

FACIAL LIPOSUCTION

What it is: Removal of subcutaneous fat from the face to improve the appearance through facial contouring.

What it treats: Best for recontouring and smoothing the lines of the face.

Common scenario: Despite diet and exercise, Margaret had always had a round, full face, which she inherited from her parents. But as she aged, the amount of extra subcutaneous fat in her face made her look excessively chubby. Facial liposuction was a fast and effective solution, instantly yielding a more angular profile.

The procedure: Less invasive, simpler, and safer than a face lift, facial liposuction can help in smoothing wrinkles, especially when done in conjunction with laser resurfacing or a chemical peel. Very small incisions, hidden in the hairline, are made in the face to remove small amounts of excess fat from the upper face using a small cannula device. Because only local anesthesia is used and incisions are small, downtime and the risk of scarring are minimal.

Investment: $ **Recovery:** RR

Patients are generally required to wear a compression garment for 18 to 36 hours after surgery. Patients may have some discomfort for a few days, which usually can be managed with over-the-counter pain medication. Visible results of the surgery will be more apparent each month after the surgery.

Margaret
Facial Liposuction

At age 58, Margaret felt she had the round, full face of her mother. After surgery, she was more confident with the improved angularity and felt her features were more consistent with her youthful appearance.

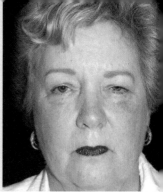

AFTER ▼   ▲ BEFORE

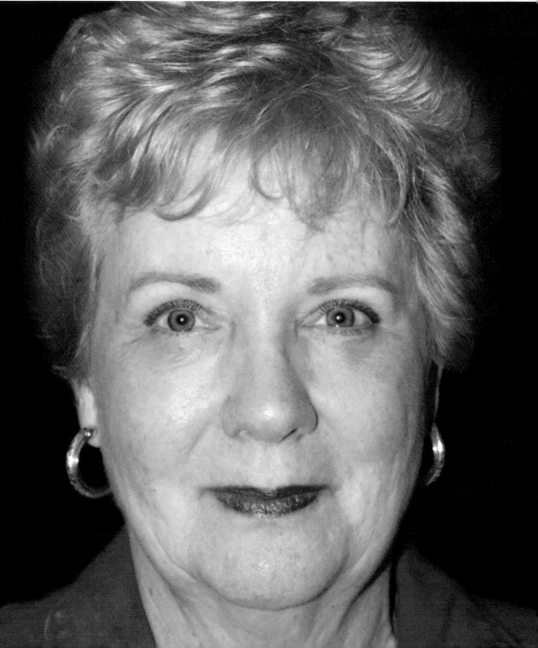

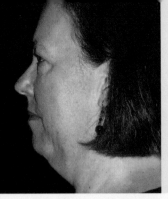

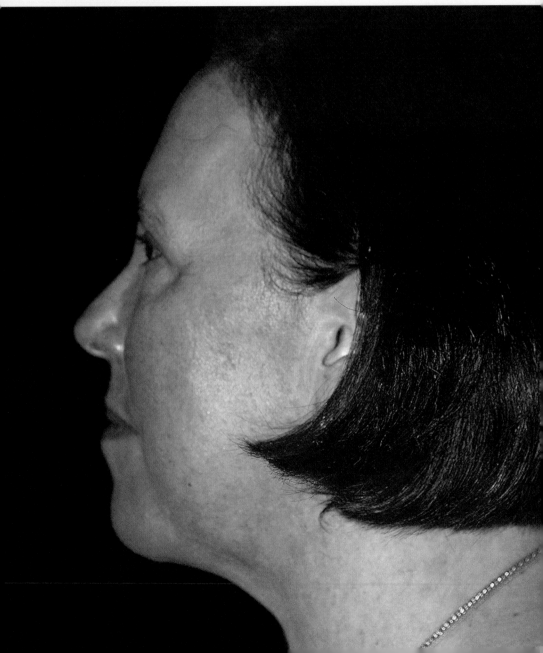

Jacqueline Neck Liposuction

At age 48, Jacqueline was very bothered by her neck — especially the side profile. After surgery, she loved the improved side view. Although this technique only minimally improves the frontal view, she was very happy because she could not afford the time off or investment for a face lift.

BEFORE ▲

▼ AFTER

NECK LIPOSUCTION

What it is: Suctioning of fat from the neck area, often below the chin.

What it treats: Reduces localized fatty deposits. Often done in conjunction with a platysmaplasty.

Common scenario: As she aged, Jacqueline had noticed an increase in loose skin extending past her jaw onto her neck, which created a lack of definition between chin and neck. Despite frequent exercise, the baggy skin made Jacqueline look less athletic (and certainly older) than her age. After surgery, she reported feeling renewed confidence at work and at home, thanks in part to her stronger jawline.

The procedure: Neck liposuction is often performed in conjunction with a neck lift/ platysmaplasty, so that fat is removed through the same incision. To conceal the incision, it is generally made beneath the chin.

Investment: $ **Recovery:** RR

Recovery time is minimal, with most patients returning to work after three to five days. A compression garment may be worn. Some bruising and minimal pain have been reported.

LIP AUGMENTATION

What it is: The implantation of a synthetic material to add volume to the lips.

What it treats: Used to treat thin lips or those that have narrowed or descended with age.

Common scenario: Though Kimberly had lush, expressive features — including high cheekbones and large eyes — her very thin lips seemed out of place. Having used hyaluronic acid fillers for years, she was in the market for a more permanent solution. After an outpatient lip augmentation, Kimberly marveled at her fuller, more sensual lips (as did her husband).

The procedure: Hyaluronic acid fillers and/or injections of the patient's own fat can give temporary fullness to thin lips. But only a surgical treatment achieves permanent results. Surgical lip augmentation uses a special needle to infuse the lips with a synthetic material.

Investment: $ **Recovery:** R

The surgery requires only local anesthetic, so there is generally very little or no bruising, and patients can resume their normal routine after one week.

Rachel

At age 44, Rachel wanted a very subtle improvement in her upper lip. Her main goal was to give balance and improve the fine lines from her early years of smoking. Afterward, she was thrilled.

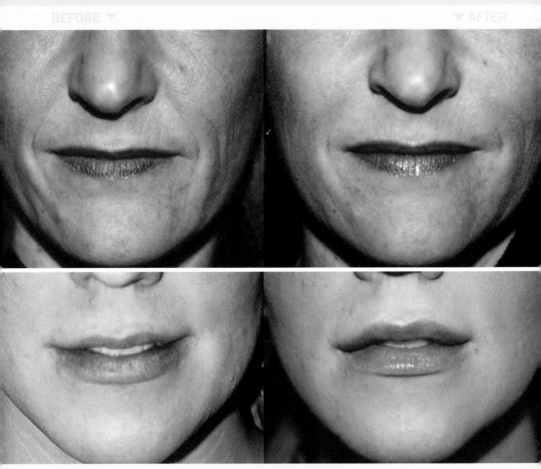

Kimberly

At age 32, Kimberly had been a model for years and was very specific about her goals. She tried temporary fillers for years and wanted a permanent solution. After her lip implant, she started modeling again. Her husband was amazed, because he was hesitant before the procedure.

CHIP'S TIPS

BLEPHAROPLASTY (AKA EYELID LIFT) **What it is:** In this procedure to tighten sagging eyelid skin, either fat or skin is removed, most often using a laser. **What it treats:** Sagging and/or puffy eyelids.
Investment: $ **Recovery:** R **Case Study:** page 192

ENDOSCOPIC BROW LIFT **What it is:** The surgical lifting of the brow, using the less-invasive endoscope technique. The key concept is to stabilize the brow so it does not drop postoperatively. **What it treats:** Drooping eyebrows and worry lines.
Investment: $ **Recovery:** R **Case Study:** page 194

ENDOSCOPIC CHEEK LIFT (AKA MIDFACE LIFT) **What it is:** A sagging cheek region is lifted for a more youthful appearance. **What it treats:** Drooping cheeks, skin laxity, hollowing where the eyelid and the cheek meet.
Investment: $ **Recovery:** RR **Case Study:** page 196

LASER LIGHT (ACTIVE FX) TREATMENT OF THE EYES **What it is:** A high-energy beam of laser light is applied in a fractional pattern, leaving some areas of skin untreated, yielding a faster recovery time. New collagen formation plumps the skin. **What it treats:** Fine lines, wrinkles, skin laxity and dyschromia (unusual skin pigmentation, such as brown spots).
Investment: $ **Recovery:** R **Case Study:** page 198

EYELIGHT BLEPHAROPLASTY™ **What it is:** In this proprietary Oculus treatment, a combination of endoscopic and laser surgery is used to treat sagging eyelid skin, as well as fine lines and crepiness (crepe paper skin) in the cheek area. This may include a combination of any of the following procedures: endoscopic brow lift, upper-eyelid blepharoplasty, lower-eyelid blepharoplasty, endoscopic cheek lift, or laser skin resurfacing of the eyes. **What it treats:** Loose and baggy eyelid skin and eyelid hooding, in which the eyelid skin sags enough to occasionally interfere with vision and makeup application. Can also be combined with other procedures to treat midface descent.
Investment: $ **Recovery:** RR **Case Study:** page 200

LOWER FACE LIFT **What it is:** A surgical procedure performed under general anesthesia to tighten loose skin and lift descending facial features. **What it treats:** Facial descent, jowling, excess skin and fat in the neck.
Investment: $$ **Recovery:** RR **Case Study:** page 202

NECK PLATYSMAPLASTY **What it is:** Repair of the underlying neck muscle (platysma). **What it treats:** "Turkey neck," sagging skin.

Investment: $ **Recovery:** RR **Case Study:** page 204

LASER (CO2) SKIN RESURFACING (DEEP FX) OF THE FACE **What it is:** A fractional CO2 laser microbeam is used to target the deep dermal layers of the skin and vaporize the superficial layers of the skin. **What it treats:** Scars, wrinkles and undesirable skin texture. The treatment is especially effective for aging, sun-damaged or scarred skin.

Investment: $ **Recovery:** R **Case Study:** page 206

CHEEK IMPLANTS **What it is:** Implantation of either a surgical-grade synthetic material or fat transplanted from other areas of the patient's body to give height and youthfulness to a descending midface region. **What it treats:** With age, the fat pad and soft tissues in the cheek area begin to slip. Hollow depressions can form beneath the cheek, and deep folds can develop around the mouth. Cheek implants can also enhance facial harmony, reducing a prominent nose or chin.

Investment: $ **Recovery:** RR **Case Study:** page 208

CHIN IMPLANTS **What it is:** The insertion of a surgical-grade implant material like silicone, or the patient's own bone or fat, are used to strengthen a weak or receding chin. **What it treats:** A weak chin, or a less-pronounced one, can cause the nose to appear more prominent. A chin implant can give balance to a less defined face and is often done in conjunction with rhinoplasty.

Investment: $ **Recovery:** RR **Case Study:** page 210

FACIAL LIPOSUCTION **What it is:** Removal of subcutaneous fat from the face to improve appearance. **What it treats:** The recommended treatment for recontouring and smoothing the lines of the face.

Investment: $ **Recovery:** RR **Case Study:** page 212

NECK LIPOSUCTION **What it is:** Suctioning of fat from the neck area, often below the chin. **What it treats:** Reduces localized fat deposits. Often done in conjunction with platysmaplasty.

Investment: $ **Recovery:** RR **Case Study:** page 214

LIP AUGMENTATION **What it is:** The implantation of a synthetic material to add volume and contour to the lips. **What it treats:** Used to treat thin lips or lips that have become thinner or descended with age.

Investment: $ **Recovery:** R **Case Study:** page 216

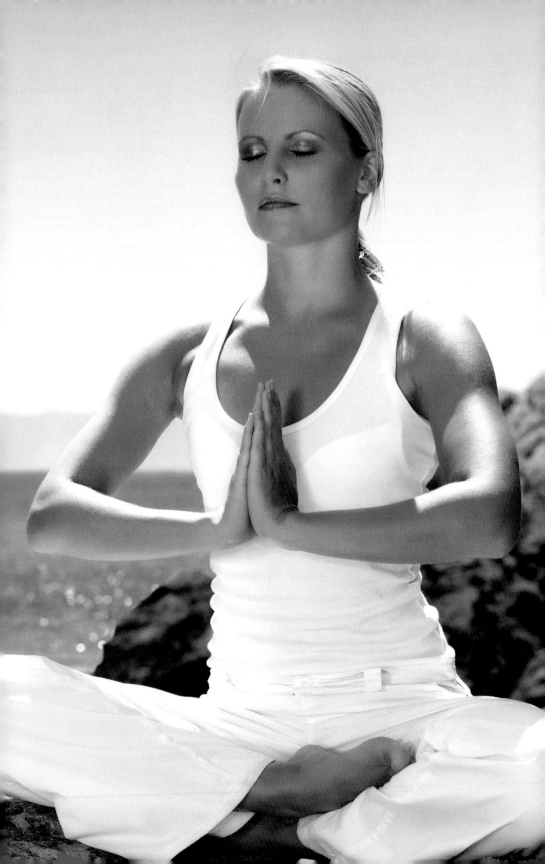

CHAPTER 10

* * *

FIND BALANCE, AND
GOOD HEALTH WILL FOLLOW

Driving to work one crisp fall morning, I was listening to a great talk-radio piece that spoke to the importance of turning off the phone once in a while, stepping away from the computer, and engaging with your family. This really hit close to home for me.

A phrase we often use around the house is "U.P." It's one way my wife and I remind each other to *unplug.* It's not enough for us just to be present; we want to be fully engaged. Doing so often means breaking away from the technology that so often separates us from the truly meaningful things — and people — in our lives.

Who among us can't appreciate this sentiment? Instead of technology liberating us, it often enslaves us. The most precious commodity in life is time, but we squander it with endless emails, text messages, and web surfing. We barely have time for the old-school pastime of watching TV.

I had an epiphany that morning, listening to this very 21st-century lament: We could all use a wake-up call — an alarm to remind us that perhaps the most important things in life are indeed our family and friends, our health, and our connection to community and nature.

These essentials often get lost in the frantic pace of daily life (and our quest to look better and work harder). As I've learned the hard way over the years, you can work with a feverish passion to get ahead, but you can't bring back your kids' childhoods, or the time you spent away from your family and friends.

Thankfully, things may be changing. It seems we're beginning to re-prioritize, to reflect on our lives and what we can do to make them more rewarding. I see more and more of my friends putting attention into their families that they used to funnel exclusively into work.

Much of this change was sparked for me in the wake of September 11, 2001. The tragedies of that day helped remind us how precious life is, and how vulnerable we all are. For many Americans, the focus shifted inward, and I think that's an immensely positive result of an otherwise unfathomable catastrophe. In a deep and soulful way, Americans now are addressing how they really want to lead their lives. With the devastation of 9/11, followed by Hurricane Katrina (a disaster that hit closer to my hometown), the financial collapse of 2008, and the subsequent recession, many people are beginning to reassess what makes them happy and what constitutes a satisfying life. It's not always about the accumulation of material wealth. More vital, perhaps, is to access intangibles like freedom, love, and a positive self-image.

In our industry, assessing people's appearance and discussing their anxieties provides a certain window into life in general, and I've come to understand that the essence of true beauty doesn't come from fuller lips or a face lift alone, but from a rich inner life. I don't claim to have found the path to enlightenment or the secret to eternal life. I am not Deepak Chopra or the Dalai Lama, or even Dr. Phil. But I can certainly share some things I've learned along the way, as a 50-something longtime denizen of planet earth.

Around the office, our mantra is "BE." It's what we say to remind each other when someone needs extra help, has difficulty with a project or has to stay late. It stands for "Beyond Excellence," and it's what we all strive for — from prepping a patient for surgery to cleaning the break room. No one is perfect, and I'm no exception, but here are some of the things I've learned from my patients, family, and friends along the way that help lay a foundation for going Beyond Excellence:

> My recipe for a happy, healthy life is really pretty basic: honor yourself and strive for meaningful relationships. Like most things in life though, simple does not necessarily imply easy. It takes momentary willingness over the course of a lifetime to be able to relax into the basic truths of love and connection.

BE ACTIVE

Exercise — and the endorphin release that accompanies it — creates a feeling of bliss and well-being, boosts the immune system, and delays the aging process. People who regularly exercise are less prone to stress, anxiety and depression, which so often lead to 11s between the eyes (those furrows in the brow). Exercise is one important antidote for the angst of modern life. It's a proven investment in your health, longevity, quality of life — and even your work productivity.

It's easy to look at exercise as a chore, but there are countless ways to weave regular activity into the fabric of our lives and make it a pleasure rather than an inconvenience. For example, I never have been able to get into golf, even though some of my best friends swear by it. (Why force something you're not into when there are endless avenues for movement?) For every personality, there's an exercise that is fun and enjoyable.

I try to get back to the place I remember as a child, where going to the park or the playground was the absolute best thing in life. It helps me to vary my activities: swimming one day, biking with a friend the next, lifting weights another. One way I associate exercise with pleasure is by linking it with my relationships, by involving a workout buddy or my wife. Susan and I like to play a lot of tennis together, which is perfect because it's physically beneficial and it gives us quality time together. I often get up early before work and go swimming, lift weights, or play tennis for a couple hours with a friend. Exercising early in the morning works great for me, because I get it out of the way early, freeing up the rest of my day.

Some other exercises my wife and I enjoy aren't that rigorous at all, such as walking and hiking. We walk along the Chattahoochee River with our dogs or take hikes around the North Georgia mountains. It's so fundamentally soothing, pleasurable, and relaxing that I look forward to it with the same sense of delight that so often accompanies our childhood memories of play. Another great avenue for taking care of the body is Pilates. Susan tells me she doesn't want to be tying my shoes for me in a few years, so I stepped up and took the challenge.

Exercise should be functional too. I lift weights to help with my posture and alignment, not to try and look like someone out of a testosterone commercial. Because I spend so much time with my back bent during surgery, I need the additional help to keep me standing upright. I want to be able to keep up with my grandkids.

Doing some sort of weight-lifting or weight-bearing routine to increase back strength is probably a good idea for anyone, considering how much time many of us spend at a desk. And for women who are at risk for osteoporosis, it can even help build bone strength.

BE SOCIAL

Human interaction is fundamental, and something we often lose sight of in our hurried lives. One way Susan and I try to stay socially plugged in is through a life group at our church. Eight couples get together every other Sunday to talk about our kids, work, financial issues — really anything of interest to us.

But having a group of like-minded peers doesn't have to be faith-based. Just making time to be with friends, to have quality conversation and share one another's wisdom and life experience, taps into the deep need for social bonds, which is so vital to a healthy, balanced life. Family can be a great social outlet as well, but many of us are not fortunate enough to be around our families. Speaking of families...

BE FAMILIAL

Rooted in Southern tradition as I am, family has been an especially big deal to me from the start. Susan and I have always put family first. We taught our kids early on that friends will come and go, but family is forever. Now that all three of our children are well into adulthood, it's great to see this investment in our kids pay such rich dividends. While some adult children can't seem to get far enough away from their families, Susan and I are thrilled to see our children migrating back home after striking out on their own after college. We trust that even if they don't stay close, they'll always stay in close contact.

Our eldest, Chris, is married to a wonderful young woman named Taylor. In developing his passion for psychology and holistic medicine, Chris has returned to Georgia to attend chiropractic school. He and Taylor live a few houses down the street from us, and it has been great fun watching them as new parents. They delivered our first grandchild, Cannon Forbes Cole, on leap year day, 2012. We're now called G-Pop and G-Mom. Susan and I enjoy being able to help them in ways our parents were able to help us, and we hope to always play a major role in Cannon's life.

Our daughter, Allison, after graduating from nursing school, came back home to roost, and now she works in our office. She is married to Tyler Perkins, and they are the proud parents of Gavin Alexander Perkins, our second grandchild. We feel so blessed to be able to watch as our family grows, and it only affirms for me that family is and will always be the most important aspect of my life.

Our youngest son, Tyler, recently graduated from Colorado University and is heading for Los Angeles to become an actor and comedian. While I wish him well in his showbiz pursuits, I hope that one day he, too, will return to the homestead (and not just because Georgia is the new film boomtown). He is a true highlight of our family, providing a comic spark and creative inspiration for us all.

My own parents live down the same street in the opposite direction from Chris's family. We get together for dinner as often as possible, and they're included in many of our travels. Every New Year holiday, we all go on a ski vacation — a family tradition — and when we return to the warmer climate of Atlanta, we get together with all of our extended family and friends to share in the holiday fun. There's drink, food and merriment as we gather around and catch up on another year passed.

I don't necessarily think our experience is so unusual, since we all have our own traditions. Most Americans yearn for greater family connection, and Susan and I are lucky to have children who seem to enjoy their parents' company. I believe more and more families are seeing the benefits of staying physically and emotionally close. Even if we are not geographically close, technology has provided awesome opportunities for connection with the advent of Skype, Facebook, and all those other spacefacethings I haven't quite mastered yet.

Evidence of a return to familial values is everywhere. Instead of sending aging parents to nursing homes, for example, there is a growing trend to create mother-in-law and father-in-law suites in homes. The economy has definitely played a part in some of these changes, but the advantages are legion — not just for the aging parent but for their children and grandchildren, who can benefit from the wisdom and life experience of having an older relative nearby. Americans can sometimes be seen as cautious about too much closeness, but extended families living in one home is a long-standing European tradition. We're seeing an evolution away from the fractured, dispersed families of recent American history and seem to be revaluing a return to our roots.

Inspired by the cultural phenomenon captivating the hearts and minds of men everywhere, I recently created a man cave in our basement, for football games and other sporting events. We've always tried to be the house where our kids and friends could join together, and there is something that feels so satisfying about having a house full of people enjoying themselves.

When our kids were growing up, I tried my best to participate in any way I could. I would shuttle them to their team practices or the movies, make space for them to study at the house — anything just to be able to soak in the splendor of their fleeting youth. After a long week of consultations and surgeries, even just being a fly on the wall was a reminder of the real reason I work so hard. Driving them around town was such a delight — a weather report that foretold storm clouds brewing or sunny skies ahead. I wouldn't have traded that access and insight for the world.

I felt the same way recently when my wife and some of her girlfriends, all having milestone birthdays around the same time, had a reunion. I relished the opportunity to play chauffeur and margarita maker, and just to lend a hand. It was quality time for me, too — a bird's-eye view on these exceptional women who were having an amazing time together. It made me feel closer to my wife and let me see how much joy she gets from her friends.

It's a notion I'm reminded of daily — the need to really engage with life, to take risks and get involved and be the designated driver sometimes. As the wise man once said, it's not about the destination, it's about the journey.

BE AVAILABLE

Simply making ourselves available to our spouse, our kids, our friends, and the people we care about is so important. Speaking of family and friends, as my dad always says, no one cares how much you know until they know how much you care. A simple way for me to show care and find balance in my life is to make myself available. Everyone — our partners, spouses, kids, friends, all the people we care about — all feel the love of our willing presence.

Recently, my son wanted to see a late movie with me. I was tired, and it had been a long, eventful day. Even though I definitely would not have gone to the movies on my own, I welcomed the opportunity. As corny as it is, that song "Cat's In the Cradle" always plays in my head whenever I start to say no to time with my kids. Harry Chapin's poignant song, about a father who never had time for his son, resonates with me because perhaps we all struggle with guilt, justified or not, about not spending enough time with our families. My son really wanted to go to that movie, and so even though we'd be getting home well after midnight, it was worth it.

Anyone who's in a committed relationship knows how important being available is to maintaining lasting love. One night a week my wife and I make sure to have a date night. Yes, it's hard sometimes to squeeze it in, but we figure out a way to make it happen, and we're always happy we do. I recommend to everyone, even my children with those time-consuming newborns, to commit to this weekly ritual. You'll be glad you did.

Now, when you're in your fifties and have been married as long as we have, date night becomes a somewhat flexible concept. For us, it could be as simple as barbecued chicken in the backyard and talking about our kids. Date night doesn't have to mean getting dressed to impress and going out to a fancy restaurant. Just being present, spending time together, and slowing things down is the important thing for us.

BE OUTWARD-BOUND

As a kid growing up in Louisiana, the heralded "sportsman's paradise," I was perpetually outside on the water, fishing, swimming, water skiing, or riding my bike for miles. As adults we sometimes lose that connection to nature. We get trapped inside our steel horses and air-conditioned houses and forget how healing, peaceful, and soothing it can be simply to walk in the woods or drift along a glassy lake in contemplation. When we lose that connection, we lose an essential part of ourselves. And connecting with nature doesn't have to mean trekking vacations or

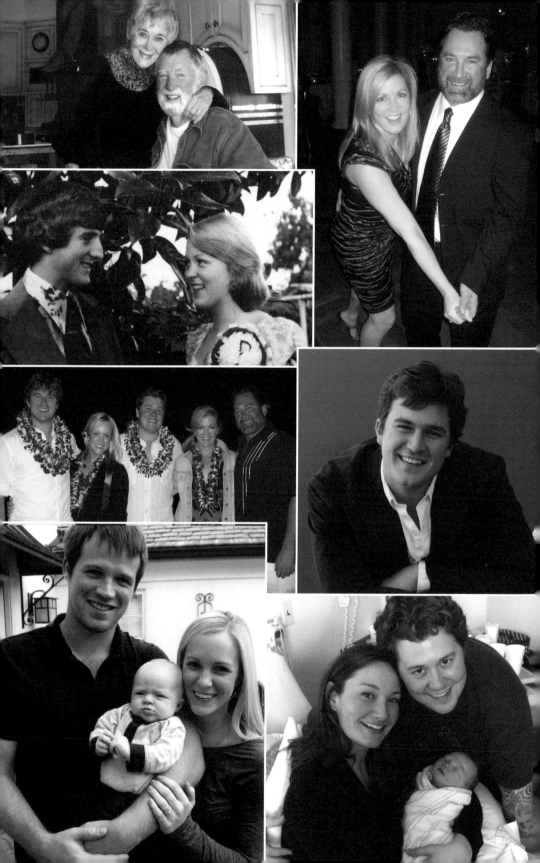

expensive time-shares on the beach. Nature is all around us, accessible as a city park or a stroll around the neighborhood. It's just a nice walk or bike ride away.

Reflecting on the time of our forefathers, before all this technology became a part of our daily lives, can help us live a more natural life today. And it's something that happens a lot when we reënter the realm of the forest and the ocean. It's a lesson I would also stress as a scoutmaster when my sons were Cub Scouts, trying to instill in them an awareness of the vital relationship between humanity and this planet.

Spending time in nature was part of all of my kids' upbringings, I'm happy to say. Every summer when the kids were little, we would go to a Colorado dude ranch camping, where there was no television, no video games, no alcohol, and no distractions from the outside world. This gave us a chance to really bond as a family, and perhaps my fondest vacation memories are from here. It was good old-fashioned fun: family horseback rides, hikes, skits and campfire stories. When you're outside you can't retreat into your iPhone or YouTube or Twitter. Nature requires engagement with each other and with ourselves.

Besides, being outside just *feels* good. It makes you feel connected and grounded. Personally, I like to encounter nature in the raw and explore it on my own terms, with no guide or gear necessary.

Communing with nature makes us more conscientious, too. As humankind continues to encroach on wilderness areas and threaten entire species of animals, it becomes more and more critical that our children have a baseline understanding of what the wild even *is*, so they have a scale against which to measure that destruction.

Throughout history, schools of philosophical thought, both East and West, have spoken of the soul of the earth — *anima mundi* — a deep connection between the natural world and ourselves. How else to explain the remarkable connection so many of us have to animals? The joy we get from gardening? Or the feeling of pure contentment that sweeps over us when we walk through the woods or gaze out at the sea?

The healing benefits of spending time outdoors in quiet contemplation are undeniable. By the same token, if we're going to be good stewards of the earth, we need to appreciate its gifts and allow our children to appreciate them too.

BE SPIRITUAL

No matter what faith or denomination — Buddhist, Muslim, Hindu, Christian, Jewish — having some connection to a higher power outside ourselves is vital

in helping us lead a healthy, balanced life. My wife was raised Mormon and I was raised Catholic, but we go to a non-denominational church where what is most important is *that* we believe, rather than *how* we believe. For us, we think it's important for children to witness their parents' values in action: having compassion for others, knowing right from wrong, and honoring qualities beyond surface beauty or material possessions.

It has always been easiest for me to think about spirituality as connection to self, others, and some higher natural order. Watching my kids go through their trials has taught me that there are many walks of life and many ways of viewing the world.

BE GENEROUS

For me, charity begins close to home. I've always made it my policy that no patient will ever be turned away for financial reasons. People may have preconceptions about plastic surgery as a frivolous business, but I know it changes lives; and I would hate for someone to be denied the opportunity to improve their life because of the inability to pay. Pro bono work is an important element of our practice, and I'm on call to do facial reconstruction for the kinds of orbital fractures and other horrific damage done in domestic-abuse cases. Giving our time and our talents provides a sort of nourishment for the soul that always pays us back tenfold. Early on, I witnessed that altruistic spirit in the caregivers in my own life, from my mother to my wife to my own daughter — all nurses and all committed to helping others in times of trouble.

We have tried to impart to our own children that no matter what you have, 10 percent should be invested for emergencies and 10 percent should go toward helping mankind without expecting a penny back. To us, generosity and empathy yield a more thoughtful and evolved way of living.

BE COMMUNITY-MINDED

Something more people are becoming attuned to, in our culture of sprawl and endless driving, is a desire to find value closer to home. Just as the locavore movement has captivated the food world — with foodies advocating for regional, seasonal, and sustainable ingredients — that same philosophy is being applied to community as a whole.

Susan and I make a real effort to find our entertainment and spend our downtime close to home. We try to see movies at the independent theater down the street and we pride ourselves on frequenting locally owned restaurants. This is the

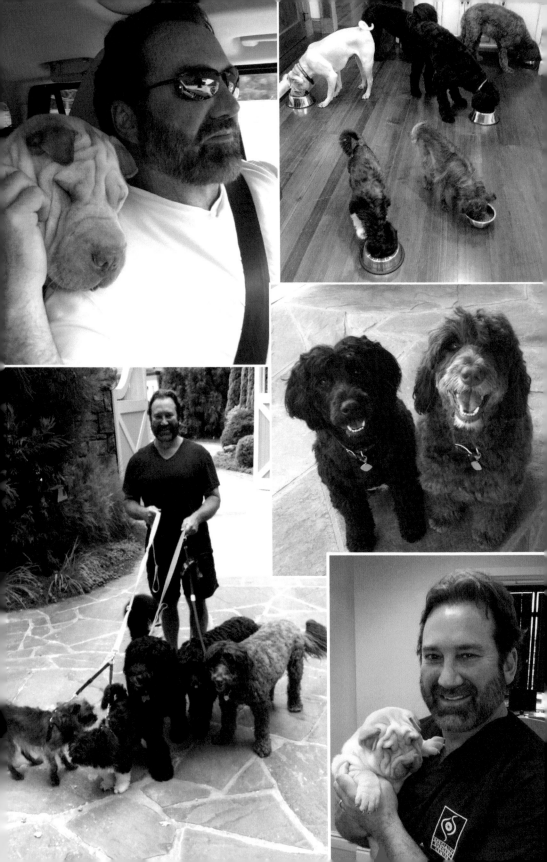

way people used to live, when nearly every business was homegrown, and the community grew and prospered with the success of each of its members.

This ethos becomes especially critical in times of economic stress. I call it the 10-minute lifestyle: trying to support everything within 10 minutes of my house, whether it's the hardware store, the dry cleaners or the gym. It's efficient and easy for me, but also beneficial to the community. And when we do inevitably push out beyond that 10-minute zone for a concert or a special meal at a destination restaurant, it can feel like a little mini-vacation.

BE ANIMAL-FRIENDLY

You don't need to have a menagerie, but you might be surprised by the many health benefits of animals. Just as being in nature soothes the mind, nothing yields the emotional dividends of spending time in the company of animals. We have two Portuguese water dogs — Bruno and Hootie — and are always happy to doggysit. Allison and TP have a Portuguese water dog, too, named Gomez. Chris and Taylor have two little rescue dogs, Lux and Marley. Our son Tyler's shar-pei, Roddy, is named for Tyler's favorite Falcons' player, Roddy White. It's not uncommon to find six or more dogs running around the yard — and, to my wife's dismay, through the house — especially when my parents bring their little rescue dog, Tiger, over to play with the pack.

Having those animals is one reason I wake up happy every morning, because the dogs are so excited to get up and go. First thing in the morning I'm hugging and kissing dogs. You just can't beat that. My favorite bumper sticker is, "Go home and try to be half the person your dog thinks you are." I often think about that. It doesn't matter if you've had a good day or a bad day, your dog thinks you've just hung the moon. To have that kind of affirmation all the time? I think it's just great.

Even if you're not sold on the idea of pet ownership, it's hard to argue against the physical and psychological health benefits of owning a dog (or a cat, or a bird, or whatever animal your lifestyle can accommodate). I strongly support pet ownership as a lifestyle enhancement, but I must admit that I'm especially an advocate for the benefits of a dog: they get you out in the world, exploring your neighborhood and engaging in the simple pleasures of sunshine, exercise, and community. If only we could all assume the best in each other the way our eldest, Bruno, does.

BE WELL-RESTED

Sleep is vital to our well-being and happiness. Getting seven or eight hours of good solid rest is absolutely essential for staying crisp, clear, and on our game. Getting the right amount of sleep slows the aging process and increases memory. It also decreases depression and stress, which in turn lowers inflammation associated with cancer, arthritis, diabetes, and heart disease.

The benefits of being well-rested can extend from getting a good night's sleep but also from taking mini-breaks throughout the day, like standing and stretching, or taking a break from work to eat lunch away from your desk. Recent studies have shown a disturbing link between our sedentary habits and the development of back problems, heart disease, and obesity. Some kind of decompression on an hourly basis is important. Standing up to get a drink of water, making a few phone calls on our feet, or taking a brisk walk on a lunch break all get the juices flowing.

Even though we need to get on our feet, we also need to kick them up, so it's just as important to find a release from the stresses of the day. Seeing a film or visiting a museum, reading a good book or doing some gardening — it's a totally personal thing. Whatever relieves mental and psychological stress also improves your overall health and outlook.

When I was doing my fellowship at Vanderbilt, with three small children back home and a wife working as a neonatal nurse, it would be an understatement to say we were feeling some pressure. At one point, our day-care provider told Susan that she spent more time with our children than their own parents did. This was not especially pleasant to hear, and it was our first moment as parents that we felt the call to make sure family was at the top of our list of priorities.

Thinking back, new parenthood and pushing through medical school was a very stressful time. Knowing how much anxiety my wife and I were feeling, Ralph Wesley (the preceptor I was training under) brought me into his office one day. He sat me down and told me he was giving me a week off and tickets to stay at a resort in Florida. He not only paid for the trip, but he covered for me in my absence. That was so meaningful to us, to have his support and for him to recognize that we needed a break. I've never, ever forgotten that. So I take that lesson and try to duplicate the spirit of it in my own life. I've always remembered Ralph's insight — that we all need an enforced break every now and then. People like Ralph make this world such a beautiful place, giving without expectation, and I do my best to recognize that whenever possible. My mantra: "Be like Ralph."

BE AUTHENTIC

Knowing who you are, and being comfortable in your own skin, helps you have better relationships with other people. To me, therapy can be an incredibly useful tool for growth, allowing us to look at the road ahead, rather than in the rearview mirror. Therapy can be a framework for viewing things from a different perspective and deciding on a plan of action. I look at it this way: I can play tennis without a coach all day long, but if I want to improve my game, I'm going to seek out the help of a tennis pro. The same logic applies for our internal selves. We can slog through life and cope with trauma or anxiety by ourselves, but to truly move forward, sometimes the best thing to do is talk it out with a professional you trust.

BE GIVING

I have traveled across the country to teach other doctors about the medical techniques I've worked with and perfected. There is a powerful feeling in sharing something we know with other people. If you can find a way to share your personal knowledge, it can be an incredible source of life satisfaction. Almost everyone has some level of expertise to share, whether it extends from their profession or just a favorite hobby. For example, a successful entrepreneur has the ability to teach kids business skills; homemakers may choose to help pregnant teenagers understand the value of caring for their homes and children.

Just giving of one's time can often be the biggest gift to a worthy cause. Spending time with the elderly or the lonely, or helping care for abandoned animals at the local shelter, can be immensely rewarding. There are so many kids out there with no quality role model to teach them the most basic things our parents taught us that we take for granted: things like hard work, self-reliance, kindness, and consideration for others.

I'm very fortunate to have such outstanding role models for parents. They have sacrificed and worked hard to establish and preserve our family. And I feel it's our duty and our privilege to pay it forward.

An important part of teaching for me is preparation, and in the very act of reviewing what I already know in order to express it, I find that my own ideas become clearer. By teaching other doctors, I become more proficient myself. It is a win-win scenario. It's also energizing and rewarding to deliver the material. Whatever way you choose to share your expertise, your time, or your companionship, I know you'll find great value in the process.

BE HANDS-ON

It may sound silly, but doing something creative with your hands is an often overlooked, wonderful exercise in de-stressing and relaxation. Whether it's painting, pottery, embroidery, or building model airplanes, making something out of nothing is relaxing and satisfying. We spent a huge portion of our childhoods doing crafts and making art, never being afraid of or embarrassed by the outcome. Unfortunately, when we grow up, we often lose touch with this experience. It's a shame too, because there's something uniquely satisfying about seeing a creative task through from beginning to end.

Taking the kids to the YMCA to make a basket, or having date night at Sips and Strokes, where couples can drink a glass of wine and make a painting together, are just a couple of ways we can enjoy this experience. My daughter, Allison, told me the other day that she needed curtains for her new house. I remembered how, when Allison was little, her mother used to take sheets and make them into curtains. Do you remember that old Carol Burnett *Gone With the Wind* parody? Scarlett O'Hara comes down the stairs wearing curtains and a curtain rod as a dress, and says, "I saw it in a window and I just couldn't resist it."

I told my daughter she didn't realize just how talented a seamstress her mother was, to transform simple department-store sheets into beautiful curtains. So Allison learned a new skill the modern way: she went onto YouTube and found a video that showed how to make curtains using glue instead of sewing. I thought it was the coolest thing. And I suspect that the feeling of accomplishment she got from the project was equal to the satisfaction my wife must have felt all those years ago. With a craft or an artwork or a weekend project, you have a tangible, physical reward for your efforts.

My mother is an immensely talented artist, and I grew up watching her spend hours giving form to her creativity. If it weren't for her artistic influence, I would not be the surgeon I am today. My hands and my vision are translations of the many lessons she taught me over the years.

In short, good health, as well as a glowing appearance, naturally extends from a balanced, integrated life. Our minds automatically tune out the humdrum day-to-day normal activities, so we need fresh input to stimulate our soul, body, and mind.

CHIP'S TIPS

ONE BAKER'S DOZEN OF "BE'S" PLEASE

1 **Be Active** — let those endorphins flow.

2 **Be Social** — people need people.

3 **Be Familial** — friends will come and go, but family is forever.

4 **Be Available** — give of self and make time for others.

5 **Be Outward-Bound** — embrace nature.

6 **Be Spiritual** — connect with a higher power.

7 **Be Generous** — share your gifts.

8 **Be Community-Minded** — give back to your community.

9 **Be Animal-Friendly** — try to be who your dog thinks you are.

10 **Be Well-Rested** — vacation is a state of mind.

11 **Be Authentic** — stay comfortable in your own skin.

12 **Be Giving** — share your knowledge and skills.

13 **Be Hands-On** — never lose the child inside.

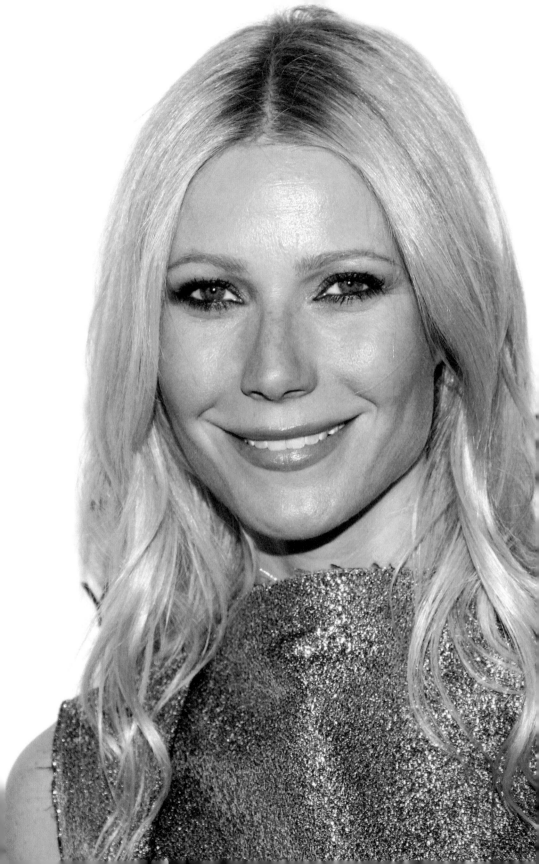

CHAPTER 11

* * *

PRETTY IS AS PRETTY DOES:
CELEBRITY SURGERY

**"I've had so much plastic surgery, when I die they will
donate my body to Tupperware."** — Joan Rivers

**"I wish I had a twin, so I could know what I'd look like
without plastic surgery."** — Joan Rivers

If you need evidence that beauty norms are not fixed, then history is a useful tool.
The impulse to modify the body to fit cultural standards is hardly a recent invention, as illustrated by the instructive case of Chinese foot-binding, one of the most bizarre instances of a beauty standard that now seems utterly barbaric.

From the time of the Song Dynasty (around AD 960), young Chinese girls' feet were contorted and restrained in pursuit of the ultimate sign of social status and beauty: unnaturally shrunken feet. Those tiny feet were the only way for a girl from a humble background to marry into money, and they set the standard of aristocratic beauty for the day. Though the practice was ultimately banned when the Communists came into power, foot binding is one historical footnote in what is often a sadly extensive list of body modifications done in the name of greater female beauty and, sometimes, female control.

But Chinese foot binding is also just one of many examples of where one century's beauty standard is another century's horror. Over the millennia, and in some cases even today, a host of strange and destructive practices have endangered the health and well-being of men and women trying to keep pace with shifting cultural notions of attractiveness. In some African and Middle Eastern countries, children and teenagers undergo horrific genital mutilation that leaves them prone to infection, death, and lifetime disability — all because someone decided centuries ago that this was a requisite step in the transition from girlhood to womanhood.

In certain parts of Asia and Africa, including among the Dinka people in the Republic of South Sudan, a beauty standard of elongation is achieved by stretching the neck with stacks of metal necklaces. In some cultures, filed-down teeth, wildly enlarged lower lips, and dramatically elongated ear lobes have all been considered ideals of beauty. During the Renaissance, women pursued porcelain complexions by whitening their skin with toxic chemicals including mercury or Venetian ceruse, made from a mixture of lead and vinegar. That pursuit of a whiter complexion with dangerous chemicals continues even today. In 2002 thousands of women in Hong Kong were sickened with mercury poisoning by the face creams they had purchased to lighten their skin. In the often culturally determined definitions of beauty, white skin is overvalued in Asia. But in America many still risk skin cancer and premature aging in pursuit of the opposite effect: darker skin. These shifting standards of beauty can at times seem almost comical, as half of the world pursues aristocratic white skin and the other half yearns for aristocratic dark skin.

The layperson's pursuit of beauty through the ages is nothing compared to some of the more unusual attempts made by early plastic surgeons to improve or correct their patients' appearances. In the earliest, experimental days of plastic surgery — beginning in ancient India and continuing into ancient Rome — features marred in battle were often repaired using skin removed from other parts of the body. In the 16th century, Italian surgeon Gasparo Tagliacozzi performed skin grafts to replace noses and ears lost in duels, and to repair the all-too-visible ravages of syphilis.

Beginning in the 19th century, American doctors began to employ surgical techniques to correct maladies like cleft palates. The first cleft palate operation was performed in 1827 by Virginia doctor John Peter Mettauer, with specially designed instruments, despite the fact that in these early days of plastic surgery many still considered such efforts to be meddling with God's grand design. The horrific injuries experienced by soldiers during World War I meant a great leap forward in plastic-surgery advances. Doctors attended to the disfiguring injuries of modern trench warfare, where slashed-off noses, shattered jaws and massive head wounds created a demand for new innovations in surgical repair.

In 1921, the American Society of Plastic Surgeons (ASPS) was formed. This professional organization gave plastic surgery a new credibility and sense of purpose, resulting in rapid advances in skin grafting and limb reconstruction techniques. Post-war, ordinary people witnessing the extraordinary transformations made possible with these cutting-edge surgeries sought out their own plastic-surgery corrections. Pioneers in the field like Dr. Charles C. Miller performed early rhinoplasties and could even create dimples in his patients' faces. There was an enormous demand among plastic surgeons of the day to correct conditions such as "saddle nose" — a depressed nose that often occurred with untreated syphilis. Without correction, a patient's social station and earning potential could be greatly affected.

Some of the early techniques for correcting such conditions were experimental, and often tragic, failures. Paraffin — frequently used in combination with Vaseline, grease, or olive oil — was adopted as an injectable for the reshaping of noses. Such substances were used to build these up in lieu of prostheses and bone grafting. Dreadful complications resulted. The paraffin would gradually shift, causing cancers that could migrate throughout the body, especially if the patient spent too much time in the sun.

Celebrities began employing plastic surgery around this time, greatly raising the profile of the plastic-surgery profession. When comedienne Fanny Brice had a much-heralded rhinoplasty in 1923, it became a cause célèbre that foreshadowed the present high-profile surgeries of stars like Pamela Anderson, Kim Kardashian, and Melanie Griffith. In 1934, the notorious Depression-era bank robber John Dillinger employed the services of a plastic surgeon for a rhinoplasty and face lift to disguise his looks and abet his escape from justice.

In the period following World War II, plastic surgery's prominence shifted dramatically, jumping more definitively into the public sphere, where it was increasingly marketed for cosmetic, rather than reconstructive, purposes. But here began a new wave of desire for self-improvement, yielding some not-so-great moments in plastic surgery history. One procedure involved the injection of liquid silicone into breast tissue to enhance the figures of dancers and performers. This commonplace practice resulted in drifting implants, disastrous infections and even loss of tissue, necessitating mastectomies.

In contemporary culture, it's often movie stars (rather than the royalty of the past) who drive our standards of beauty, whether good or bad. These aristocrats of 21st century life — the Madonnas and Angelinas of the world — establish the beauty trends we emulate. The entertainment industry is arguably the most looks-obsessed field. It's fair to say, the growing prominence of celebrity culture has stoked the popular desire for movie-star looks.

The beauty standard has gotten so far out of control, even for the celebrities themselves, that some have chosen to rebel. In the fall of 2011, British actress Kate Winslet and a group of like-minded British performers, including Rachel Weisz and Emma Thompson, formed the British Anti-Cosmetic Surgery League to resist plastic surgery. Easy to do, of course, if you happen to be born beautiful. But I don't disagree with the sentiment. So many impressionable young people are measuring themselves against a cosmetically enhanced, Photoshopped ideal. Having a group like Winslet's making a stand against perfection extremes may be a step in the right direction.

Even today, it's easy to find evidence of extreme plastic surgery that mirrors even the most bizarre historical aberrations, like the aforementioned foot binding and paraffin injection. In recent years, a number of cases have emerged involving women self-injecting substances — from cooking oil to low-grade silicone — in the dangerous pursuit of eternal youth.

> The best plastic surgeries are the ones you don't know about. If I've done my job, the best compliment you can get following a procedure is, "You look great, really well rested and relaxed."

Unscrupulous predators have done terrible damage in the name of beauty, as illustrated by the case of Priscilla Presley. Presley bravely admitted to falling prey to plastic surgery quack Dr. Daniel Serrano. Though not licensed to practice medicine in the United States, the South American doctor managed to make a small fortune hoodwinking a number of prominent celebrities into black-market facial injections.

Serrano's clients — including Larry King's wife Shawn King, and Lionel Richie's ex-wife Diane Richie — would get together for parties, during which Serrano would inject his victims with industrial-grade silicone and other substances smuggled into the United States from his native Argentina. He would tout these volatile materials as widely used by the Europeans for restoring youth and permanently removing wrinkles. Instead, the good doctor left his patients' faces lumpy, paralyzed, and cratered. Like the rest of us, celebrities can fall prey to bad medicine, losing sight of what is pretty and natural when plastic surgery becomes more of a fad than a fix.

The sad case of Presley being manipulated by a snake-oil salesman shows that even celebrities aren't immune to the relentless hunger for beauty that infects our society.

Another example most plastic surgeons are familiar with is Jocelyn Wildenstein, the Manhattan socialite who's been nicknamed the Cat Woman of New York due to all the dramatic procedures she's undergone. Her distinctive appearance stems from lip augmentation, chin augmentation, cheek implants, eyelid surgery, face lift, brow lift and canthopexy, which gave her eyes that cat-like appearance. She's literally spent millions to achieve that scary look.

We also find unfortunate cases among mainstream figures like Pamela Anderson, whose fluctuating breast augmentations have become a much-emulated aspect of her celebrity persona. Encapsulation (a formation of scar tissue around the breast) caused her implants to ride higher and higher in her chest, resulting in an unnatural positioning close to her collarbone. Rather than reacting with horror, American women started asking their doctors for breasts like Anderson's. What they were copying was, in essence, a medical complication.

We often don't see the results of a badly set leg or a slipshod appendectomy, but when plastic surgery goes wrong it's readily apparent. The Internet is filled with sites that chronicle misguided efforts to preserve youth and confused notions of what's beautiful. Just Google "plastic surgery gone wrong" to see some examples of vanity met with unscrupulous surgeons, who won't tell their clients "Enough!"

If you're only getting your cosmetic surgery tips from Hollywood red carpets and celebrity magazines, chances are you're going to want your work to be really dramatic, chiseled, or angular. My goal is to educate consumers about more naturalistic options. The best plastic surgeries are the ones you *don't* know about. If I've done my job, the best compliment you should get following a procedure is your friends telling you, "You look great, really well rested and relaxed."

CELEBRITY SURGERY

Whenever I host a cosmetic surgery seminar for prospective patients, I always flash two famous Hollywood actors up on the screen: Michelle Pfeiffer and Meg Ryan. For me, the cosmetic surgery work these two Hollywood stars have had over the years brilliantly illustrates the difference between my philosophy and that of some other docs in the business. When you look at both actors side by side, most women tell me they might rather look like Michelle Pfeiffer, not Meg Ryan, and Pfeiffer's is the approach I most often recommend.

Visually speaking, it comes down to the difference between her fresh and natural look as opposed to Ryan's more dramatic, altered appearance. Even if you're not a plastic surgeon with a medically trained eye, you can pick out the major differences in the actresses' features. With Pfeiffer, you know she still looks great but you don't see

WANT TO KNOW WHERE THE CELEBRITIES GO?

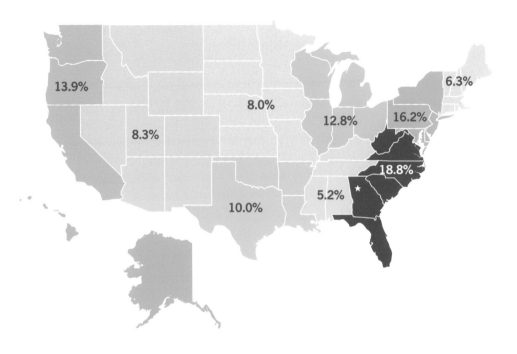

Practice Locations by Region

	Region	%
■	**South Atlantic** (DE, FL, GA, NC, SC, VA, WV)	18.8%
	Middle Atlantic (MD, NJ, NY, PA, DC)	16.2%
	Pacific (AK, CA, HI, OR, WA)	13.9%
	East North Central (IL, IN, MI, OH, WI)	12.8%
	West South Central (AR, LA, OK, TX)	10.0%
	Mountain (AZ, CO, ID, MT, NV, NM, UT, WY)	8.3%
	West North Central (IA, KS, MN, MO, NE, ND, SD)	8.0%
	New England (CT, ME, MA, NH, RI, VT)	6.3%
	East South Central (AL, KY, MS, TN)	5.2%
	Other	0.5%

★ =(Highest Density of Plastic Surgery in the United States)

Americans Spent Nearly $11 Billion on Cosmetic Procedures in 2012. Percentage of Procedure Based on Expenditures.

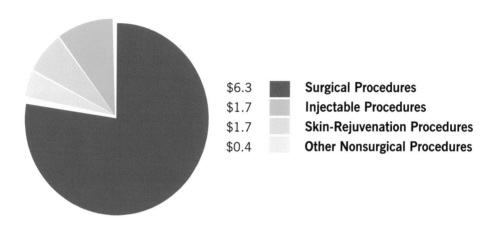

$6.3 — Surgical Procedures
$1.7 — Injectable Procedures
$1.7 — Skin-Rejuvenation Procedures
$0.4 — Other Nonsurgical Procedures

Source: American Society for Aesthetic Plastic Surgery
$ amounts in billions

Percent of Total Procedures by Race/Ethnicity

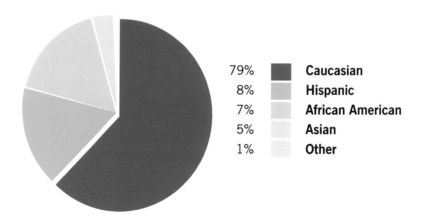

79% — Caucasian
8% — Hispanic
7% — African American
5% — Asian
1% — Other

Source: American Society for Aesthetic Plastic Surgery
Total ethnic minority population (rounded) = 21%

the physical evidence of a procedure. You can't *quite* put your finger on it. That's the sign of excellent work. That fresh and natural look is the result of a careful process. It's not a quick fix. It's not a total overhaul. It's a staged series of treatments.

In my industry, stars like Halle Berry, Sophia Loren, Raquel Welch, and Denzel Washington are the celebrities we point to as positive examples of successful treatments that fly under the radar. This subtle, incremental approach that I specialize in is a big reason patients fly in from Beverly Hills and New York to have their work done here in Atlanta. Just as traits like discretion, hospitality, and kindness are favored in the South, Southern women also value the understated changes that make them look refreshed, instead of inspiring one of those *poor thing* moments at a charity gala. Over-the-top, visible, gaudy surgeries are out. (At my seminars, I'll even use a photo of Joan Rivers, bless her heart, as an extreme example to explain what she's had done and what patients can learn to avoid).

The emphasis now is on the preventive and the minimal.

My approach is to arm patients with education whenever possible. It's part of my job to be a resource in the conversation around aging and its effects. I can show you how you've aged and what may have exacerbated that, and how you came to look the way you do. If a patient understands the process, I'm a big believer that she will choose what's right for her.

In studying the science of skin care over the years, you learn a lot about true beauty as an internal phenomenon, not just an external one. Part of my job is to explain to patients the science of beauty…why success stories appear beautiful and how my patients can achieve that beauty as well. What helps me in this job are the prospective patients who are now a lot more sophisticated than they used to be, because there's a lot more information out there now and patients really do their homework. They read everything.

Ten years ago, patients would rarely approach me with an already-sophisticated understanding of plastic surgery. These days, with the power of the Internet, that's all changed. My clients are savvy enough to know that skin doesn't just stretch and fat doesn't just disappear. It's all there, waiting to be restored. If you can maintain someone's eyes and mouth and change their facial framework, then the results still look very much like them, but an improved, refreshed version of them.

WINNERS' CIRCLE: THE SUCCESS STORIES

There's a good reason movie stars are so often emulated by us mere mortals: Many appear to possess the secrets of eternal youth. These women and men are the success stories, the eternal beauties who inspire so much copycat surgery. The reason many of them look so good, with few telltale signs of plastic-surgery excess, is their gradual and moderate approach to surgery.

We could learn a lot from their example. Most pay extraordinary attention to not just how they look, but what goes into their bodies. Many extraordinarily beautiful women follow a vegetarian, vegan, or macrobiotic diet, and the results appear very clearly on their radiant, clear skin and healthy physiques. Alicia Silverstone has advocated for the health benefits of a vegan diet in her book *The Kind Diet: A Simple Guide to Feeling Great, Losing Weight, and Saving the Planet*. And Madonna has maintained a clock-stopping trimness through her longtime macrobiotic diet and a relentless exercise routine that has been rumored to include even birthday and Christmas workouts.

But as I tell my patients, these are also people who get paid to look good for a living. Many of them spend a fortune far beyond what any of us can imagine in their ongoing, lifelong maintenance and pursuit of perpetually camera-ready beauty. A recent article in *Allure* magazine estimated that the array of procedures needed to maintain Demi Moore's astounding, youthful beauty — from hyaluronic fillers to Botox, veneers and Thermage — would likely cost somewhere in the neighborhood of $49,900 a year.

While we may not all have the cash or even the desire to attain that level of perfection, we could all learn a lesson from Demi. What most of these stars understand, and the nature of their job demands, is that rather than suddenly hitting 40 or 50 and rushing in for a full face lift, they have been making small, incremental changes, probably beginning in their 20s. That is the secret to looking great: doing little things along the way instead of a dramatic, jarring change.

As just one example of what I'm taking about, consider the skin around the eyes, the thinnest skin on the body. Though I often recommend that patients take a comprehensive rather than segmented approach, there are benefits to occasionally focusing in on one key feature for correction. For instance, most people should have their eyes done before they take other approaches to maintaining facial harmony, so that later, when they adjust other features, they can just go back and have a little laser resurfacing to freshen it up. If someone waits too long to have eye surgery or a cheek lift or a neck lift, they will find that just targeting one feature at this late date will look unnatural. So the best lesson the stars can teach us is maintain, maintain, maintain.

Stars like Madonna, Demi Moore and Halle Berry — the masters of natural beauty maintenance — all share a secret. It's one that I, too, have advocated in my own practice. Instead of stretching their faces tight, these stars use fillers to plump up and recreate a youthful face. Instead of taking a segmented approach and tackling the nose one year and the eyes the next, they work holistically to balance their features and leave no glaring traces of "work."

These are some examples of stars who have approached plastic surgery with restraint, with the help of a skilled doctor. This isn't to say that women can just plop Madonna's eyes or Demi's mouth on their face and achieve the same results. Anatomy varies from person to person, and a feature that works on one woman's face might not work on another's. What I recommend — instead of simply asking your surgeon for "Pam's breasts" or "Lindsay's lips" — is to take a cue from the following beauty success stories, and to trace their steps to achieve a consistent and ongoing beauty practice. Let's examine some of the most prominent…

Like her mother Blythe Danner, **Gwyneth Paltrow** — a darling of both indie and mainstream movies — is a case study in aging gracefully. Perhaps some very careful use of Botox and maybe some filler in the temple area, rather than the usual overinjected cheeks, have given this actress the appearance of stopping time. She is today's poster child for "natural" beauty.

A possible cheek lift, liposuction on the neck and a very subtle "sow as you grow and no one will know" approach to aging has meant **Michelle Pfeiffer** looks great and incredibly natural. Miraculously, she looks as good now as she did when she famously lounged on a grand piano in *The Fabulous Baker Boys* in the late '80s. As you get older, making small changes over time is far better than waiting (which would mean having to do much more to get the same effect). Pfeiffer is maybe proof of the need for consistent, long-term nips and tucks.

Throughout a wildly dynamic career spanning the performing arts — from music to dance to film — **Madonna** has taken it all in stride. She has likely had a cheek lift, but most important, while undergoing multiple procedures she has held on to the essential architecture and angularity of her face. Her cheeks are high and defined, rather than having that overinflated look. Her jawline is distinct. Careful attention to small procedures over time, combined with what some have described as an obsessive devotion to good health, may have kept Madge looking phenomenal.

"I tried for modeling work, but it was a bit slow, and that's when I took a part-time job at McDonald's. It gave me income while I was waiting for my big break, and at the very least I could eat." Hard to imagine that this quote came from one of the most beautiful women ever to grace the silver screen. **Sharon Stone** has managed to look extraordinary throughout her career, without obvious signs of surgery (apart from a less-than-subtle breast augmentation some time back). Stone had a brief romance with "trout pout" following her divorce from newspaper editor Phil Bronstein.

As she told *More* magazine of her rash surgery to correct a broken heart, "Nobody loved me. I'm a hundred and three. My life would be better if I had better lips." Stone quickly realized magnified lips don't equal magnified beauty, and she has since lost the trout pout and taken a more moderate approach to looking beautiful.

An amazing-looking woman, **Halle Berry**, a former beauty queen and an Academy Award–winning actress, most likely has had a little help with a very discreet rhinoplasty, some Botox, and veneers, procedures that have been helped by Berry's fortunate genetics. She has some truly remarkable skin. She's a shining example of how doing only minor tweaks over time can lead to a look of unmodified youthfulness.

Dewy, voluptuous, and seemingly perpetually youthful, **Salma Hayek** is an instance of a star who possibly did some slight, very subtle modifications to the width of her nose early on in her career. But she's managed to keep subsequent procedures minimal, with attention to scrupulous skin care.

We all remember that scene from *Ghost* with Patrick Swayze and the potter's wheel. Hard to believe we first saw it over two decades ago and that **Demi Moore** still looks so great, appearing to have stopped time. Want to know how she's done it? She doesn't concentrate on any one or two features for anti-aging, but has taken a holistic approach. It's likely that a consistent combination of hyaluronic fillers, fat injections, veneers, Botox, Juvéderm, and IPL (intense pulsed light) treatments have helped keep Moore looking practically ageless.

For some time, **Christie Brinkley** appeared to have the overfilled cheeks that can detract from the contours of a naturally beautiful face. But more recently, she has perhaps undergone an elegant face lift, which has nicely stabilized her brows without sacrificing facial fullness. Personal travails aside, she has enjoyed a more enduringly youthful appearance than most of her contemporaries.

Wrinkle-free but still extraordinarily natural looking, **Cindy Crawford** is a former prom queen and pioneer supermodel who has admitted to having injections of collagen, vitamins, and Botox. But she has maintained her all-American natural good looks by exercising restraint and keeping any procedures to a minimum. Definitely another example of "sow as you go and no one will know."

"She was unquestionably gorgeous. She was lavish. She was a dark, unyielding largess. **Liz Taylor** was, in short, too bloody much." What can you say about a woman who was so impossibly, exquisitely beautiful that her future husband Richard Burton admits to laughing out loud upon first laying eyes on her? Until her death in 2011, Taylor's tendency toward weight gain paid off when it came to her looks. She had plump, glowing skin, and her beauty was undoubtedly enhanced by her joie de vivre and embrace of social causes that surely contributed to her long, fruitful life.

The first *Friends* actor to get a star on the Hollywood Walk of Fame, **Jennifer Aniston**, the quintessential girl-next-door, has probably used fillers to maintain her healthy good looks and youthful mid-face region. But like so many in the new generation of younger stars, Aniston clearly understands that less is more.

In **J.Lo** we find an instance of a woman who has aged gracefully by perhaps having a number of small procedures over time. This has proven a major advantage for someone who's equally comfortable cutting Grammy-nominated records and starring opposite George Clooney. A very minor nose refinement may have helped draw more attention to her lovely eyes, and a rumored lip reduction and cheek implant may also have led to honors like *People* magazine's "World's Most Beautiful Woman." Whatever Lopez has done, she has a very skilled surgeon with a talent for making inconspicuous alterations. Some weight loss has also created Lopez's more chiseled features.

Who knew that the idiosyncratic and wildly talented co-star of *Girl, Interrupted* would become the poster girl for American beauty? Though **Angelina Jolie** was born beautiful, she has possibly become even more so with some subtle alterations to the face, including a very discreet slimming and refinement of her nose early in her career and, perhaps, the use of Botox, fillers, and subtle upper-lip augmentation to maintain her beauty.

Sophia Loren, the classic Italian bombshell and icon of feminine charm, has denied having plastic surgery; perhaps she's just very discreet in using a surgeon who has bestowed an exceedingly natural look, without too much tightness, through what I would wager has been at least one face lift.

Despite a family legacy of troubled silver-screen stars, **Drew Barrymore** has become an enduring fixture of our pop-culture landscape. She has also been public about undergoing breast reduction early on, because of both physical and psychological discomfort with breasts that were too big for her frame. Since that surgery in her youth, Barrymore has likely used Botox to smooth her forehead and some fillers to plump up her cheeks and lips, coupled with facial liposuction. Barrymore has nevertheless tackled facial changes with such restraint that she just looks great rather than altered.

Corrective or not, **Bristol Palin's** jaw surgery (which looks very much like a chin implant) has helped refine her jawline, giving her more definition. Combined with a possible rhinoplasty and injection of Botox in her forehead, Palin has traded her baby fat and facial fullness for a more-chiseled look.

The hallmark of really good plastic surgery is that you can't quite pinpoint what's been done. Instead, there is just a consistent, beautiful appearance. No single detail — such as overfilled lips, too-tight face lift, or aggressive rhinoplasty — gives away a surgeon's handiwork. **Raquel Welch** is the perfect example of a woman who has probably had work done, but while retaining a natural look. She still looks age-appropriate, with slight crinkling around her eyes, remaining an incredibly stunning woman in her 70s. The longtime beauty has been especially smart about maintaining volume, possibly with the cautious, strategic use of fillers.

I may be bucking the system on this one, but I'm perhaps one of the few people who believes that **Jennifer Grey** looks better — not worse — after her career-defining rhinoplasty. The actress, best known for her star turn in *Dirty Dancing*, was an unfortunate example of plastic surgery's double standard. When stars like Angelina Jolie and Halle Berry get nose jobs, no one bats an eye, but Grey's rhinoplasty was a cause célèbre that unfairly singled her out as a representative of the hazards of cosmetic surgery. In the irony of ironies, she was crucified for being vain in an industry founded on vanity. Grey became the symbolic whipping girl in a business in which modification is the norm, and it was that vilification, rather than the nose job, that probably led to her later difficulty finding work in Hollywood.

Grey's case also points to another ugly trend in the public response to beauty and celebrity. Though I have talked in this book about how less-attractive people can often suffer in the workplace, perhaps attractive people just as often are viewed with suspicion and disdain. This is especially true for female politicians, whose looks, rather than their policies, can become the primary focus of media attention. On April 4, 2013, President Obama assessed the beauty of California's attorney general, Kamala Harris, calling her "by far the best looking attorney general" during remarks at a televised fund-raiser. Importantly, many experts felt this was sexist and diminished her many political accomplishments. This was a horrible example to all Americans by the highest-ranking official of the United States. America is rife with double standards, especially for women, who are criticized for not looking good and also for looking too good. Where a man's attractiveness can often help him in life and business, it's as if women have to overcome their good looks. After all, I doubt President Obama would say that about a male attorney general.

GWYNETH PALTROW (born 1972)

Shakespeare in Love

16 years later

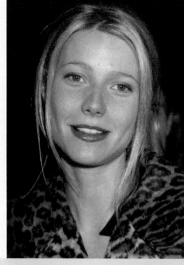
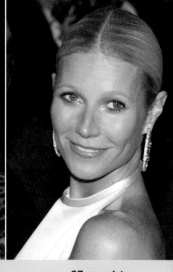

The emblem of humility and grace amid the trappings of fame, Gwyneth Paltrow is comfortable in her own skin, which makes her all the more radiant.

MICHELLE PFEIFFER (born 1958)

The Fabulous Baker Boys

27 years later

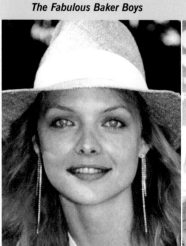
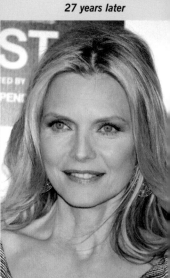

Wisdom and intelligence twinkle all the brighter now in the eyes of Michelle Pfeiffer, adding a layer of depth to her 1980s' beauty.

MADONNA (born 1958)

The Material Girl

27 years later

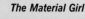
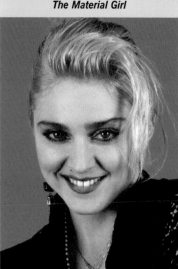
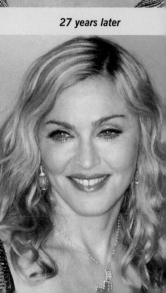

A full family life and rigorous training regimen have helped keep Madonna glowing from the inside out.

Basic Instinct

16 years later

SHARON STONE (born 1958)

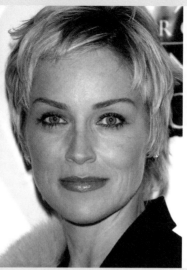

"What are you going to do? Charge me with smoking?" Probably not. A healthy lifestyle has helped keep Sharon Stone looking ageless.

Bond Girl

16 years later

HALLE BERRY (born 1966)

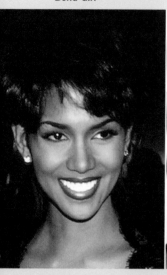

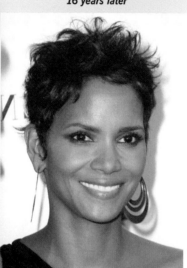

Though she's settled into her good looks with time, that wicked Halle Berry Catwoman grin is still very much alive.

Desperado

15 years later

SALMA HAYEK (born 1966)

Salma Hayek's Latin blood courses with good humor and fun...the surest way to stay looking young.

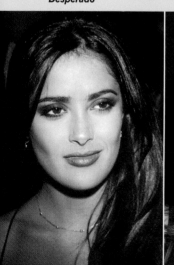

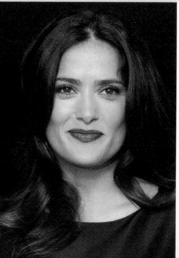

DEMI MOORE (born 1962)

The Ghost Star

21 years later

Bruce, Ashton, beyond...
Demi Moore's ever-more-
youthful beauty has been
mirrored by her choice in
men.

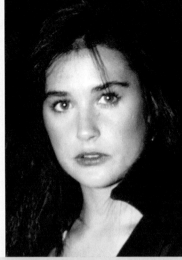

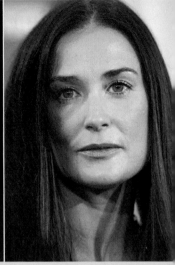

CHRISTIE BRINKLEY (born 1954)

Uptown Girl

22 years later

From left to right, almost
a quarter-century elapses,
and it feels like the blink
of an eye...

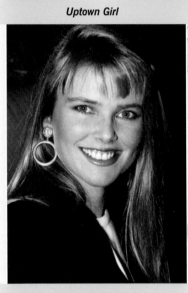

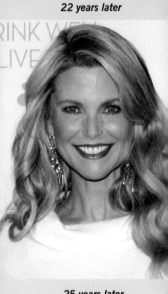

CINDY CRAWFORD (born 1966)

SI Supermodel

25 years later

Season timeless beauty with
worldliness and business
savvy, and you have the
recipe for a knockout at
any age.

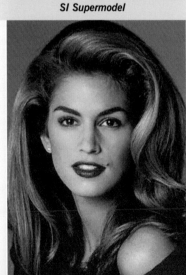

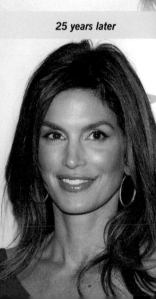

Hollywood's Golden Girl

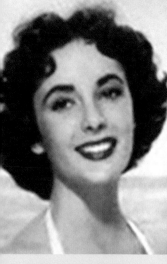

38 years later

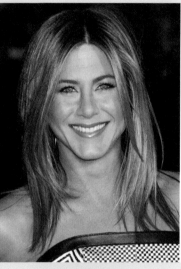

ELIZABETH TAYLOR (born 1932)

What can you say about the grande dame of elegance and self-possession? Elizabeth Taylor did everything right. In some cases more than once.

Rachel On Friends

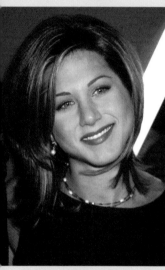

17 years later

JENNIFER ANISTON (born 1969)

That girl-next-door charm, combined with a daily beauty and health regimen, have perfectly preserved Jennifer Aniston.

J.Lo from The Bronx

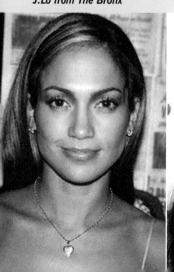

13 years later

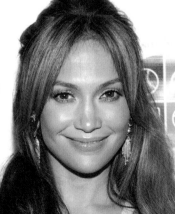

JENNIFER LOPEZ (born 1969)

She's still Jenny from the Block, and her humility and sense of roots has served Jennifer Lopez well in the beauty department.

ANGELINA JOLIE (born 1975)

Girl, Interrupted

15 years later

Whether it was that vial of Billy Bob's blood or her international human-rights work, somewhere Angelina Jolie appears to have found the secret to eternal youth.

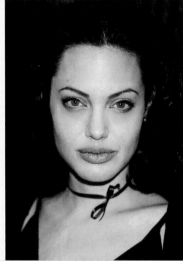

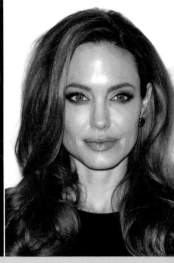

SOPHIA LOREN (born 1934)

Two Women

49 years later

In Sophia Loren, we find evidence of what a half-century can do to diminish true beauty: NOTHING.

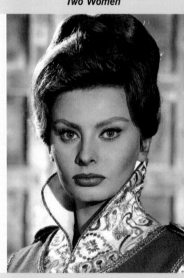

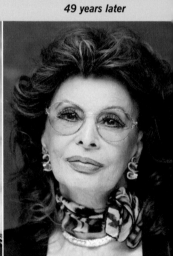

DREW BARRYMORE (born 1975)

E.T.

13 years later

Before and After...or is it After and Before? There's no telling with the girlishly charming Drew Barrymore.

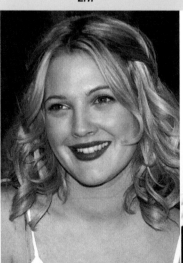

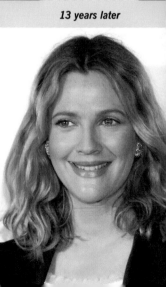

| *Reality TV Star* | *7 years later* | **BRISTOL PALIN** (born 1990) |

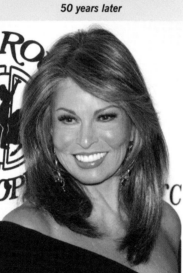

For Bristol Palin, a pretty ambitious set of procedures done with judiciousness and a sense of art.

| *One Million Years B.C.* | *50 years later* | **RAQUEL WELCH** (born 1940) |

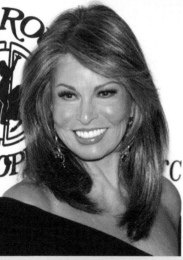

Synonyms for va va voom include sexy, voluptuous, and Raquel Welch. That goes for 45 years ago as well as today.

| *Dirty Dancing* | *19 years later* | **JENNIFER GREY** (born 1960) |

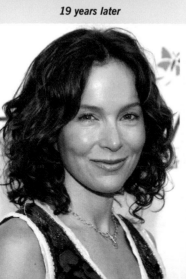

Though she's kicked off her *Dirty Dancing* shoes, Jennifer Grey is older, wiser, and more beautiful than ever.

THE TIGHT CLUB: TOO MUCH, TOO EARLY

You don't just have to open the latest issue of *People* magazine or *The National Enquirer* to see the ABCs of bad plastic surgery. The next time you're in the grocery store checkout line, pay attention to the 60-something woman with her hair in a high ponytail in front of you. See those curious scars behind her ears? This could be the sign of a bad face lift and sloppy, lazy work.

One essential principle of cosmetic surgery, applicable not just for celebrities but for ordinary folk like us, is that it correct rather than simply camouflage (which is often the case when stars like Meg Ryan or Daryl Hannah engage in filler overload). Adding too much volume without addressing the underlying anatomical effects of aging — such as drooping cheek pads — can result in an overinflated chipmunk effect. When the cheek pad begins to fall and you get a deep nasolabial fold, if you fill the hollow above it, the fold will still be present (and on top of that, now you'll have a walnut bulge in the cheeks). Overvolumizing to fill the void doesn't take into account the downward migration of the previous volume. The cheek pad is still there, it's just lower, and overfilling above only creates a displaced, unnatural plumpness. Facial volume is not lost so much as it is displaced. For that reason, I believe in restoring volume where it used to be, and moving that fallen cheek pad back to where it belongs on the cheek bone, with a cheek lift, also termed a mid-face lift.

When it comes to the stars who have made bad plastic surgery choices, or fallen prey to bad doctors, all I can say is my heart goes out to them. Their every move is clocked by a ravenous public. They're unfairly scrutinized by merciless motion-picture cameras that pack on the appearance of pounds. And they're stalked by paparazzi who can zoom in on their face to show every line and fissure. They are under unbelievable scrutiny to look great their entire lives, every day, every moment, whether walking the red carpet or simply picking their child up from school. They can never have a bad day without fear of some paparazzo recording it for posterity and featuring it on tomorrow's *TMZ* segment. And aging is definitely not encouraged. With a new crop of starlets constantly entering the Hollywood pool, the older generation is expected to compete, to stay fresh, relevant and beautiful next to men and women half their age. It's not really fair. It's only natural that many of them would overcompensate and project a fragile self-image through their bad surgical choices. The scrutiny these women and men are under is unimaginable.

But the surgical choices some celebrities have made do more than simply give them an artificial, hardened look. When their job is to emote and express vulnerability on camera, their frozen features can keep us from accepting them as fully human. Plastic surgery can be a liability not just in the movies, where it can limit emotional range, but for fans, who see an approachable, lovable persona replaced by a false one.

And difficulties on this front sometimes extend to the lives of the not-so-rich and famous. As some experts have noted, babies learn about emotions by mimicking the facial movements of their mothers. But if their mothers are so Botoxed that they can't form those expressions anymore, how will their babies pick up these cues? By the same token, if movie stars are our proxies, the people we are meant to identify with as we enter the fiction of a film or television program, what happens to pop culture behavior when their emotions don't surface from beneath a layer of Botox? The backlash against Nicole Kidman when she fell victim to an overly Botoxed forehead was evidence of the level of mistrust and even anger the public can feel when a formerly recognizable, emotionally complex face is replaced, à la *Invasion of the Body Snatchers*, with an uncanny duplicate.

> Some celebrities have made surgical choices that do more than give them an artificial, hardened look. Their job is to emote and express vulnerability on camera, but frozen features keep us from accepting them as fully human.

Hollywood is a world very much like our own, but far more intense, with more money, bigger egos, and more hype…a land ruled by copycat beauty. Stars are just as capable of emulating one another, as evidenced by the obsession with overfilled lips that can be seen on every episode of *The Real Housewives*, or the abuse of fillers that can distort and exaggerate facial features, leading to the familiar chipmunk-cheek-and-disappearing-eye combination that plagues so many former Hollywood beauties. Even younger stars like Lindsay Lohan and Kim Kardashian are falling victim to the too-much-too-soon phenomenon, erasing their facial contours and natural skin tone with fillers that can make them look old before their time. Following are a few examples of those who fall into this unfortunate category of the conspicuous.

"Heat up the clutch, set at 50 deluxe. Then we speed down the hutch, breakin' trees in the dutch." While **Lil' Kim** is clearly a master of the rhyming couplet, this hip-hop diva has nevertheless undergone some dramatic changes throughout her career — including probably breast augmentation, skin lightening, cheek implants, and a nose job. These aggressive procedures have made Lil' Kim look like a robotic copy of herself, not that that's a bad thing.

Lip augmentation, upper lids, a nose job, Botox…there is probably very little the singer and sometime actress **Courtney Love** hasn't done when it comes to plastic surgery. But one issue with surgery that isn't always anticipated is how work that is too extreme in its approach can result in facial non-sequiturs. This former wife of suicide victim Kurt Cobain went on to a formidable singing career of her own (with the band Hole), but her loose-cannon public appearances have lent her a tragicomic air. Her copious surgeries have created an odd disconnect: she still has the bearing of an impetuous rock star but with the face of an aging socialite.

It takes a lot to look so stunning, even when standing next to one of the most notoriously handsome of Hollywood's leading men, Tom Cruise. But that marriage of Hollywood royalty is over, and for a time there, **Nicole Kidman** fell victim to the notion that more Botox means more improvement. It was hard even for laypeople not to see that immobile, oddly line-free forehead and diagnose it as "too much time at the cosmetic surgeon's office."

A member of the premature alteration club, **Lindsay Lohan** has shown a desire to grow up too fast, not just in her hard-partying, club-hopping life, but in her approach to beauty. Overly-inflated lips and cheeks have aged her and distorted her beauty, to leave her looking flat and harsh. Beauty is supposed to be soft and cuddly, not hard like a mannequin, a fact that many plastic-surgery addicts have lost sight of. Probably as the result of too much filler, her eyes have receded. It makes you wonder why, when you already have youth and beauty, you would choose procedures that only harden and age you. Perhaps for members of this young Hollywood fast track, getting fillers or Botox early on is just another way of feeling older and more sophisticated. It reminds me of that topsy-turvy beauty culture in which Asian girls want to have whiter skin and Caucasian girls want the reverse. Though in this case, older women want to look younger and younger girls seem to want to look older, all of them meeting at some bizarro nethersphere in between.

A telltale sign of too many fillers is a waxy sheen like the one seen in **Meg Ryan's** skin, a phenomenon that can also occur with the use of aggressive chemical peels like phenol, which can give an unnatural alabaster tone to flesh. Too much filler stretches the skin like a water balloon, resulting in an unnatural tone and texture. People lose the soft, gentle feel of their preëxisting skin tone. A possible face lift in combination with the overinflation of Ryan's cheeks with fillers (and the corresponding shelf under her eyes) has also led to her unusual look. She's still cute as a button, though perhaps a little more *Sleepless* looking than one might prefer at her age.

Working with the nose and the lips is an art form (as is soap-opera acting, some would say, but that's a subject for a different book). Every set of lips and every nose is unique. And losing sight of the essential anatomy of these features can lead to distortion of the face. These are places where very small changes can yield enormous results. I tell patients not to go more than 30 percent larger when they are doing lip filler. But people want to go 100 percent larger, making their lip twice as wide. Well, the human eye notices that sort of monkeying around with facial symmetry. We can naturally tell when something is that out of balance. Going too heavy on the filler can lend a cartoonishly exaggerated quality. Balance is important too. In addition to overinflated lips, **Lisa Rinna** has also admitted to going too far with Juvéderm and permitting too much of the injectable in her cheeks, giving her face a patently artificial look. Fortunately, she underwent surgery to reduce her silicone lip injections. "My lips started to define who I am," she stated, "and that bothered me."

Where to start? **Joan Rivers** is brilliant and wickedly funny, but she'll be the first to admit she's a bit of a surgery addict. You have only to pick up her uproarious (and quite useful) guide to plastic surgery, *Men Are Stupid…And They Like Big Boobs*, to realize this woman knows her way around the surgeon's scalpel. You have to love someone this unapologetic about the various face lifts, nose jobs and skin treatments she's undergone. Like some women who don't know when to say when, Rivers has traded natural, age-appropriate beauty for a mask of surface prettiness. She's also an example of another era's face lift, in which tightening was the primary concern, rather than an approach to facial musculature that distinguishes current lifts. This anatomical approach actually raises fallen features and corrects the musculature under the skin, rather than simply tightening the surface.

Cher has always had an air of authoritative beauty about her, with commanding performances in movies like *Mask* and *Moonstruck*, among many others. But she has become an emblem of a now-passé approach to surgery, where skin is stretched rather than musculature restored. Cher has let this sort of aggressive surgery, including rhinoplasty that doesn't suit the lines of her face, remove some of the character and distinctive lines of her face.

It's sad to see a lovely woman like **Melanie Griffith**, who could have aged so much better, go in for faddish "improvements" like the inflated lips that have now become synonymous with bad 1990s-era plastic surgery. Enough said.

KIMBERLY DENISE JONES (born 1974)

Rapper Lil' Kim

8 years later

Not to worry, that's someone standing behind her, not an ear implant. Her other procedures, though, have proven a bit overzealous.

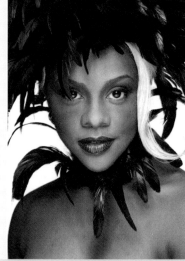
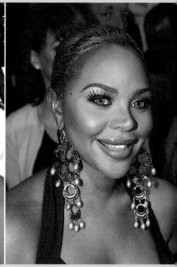

COURTNEY LOVE (born 1964)

Hole Guitarist

18 years later

Never a puppet on anyone's strings, Courtney Love did it her way. In the case of plastic surgery, though, her way wasn't all that good.

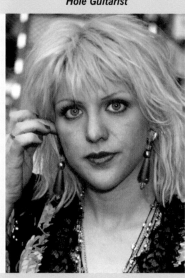
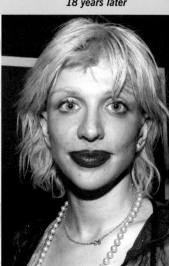

NICOLE KIDMAN (born 1967)

Days Of Thunder

18 years later

Nicole Kidman's surgical interventions may not have accentuated her natural beauty, but she's still a statuesque presence.

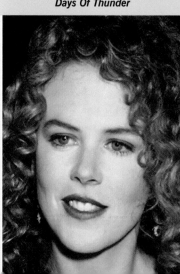
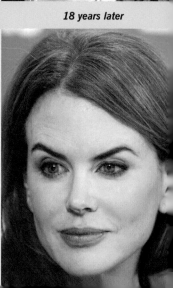

| *Disney/Mean Girls* | *6 years later* | **LINDSAY LOHAN** (born 1986) |

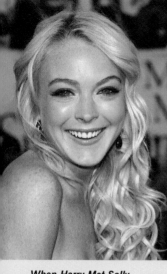
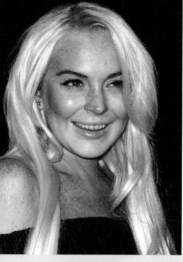

Lindsay Lohan shows us that inopportune lifestyle choices — not just in the things we do but how we care for ourselves — can come back to haunt us.

| *When Harry Met Sally* | *16 years later* | **MEG RYAN** (born 1961) |

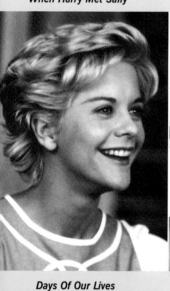
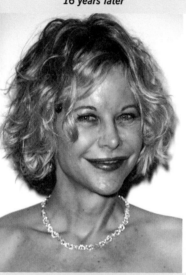

Meg Ryan still casts off the glow of a free spirit, though more-skillful cosmetic surgery might have accentuated it better.

| *Days Of Our Lives* | *16 years later* | **LISA RINNA** (born 1963) |

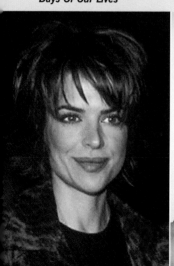
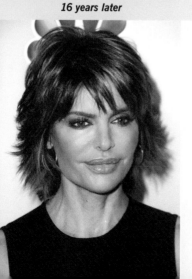

Lisa Rinna's playfulness and class have kept her looking gorgeous, through the ups and downs of cosmetic procedures.

JOAN RIVERS (born 1933)

E! Red Carpet

31 years later

She's Lady Jane Grey
meets Don Rickles, and her
wonderfully self-effacing
humor will always temper
any imperfections in
her look.

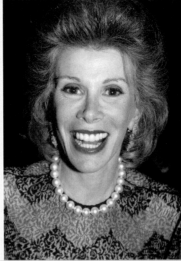
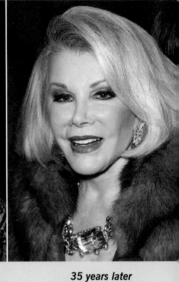

CHER (born 1946)

Goddess of Pop

35 years later

With a career spanning
over five decades, Cher
can still belt it out, and her
philanthropic work has only
added to her beauty.

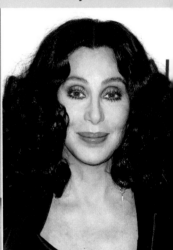

MELANIE GRIFFITH (born 1957)

Working Girl

37 years later

Though she may appear
somewhat over-maintained
of late, Melanie Griffith has
kept her sense of humor,
which is the real fountain
of youth.

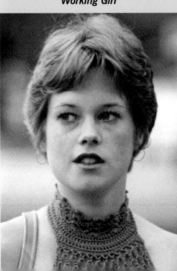
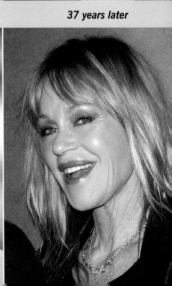

GUYS: THE GOOD, THE BAD, AND THE OH-NO!

For guys, skin treatments and surgery can be an even more delicate process. As women desire, and are even expected to undergo, maintenance of various kinds, men are expected to look like themselves and age gracefully (as the saying goes). And though many men mature and look better with age, it doesn't hurt to give nature a helping hand every once in a while. Just remember — a little can go a long way, and with no makeup to hide mistakes, sometimes it goes a longer way than it should.

Following are a few examples of men who have undergone procedures — some that helped and some that, well…see for yourself.

The Good
As spokesperson for Boys' and Girls' Clubs of America, **Denzel Washington** is a class act (he also supports American troops with morale-boosting base visits). And he's shown a real discretion in terms of keeping his cosmetic improvements close to the vest. Washington couldn't possibly look as good as he does in his 50s without some cosmetic modifications, including some not-so-great veneers that are a bit out of proportion with his mouth, combined with other, more successful, procedures. Unlike some stars, he has always kept procedures like fillers and Botox subtle, and they've never interfered with his acting ability or integrity. Age-appropriate and masculine, Washington is a cosmetic surgery "do" in a field of "don'ts."

Those in the know suspect that **Robert Redford** has undergone an eye lift to correct drooping eyelids, a common complaint among men in their 70s. But who can blame America's poster boy for wanting to maintain his celebrated looks and rugged masculinity as long as he can? There's nothing wrong with that, but with a more skilled surgeon doing his eye surgery, chances are he could have looked better.

Some men, despite growing older, hold on to a sense of virility and style, and **Tom Cruise** is certainly one of them. Still sleek and handsome well into middle-age, it's possible Cruise owes his youthful good looks to chemical peels and the occasional injectable, but either way, he has never looked "maintained," just manly.

The Bad
You gotta love **Bruce Jenner**. A gold-medal-winning Olympic athlete and father to an enormous clan of very opinionated women, the man has stamina! Unfortunately,

DENZEL WASHINGTON (born 1954)   *Training Day, Malcolm X*   *27 years later*

For 40 years on film, Denzel Washington has been like a movie-house pretzel: tough and salty on the outside, soft and warm on the inside.

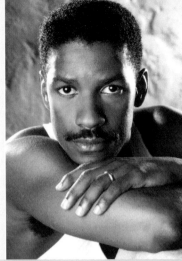

ROBERT REDFORD (born 1936)   *Butch Cassidy, Sundance Film Festival*   *27 years later*

Butch Cassidy may have ridden on to greener pastures, but the Sundance Kid is still with us, and as striking as ever.

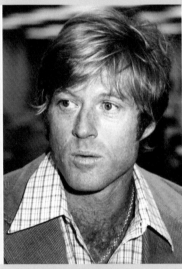

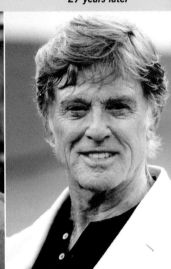

TOM CRUISE (born 1962)   *Top Gun, Risky Business*   *27 years later*

Though he's clearly had some work done, Tom Cruise still has the boyish good looks that made him a male icon more than 25 years ago.

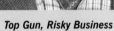

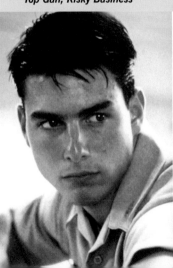

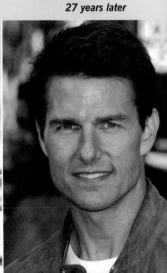

| '76 Montreal Olympics | 33 years later | **BRUCE JENNER** (born 1949) |

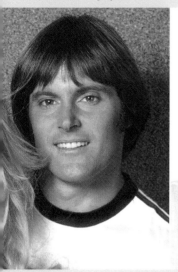 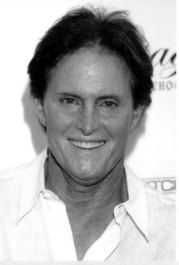

From the cover of a Wheaties box to the cover of the *Keeping Up with the Kardashians* Box Set — what a long, strange trip it's been.

| 9½ Weeks, Sin City | 26 years later | **MICKEY ROURKE** (born 1952) |

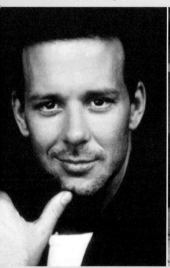 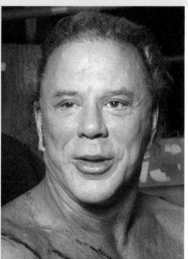

Fortunately, no amount of plastic surgery or blows to the face can beat down Mickey Rourke's big heart and on-screen talent.

| Comedian Carrot Top | 5 years later | **SCOTT THOMPSON** (born 1965) |

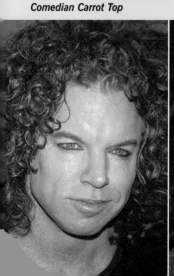 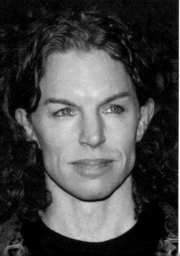

Anyone who can survive years of stand-up and Friars Club Roasts can certainly survive a — shall we say — ambitious surgical approach.

Jenner has not always shown the same comfort in his own skin when it comes to his plastic surgery choices. But he's a good example for the men out there of how important it is to find a surgeon who has real expertise working with men, and doesn't just use the same facial rejuvenating procedures in the same way with his male patients as he does with his female ones.

Two face lifts and a nose job that has thinned his nose too much have given Jenner's face an unnatural, feminine appearance. He's obviously had a run-in with a surgeon or surgeons who don't know the difference between male and female anatomy. With some of my gay clients, choosing a more feminine look for the eyes can be a desired effect, in addition to removing the buccal fat pad in the cheek to get a more chiseled look. It's possible to maintain their masculinity while altering it favorably, depending on their tastes.

But men in general look appropriate and masculine if their nose and eyebrows have a defined T-shape relationship. Women tend to have more of a C shape, with arched, subtly expressive brows. But when you alter a man's brow, oftentimes that natural T shape can become a C shape, which brings about that strange, feminine look. Jenner has most likely had the latter brand of brow lift, giving his eyebrows a subtly feminine arch. He also had too much fat removed during a blepharoplasty, which has given him a crease and a lid platform that most men just don't have.

The Oh No!
Mickey Rourke's days in the boxing ring have taken their toll, and the movie star has undergone rhinoplasty, correction of a broken cheekbone, blepharoplasty and at least one face lift, which also erased his sideburns — a serious problem when the patient is a man — in an effort to look better. While Rourke is an incredible actor who has shown the depth of his talents in films like *The Wrestler* and *Barfly,* work done by a not-especially-skilled surgeon has ended up making him look bloated and artificial.

What looks like a brow lift, the overaggressive use of chemical peels, and Botox have had a disturbingly clownish effect on the comedian **Carrot Top's** features. With his massive weight-lifting regime, he looks all male from the neck down, but strangely female from the neck up.

My hope is, rather than providing a TMZ-style lambasting, these stories can serve as cautionary tales, to help patients better understand the pitfalls that can snare any of us. At the end of the day, they also point to the great possibilities that truly skillful plastic surgery can afford.

CHIP'S TIPS

1 Plastic surgery began in the early 1800s and was advanced considerably in World War I. Make sure you are being cared for by a surgeon who is current, experienced, and uses modern techniques, such as lasers and endoscopes.

2 The best plastic surgeries are the ones you don't know about, because they are subtle and look natural. Remember that the bizarre aberrations in the news are the exceptions.

3 The earlier you have plastic surgery, the better you will heal, the more natural it will look, and the longer it will last.

4 Follow the trends of the celebrities but don't follow them into the operating room. After all, they are human (and intensely scrutinized) and make some very poor choices (like all of us).

5 Educate yourself. Remember, skin doesn't just stretch and fat doesn't just disappear. All that you need to rejuvenate is within your facial soft tissues, just in a less desirable place.

6 Do not get "over-Botoxed" because you want every wrinkle to be gone. You risk having brows like Spock's, or a droopy lid, or mouth asymmetry.

7 The most natural appearing rejuvenation is achieved by under-going several smaller procedures as you age. Sow as you go and no one will know.

8 Remember a critical difference between fillers and surgery: fillers are always just camouflage and actually correct no anatomic changes. Surgery is the true correction and actually restores the natural anatomy.

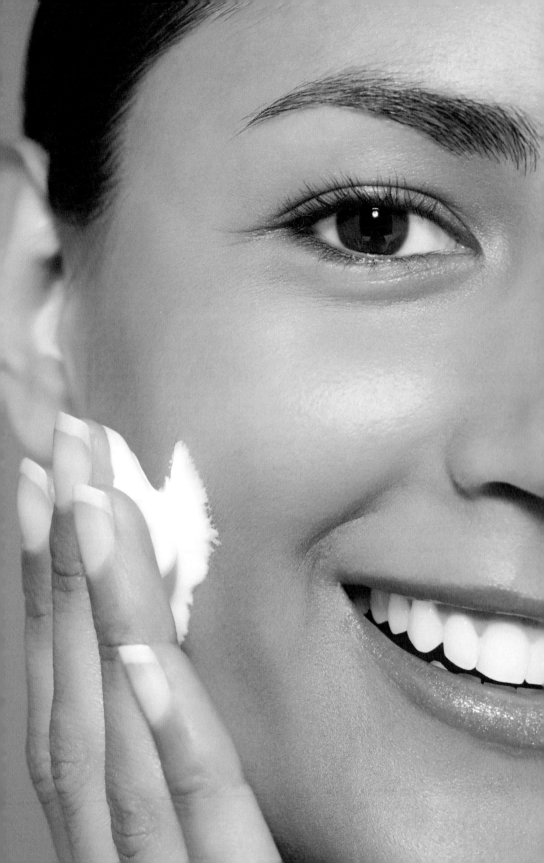

CHAPTER 12

* * *

SLOWING DOWN THE CLOCK:
SKIN-CARE PRODUCTS THAT
GET THE JOB DONE

The bottom line in this chapter is that proper, medically supervised skin care is an absolute necessity. Whether you're in your fresh and dewy teens and just looking for a great skin-care regimen, or in your 50s and looking for skin care that will prolong the results of your surgery, the right skin-care regimen utilizing the right products will make a tremendous difference in the appearance and overall health of your skin.

Skin is an organ—the largest one in the body, in fact. And as such, it encounters the harshest realities of daily life: pollution, sun, changes of weather, and the barrage of sinister products to which we subject ourselves in the quest for better skin.

The key for a proper skin-care regimen is that it be scrupulously followed and consistent, in order to maintain surgical results, especially in the period immediately following a procedure. Equally important is backing up skin care with all the everyday life choices that are reflected in our appearance. Eat healthy, exercise, and drink plenty of water. Keeping your skin hydrated will make fine lines and wrinkles less noticeable and impart that coveted glow of good health.

But first, a word of warning: beware the common misconception that you can find your wrinkle-erasing or acne-eradicating serum on the shelf. I suggest that patients instead turn to their cosmetic surgeon or dermatologist for recommendations tailored to their specific skin needs. The medical-grade products offered by doctors have ingredients that produce a more profound effect than any found in a non-medical setting. Over-the-counter cosmetics — defined as topical products (or those applied directly to the skin) — do not alter the structure or function of the skin, and therefore do not require FDA approval. But medical-grade products must be approved by the Food and Drug Administration, and their makers are held accountable for their safety and results.

SUNSCREEN

If you aren't wearing a daily sunscreen, you're asking for trouble. Trouble in the form of wrinkles. Trouble in the form of dry, ashen, lackluster skin. And trouble in the form of skin cancers of every type, which have become an increasing concern as our environment and atmosphere change (that includes depletion of the ozone layer, which has increased our exposure to dangerous ultraviolet rays).

My advice when selecting a sunscreen is to find one with SPF 30 or greater, whose texture you like. If your sunscreen beads up, turns your face into an oil slick, or adds an unpleasant white hue to your skin, you'll be less likely to use it. Find one you'll be comfortable wearing every day, come rain or come shine, since harmful UVA and UVB rays are always present.

REVISION SKINCARE INTELLISHADE

Anti-aging tinted moisturizer with sunscreen. Matches every skin tone and provides excellent protection.

> When selecting a sunscreen, find one with SPF 30 or even greater, whose texture you like. If your sunscreen beads up, turns your face into an oil slick, or adds an unpleasant white hue to your skin, you'll be less likely to use it.

SKINMEDICA ENVIRONMENTAL DEFENSE SUNSCREEN SPF 50+

An aggressively water-resistant, full-spectrum sunscreen, this SkinMedica winner — free of oil, fragrance, and PABA, and with long-lasting sun protection — provides antioxidant protection against free-radical damage.

JAN MARINI ANTIOXIDANT DAILY FACE PROTECTANT SPF 30

State-of-the-art sun protection and antioxidants are combined in this sunscreen with a light, silky finish that conditions as it protects and keeps skin oil-free throughout the day. It may be used in conjunction with other topical treatments and moisturizers.

KATE SOMERVILLE PROTECT 55 SPF SERUM SUNSCREEN

Because it's a serum, this daily sunscreen from celebrity beauty guru Kate Somerville goes on cleanly and smoothly with no residue and contains anti-aging antioxidants to boot. It also comes in a tinted version.

EXFOLIATION

The accumulation of dead skin cells leads to a variety of skin problems, from acne to dullness of complexion. Exfoliating is increasingly important as we age. Dead skin cells can take their time sloughing off, resulting in dull and tired skin. Alpha hydroxy (AHA) or beta hydroxy (BHA) acid products are especially effective for exfoliating dead skin. Whether through cleansers or creams, adding hydroxy-acid products to your skin-care routine can reveal brighter, clearer skin and result in fewer wrinkles. But both AHA and BHA can increase your sun sensitivity, so make sure you are using a sunscreen in conjunction with these products.

EXFOLIKATE INTENSIVE EXFOLIATING TREATMENT
A powerful exfoliator from Kate Somerville, ExfoliKate uses salicylic acid, microbeads, and fruit enzymes to clean pores and create a healthy glow. However, this product is best avoided by those with very sensitive skin.

SKINMEDICA VITALIZE® PEEL
This physician-grade treatment uses retinoic acid and delivers measurable results after one use, translating to significantly improved skin after several treatments.

SKINMEDICA REJUVENIZE PEEL
An advanced peel with a built-in anti-irritant, the Rejuvenize Peel uses salicylic acid to treat sun damage, pigment changes, and acne scarring, delivering visible results.

SKINMEDICA SKIN POLISHER
If you want to freshen your skin and speed cell turnover, a scrub is a great tool that will help slough away dead skin cells but won't damage your skin. SkinMedica's Skin Polisher has ultra-fine jojoba beads that are perfectly spherical and therefore do not cause microscopic tearing of the skin. This fragrance-free skin polisher lifts dead skin cells without overdrying, damaging, or irritating the skin.

JAN MARINI BIOGLYCOLIC BIOCLEAR
A powerful combination of glycolic acid, salicylic acid, and azelaic acid addresses a variety of skin concerns in this powerful product. This combination of ingredients rapidly clears acne lesions, and follicle size will appear to diminish.

CLEANSERS

This is one skin-care product even my most minimalist patients use. Cleansers are important for removing the day's accumulation of dead skin cells and pollution, but also for their ability to prime the skin — for the beauty maximalists among us — for the abundance of creams, unguents, and serums to come.

For my teenage patients susceptible to acne, I recommend cleansers with the anti-inflammatory ingredient salicylic acid, alternated with a pore-purging cleanser containing benzoyl peroxide. Salicylic acid cleans pores, and benzoyl peroxide eradicates the bacteria that helps blemishes grow.

But perhaps the most important aspect of the cleansing process is making sure you're spending the appropriate amount of time to both work the cleanser into the skin, then remove any residue. I've said it before in this book and I'll say it again: a great tool for making sure the skin gets scrupulously clean is the Clarisonic brush, whose timed cleansing cycle forces you to stand at the sink for two minutes washing your face. For extra insurance, the sonic frequency removes makeup, oil and dirt with a thoroughness that can't be achieved through manual cleansing.

OCULUS LACTICLEANSE
Our LactiCleanse is a great multitasking cleanser for women in their 40s and 50s, because it kills two birds with one stone. LactiCleanse contains the alpha-hydroxy lactic acid, which is quite hydrating to the skin, and a mild exfoliant to speed skin-cell turnover, resulting in a good, thorough cleanse.

JAN MARINI BIOGLYCOLIC FACIAL CLEANSER
A great cleanser for all skin types, this soap-free, non-irritating cleanser incorporates a glycolic acid for a substantial, deep cleanse, making toner or astringent unnecessary.

JAN MARINI C-ESTA CLEANSING GEL
Suitable for all skin types (including oily and sensitive skin), this cleanser also prepares skin for the application of other C-ESTA serums and creams. This treatment can be especially beneficial when used following chemical peels and CO_2 laser resurfacing, where cleansers with glycolic acid may not be appropriate.

OCULUS SKIN CARE MULTI-HA FOAMING CLEANSER
With 2 percent salicylic acid combined with glycolic acid, this cleanser works beautifully for patients with acne-prone and oily skin.

OCULUS SKIN CARE LACTICLEANSE

This creamy cleanser, ideal for dry skin but also useful for normal skin, moisturizes with lactic acid, petrolatum and sodium PCA. It's especially beneficial for patients experiencing dry skin as a result of products or procedures.

OCULUS SKIN CARE ROSACLEANSE FOAM CLEANSER

An extra-gentle, 100 percent fragrance-free cleanser formulated for redness-prone and sensitive skin. The cleanser contains Evodiox, a powerful redness-reducing agent derived from the Chinese *Evodia rutaecarpa* plant.

MOISTURIZERS

The greatest benefit of working with next-generation skin-care products is their ability to multitask. A good moisturizer can perform a variety of functions — from exfoliation to free-radical control and sun protection — in one bottle. Whether your skin is oily, dry, or somewhere in the middle, a good moisturizer, especially one with some SPF protection, is critical. As with a good sunscreen, finding a texture that suits your skin will encourage you to use it more often.

SKINMEDICA 15% AHA/BHA

This moisturizer for all skin types contains both AHAs and BHAs. As a value add, it also exfoliates and removes dead skin cells, allowing fresh, young cells to surface. It also nourishes and protects skin from free-radical damage with vitamins and antioxidants. A side note: because it contains alpha-hydroxy acid, realize that this product could increase sun sensitivity.

REVISION® SKINCARE INTELLISHADE® BROAD-SPECTRUM SPF 45

This daily three-in-one acts as an anti-aging moisturizer, sunscreen, and mineral tint. This product stands out because it is formulated with advanced peptides, including palmitoyl tripeptide-5, to reduce fine lines and wrinkles.

JAN MARINI TRANSFORMATION FACE CREAM

I really like Jan Marini Transformation Face Cream, which has plant growth factors that are healing to the skin but not quite as expensive as the human growth factors.

SKINMEDICA ULTRA SHEER MOISTURIZER

This oil- and fragrance-free moisturizer uses antioxidant vitamins C and E to protect against free-radical damage.

SKINMEDICA TNS BODY LOTION
This silky lotion, appropriate for all skin types, improves the quality of aging and sun-damaged skin. It's wise to treat the whole body, not just the face.

OCULUS SKIN CARE VITAMIN B3/NIACINAMIDE
This topical vitamin B product can greatly aid in promoting cellular repair. It can help create a barrier to skin aging and damage from pollutants and other irritants and can also help inflammatory skin conditions such as rosacea and acne.

OCULUS SKIN CARE NIARICHE
An intensive moisturizer, NiaRiche is blended with 5 percent of the powerful cell-repairing, anti-aging B3/niacinamide ingredient, making it ideal for dry, sensitive, and photo-damaged skin (from exposure to sunlight).

SPOT TREATMENTS

THE TANDA ZAP
The Tanda Zap is a powerful blue light that destroys acne-causing bacteria. It uses gentle vibration and warmth to open pores and kill bacteria.

OCULUS SKIN CARE BLEMERASE TOUCHSTICK AND BLEMERASE CONCEALER
In this unique two-step process, the BlemErase TouchStick rapidly resolves active breakouts and inflammation, while the BlemErase Concealer helps reduce the appearance of redness.

JANE IREDALE DISAPPEAR CONCEALER
A great multifunction concealer, this one contains green-tea extracts to help treat blemishes, even as it hides them.

TONERS

Though some consider toner an unnecessary skin-care step, many current toners perform multiple functions that can justify this addition to your daily routine. For many patients, toners are also the opportunity, between skin-exfoliation sessions, to clear the skin of clogging, complexion-dulling detritus.

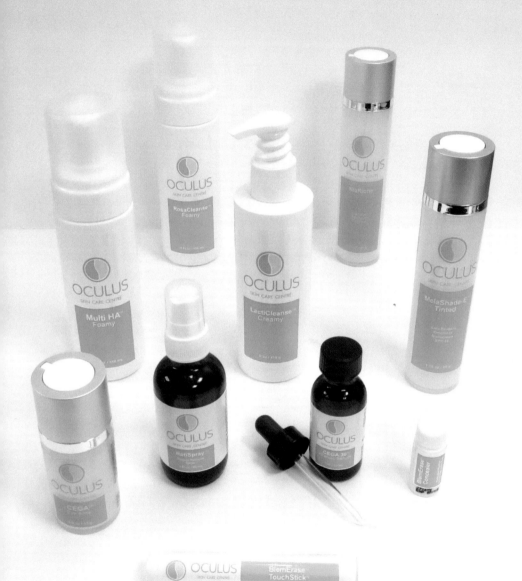

REVISION SKINCARE EXFOLIATING FACIAL RINSE

A good toner can deeply clean pores and revitalize dull skin. This concentrated product contains not only glycolic acid and salicylic acid but also aloe vera and a blend of marine seaweed.

REVISION SKINCARE SOOTHING FACIAL RINSE

This rinse is perfect to calm skin. An oil-free blend, it gently hydrates and conditions the skin with Arnica Montana, grape seed and vitamin K. Most important, it restores your skin to the correct pH level after cleansing.

RETINOLS

Retinols, which are a form of vitamin A, have become the go-to skin-care treatment for their ability — when absorbed into the skin — to speed skin-cell turnover. What that means is unclogged pores, the reduction of fine lines, and more-even skin tone. These are all tremendous pluses in making skin look refreshed, healthy, and glowing. Prescription-strength retinoids include Differin, Retin-A, Renova, Avage, Tazorac, Atralin, and Avita. If you have not yet incorporated a retinol into your beauty routine, now is the time to begin a retinol regime — ASAP. It's money well spent: the beauty of retinols is that they deliver visible results by impacting the cell architecture and not just the skin surface.

> Retinols speed skin cell turnover, which means unclogged pores, the reduction of fine lines and more-even skin tone, big pluses in making skin look refreshed, healthy and glowing.

RETIN-A

While Retin-A is an appropriate treatment for women worried about wrinkles, this topical prescription retinol is also quite useful for teenagers suffering from acne. Retin-A speeds cell turnover double-time, rapidly clearing the way for gunk to stay out of your pores. You might expect some redness, irritation and flakiness when you first begin using this product, but with time most of those side effects should go away.

Be extra vigilant to avoid the sun, making sure to use a sunscreen during the day. Retin-A will increase your skin's sensitivity to the sun, making it more susceptible to burning, so extra caution is advised. If you're older and already use Retin-A, but want to see enhanced results, it could be time to up the strength and frequency of your application, from every other day to every day, or from daily to twice daily, depending upon your skin's tolerance. Some patients are able to tolerate such frequency, while others will find it leads to greater photosensitivity, peeling, or flaking.

SKINMEDICA TRI-RETINOL COMPLEX ES

If you'd rather not use Retin-A, this SkinMedica retinol can do wonders in treating the fine lines and wrinkles that can begin to crop up as you enter your 30s. The three forms of vitamin A in this microdelivery system improve the appearance of fine lines resulting from sun damage and aging. Tri-Retinol also enhances skin texture and accelerates exfoliation.

OCULUS SKIN CARE RETISILC

RetiSilc is the first low-dose retinoid formulated for sensitive and redness-prone skin. Retinoids may help reverse certain kinds of chronic redness by promoting the growth of new collagen. Lipids are essential in cell-barrier function. The two main components are fatty acid — such as Omega-6 linoleic acid — and the restoration of epidermal ceramides (also found in a diet that's rich in linoleic acids). RetiSilc contains this unique combination of ceramides and fatty acids that help restore this essential barrier function. This product has a fragrance-free, preservative-free, silicone-based vehicle that improves retinoid tolerance.

COSMETIC AND SPECIALTY TREATMENTS

LATISSE

There are a number of steps you can take to restore thinning or sparse lashes, including using Latisse, a prescription treatment that can restore the length and fullness of lashes. Latisse is not FDA approved for use on the eyebrows, so patients are advised to discuss potential side effects (which could include darkening of the skin) with their doctor before using Latisse in this off-label way.

JANE IREDALE MAKEUP

I recommend the Jane Iredale line of cosmetics to all my patients for its non-comedogenic quality. I like this line because it's free of oil, talc, dyes, parabens, preservatives, and irritating fragrance, all of which can aggravate skin. The powders and foundations also include sun protection, which is a great added value.

SKINMEDICA REDNESS RELIEF CALMPLEX

Clinically proven to decrease skin redness without clogging pores, this Redness Relief CalmPlex offers visible results in as few as two weeks, while enhancing radiant skin.

OCULUS SKIN CARE ROSAGEL

A skin-soothing gel for those with sensitive, redness-prone skin, this combination therapy uses vitamin K, required for blood clotting, and aids in minimizing the appearance of small capillaries that have enlarged under the skin. Free of irritants, preservatives, fragrances, and emulsifiers, this product is well tolerated by patients with sensitive skin.

SERUMS

Serums are your secret weapon against aging. They add a little extra dose of protection and nurturing that skin enjoys as it ages. They protect the skin from the ravages of time, while delivering nutrients deep into the layers of the skin. Unlike moisturizers, a serum has specific tasks that it performs, from combating fine lines to brightening skin to fighting acne. It's applied after toner and before your moisturizer, so it sinks into the skin and really delivers its beneficial ingredients.

JAN MARINI C-ESTA SERUM

The importance of vitamin C increases as you grow older. A daily vitamin C supplement taken orally, as well as the antioxidant properties of a topical vitamin C serum, are both critical as we age. Known to stimulate the body's production of collagen, vitamin C can also aid healing, combat inflammation, and strengthen the skin. The best topical vitamin C is vitamin C-ester, which is more easily absorbed into the skin and will not irritate. A good option is Jan Marini C-ESTA Face Serum, applied twice a day to both face and neck, to help repair sun damage. It can visibly reduce the appearance of deep lines and leave skin looking healthier, smoother and more supple. Skin tone will also become more even. As an added plus, C-ESTA Serum is compatible with glycolic acid and Retin-A.

OCULUS SKIN CARE CEGA 30+FERULIC SERUM

Part of the Oculus CEGA line of products, containing the only form of vitamin C clinically proven to increase collagen production, this serum for normal to oily skin types is a powerful anti-aging weapon.

JAN MARINI TRANSFORMATION FACE SERUM

For smoother and more refined skin texture, this oil-free, non-comedogenic serum with hyaluronic acid is quickly absorbed and helps prevent many signs of skin aging.

REVISION SKIN-CARE HYDRATING SERUM

This 100 percent oil-free moisturizer is for all skin types, but it's especially useful for oily skin that needs moisture without greasiness. The Revision Hydrating Serum contains the anti-aging ingredients palmitoyl tripeptide-3 and hydrolyzed hazelnut protein — as well as pomegranate extract and vitamin E to protect skin from free-radical damage — all in a lightweight, water-based product. Honey and sea-kelp extract are included for skin nourishment. If used during the daytime as a moisturizer, be sure to add a sunscreen for full protection.

HUMAN GROWTH FACTOR

If you're going to spend money on skin-care products, you might as well put it where it counts, on the human growth factors that actually impact cell architecture (and not just the surface) of the skin. Originally used to aid in the healing of wounds, human growth factor originates from human tissue reproduced in a lab. Though it all sounds slightly sci-fi, the possibilities of this new technology to stimulate collagen production in the skin are amazing. Newly repurposed for cosmetic use, anti-aging human growth factors can be a great option for women in their 40s and 50s. Human growth factor tricks your skin into thinking it's younger than it is. It stimulates collagen production, getting rid of fine lines, wrinkles and brown spots. And unlike Retin-A, which can cause irritation and flaking in some women, human growth factor is healing and therapeutic to the skin. It's typically applied two times a day, in gel form. I recommend that women start using a topical human growth factor in their 40s to stimulate collagen production and get rid of fine lines, wrinkles and brown spots.

SKINMEDICA TNS ESSENTIAL SERUM

This truly essential all-in-one anti-aging serum contains human growth factor, antioxidants, and peptides. It combats fine lines and wrinkles, improving skin tone and texture.

JAN MARINI TRANSFORMATION FACE CREAM

Using a patented transforming growth factor, this cream contains hyaluronic acid, which stimulates collagen and elastin production and results in healthier, more youthful skin. It also aids in healing, making it good for post-procedure use.

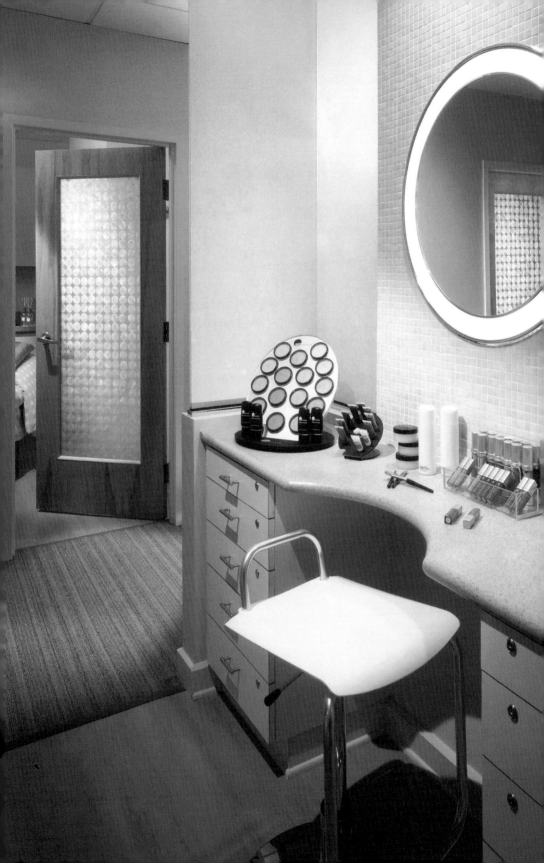

SKINMEDICA TNS RECOVERY COMPLEX

Used twice a day on the face, neck, and décolletage (fancy French for chest area), this gel utilizes human growth factors to naturally regenerate the skin. Recovery Complex enhances skin texture and strengthens elasticity, minimizing wrinkles and age spots.

SKIN LIGHTENERS

OCULUS SKIN CARE TRIPLE BLEACH

With hormonal changes, pregnancy, and aging come changes to the skin's pigmentation, which can be treated with a variety of bleaching creams in low, medium and heavy strengths. At our office, we have what I think of as a "high-tech" triple-bleaching cream, manufactured by Concord Pharmacy, which uses a combination of a steroid, hydroquinone, and tretinoin (similar to Retin-A) to penetrate the skin's surface. I also recommend the product for skin lightening, with a typical treatment cycle of four months on, four months off. This works wonders for brown spots and acne scarring.

WRINKLE TREATMENTS

With age comes wisdom and wrinkles. Whether you're concerned about the fine lines that form around the eyes or the deeper wrinkles that can affect the forehead or the skin between the eyes, a medical-grade anti-wrinkle product can plump up, smooth, and otherwise lessen the appearance of lines, in lieu of a surgical procedure.

JAN MARINI C-ESTA EYE REPAIR CONCENTRATE

This concentrate rejuvenates thin, delicate skin around the eye area to reduce the appearance of fine lines and wrinkles. It repairs free-radical damage, tightening and defining the eye area with increased collagen production.

SKINMEDICA TNS EYE REPAIR

Using human growth factor and peptides, this twice-daily eye cream helps enhance skin firmness and elasticity, diminishing the appearance of fine lines and wrinkles, and reducing the appearance of dark circles.

SKINMEDICA TNS LIP-PLUMP SYSTEM

Rejuvenating growth factors yield pillowy lips and help enhance skin texture. This two-part system includes a lip plumper with a natural lip gloss to increase volume.

JAN MARINI C-ESTA CREAM

An evening product meant to complement daytime use of Jan Marini C-ESTA Serum, this cream decreases the appearance of fine lines and moderate wrinkles, and helps to tighten and define the skin.

JAN MARINI C-ESTA EYE CONTOUR CREAM

Using topically absorbed vitamin C, this rich cream smooths the delicate eye area while lessening the appearance of under-eye circles and increasing elasticity. It's suitable for all skin types, and generally is applied every morning and evening.

Whether you're concerned about fine lines, deeper wrinkles, or the skin between the eyes, medical-grade anti-wrinkle products can plump up, smooth and otherwise lessen the appearance of lines, in lieu of surgery.

JAN MARINI AGE INTERVENTION FACE CREAM

This face cream combats hormonal imbalances and skin damage that increase the appearance of skin aging. It targets skin inflammation and boosts the skin's ability to repair damage, restoring suppleness and elasticity.

REVISION SKINCARE LUMIQUIN®

This hand cream tackles an often-neglected element of the aging-skin equation: it targets discoloration, textural changes, and skin dryness via lightening agents while dramatically improving the appearance of aged and sun-damaged hands.

REVISION SKINCARE NECTIFIRM

Nectifirm is an advanced new technology for firming and tightening the neck and décolletage, while smoothing roughness and crepey skin. It's the only product on the market that actually addresses the signs of aging on the neck. Nectifirm caters to the neck's specific needs with eight ingredients working together to help strengthen the dermal-epidermal junction. It's suitable for all skin types.

OCULUS DAILY LONGEVITY VITAMINS

These vegetarian capsules are formulated with antioxidants in a powerful fruit and vegetable base.

OCULUS SKIN CARE CEGA 30 EYE AREA

Part of the Oculus CEGA line of products, this product contains the only form of vitamin C clinically proven to increase collagen production. This eye-treatment contains vitamins C and E, green tea, and a synthetic peptide — acetyl hexapeptide-3 — used to relax muscles and smooth skin wrinkles.

OCULUS SKIN CARE TEADERMA PADS

TeaDerma Pads contain the first commercially available form of topical epigallo-catechin gallate (EGCG) the most biologically active component of green tea. EGCG is associated with a variety of biological benefits, including free-radical scavenging, inflammation reduction, and UVA/UVB photo protection. The antioxidant activity of EGCG is approximately 100 times that of vitamin C (and 25 times that of vitamin E) for protecting cells and DNA from damage.

POST-SURGERY TREATMENTS

Many patients mistakenly believe they can relax when their surgery is over and become a little complacent in their skin-care regimen. In fact, the post-surgery period is a time to be ultra-attentive to skin care. Proper skin care will extend the benefits of a surgical or nonsurgical procedure and help the skin recover from the trauma of surgery. To bring back a healthy luster to the skin, to combat scarring and to help the skin bounce back, some form of special post-surgical treatment is important. Here are a few:

BIOCORNEUM

This self-adhering, self-drying silicone cream with SPF 30 will help speed the recovery process and heal scars. If you have a tendency to form hypertrophic post-surgery scars, bioCorneum can break up scar tissue, flattening and smoothing scars and reducing discoloration when applied twice daily for twelve weeks.

SKINMEDICA TNS CERAMIDE TREATMENT CREAM

For dramatic, rich moisturizing of post-procedure skin, this combination of human growth factor and peptides restores the skin's defensive barrier and moisture balance.

SKINMEDICA POST-PROCEDURE SYSTEM

Here's a comprehensive, clinically tested post-treatment system, best used as a follow-up to laser resurfacing and chemical peels. As an added benefit, the Skin-Medica Post-Procedure System can help patients who tend to suffer acne breakouts following skin procedures. The system, which should be used only under the watchful eye of your doctor, includes a Sensitive Skin Cleanser, Restorative Ointment, TNS Ceramide Treatment Cream, and Environmental Defense Sunscreen SPF 30+.

OCULUS SKIN CARE SOOTHING BALM

With the healing benefits of .7 percent hydrocortisone in an emollient, silicone-elastomer gel base, this ointment feels like a silky cream but has the purity of an ointment. The balm is ideal for post-care following in-office peels, microdermabrasion, and light, non-ablative laser treatments. The Oculus Soothing Balm is also preservative, solvent, and fragrance free.

BALANCE

In many ways, balance has been the theme of this book — balancing your nutrition, your time, your features, your healing. This ethereal balance can be considered the link between "turning back the clock" and "slowing it down going forward," an approach that ultimately leads to what I call true facial harmony.

CHIP'S TIPS

1 Skin care is like brushing your teeth: you need to do it consistently and effectively to get the best results.

2 Sunscreen (SPF 30 or more) is not an option. We all need to salvage our skin from the poor choices we made as teenagers, when we applied the baby oil and the iodine — then baked on a reflective blanket!

3 Retinols, which are a form of vitamin A, are the go-to skin-care treatment. They speed skin-cell turnover, which reduces fine lines, unclogs pores, and evens out skin tone.

4 Latisse is FDA approved for sparse lashes and will thicken, darken, and lengthen your lashes.

5 Human growth factors are the most significant advancement in skin-cell architecture. These gel products are pricey but worth the investment.

6 With age comes wisdom and wrinkles. Physician prescribed skin care will reduce the wrinkles. Laser surgery will essentially eliminate the wrinkles. Both allow you to keep the wisdom.

7 Surgery can "turn back the clock"; skin care is perfect for "slowing it down going forward." Both will give you true facial harmony.

8 "You are what you eat." Your skin needs proper fuel (like the rest of your body). Those moms just get smarter as we get older!

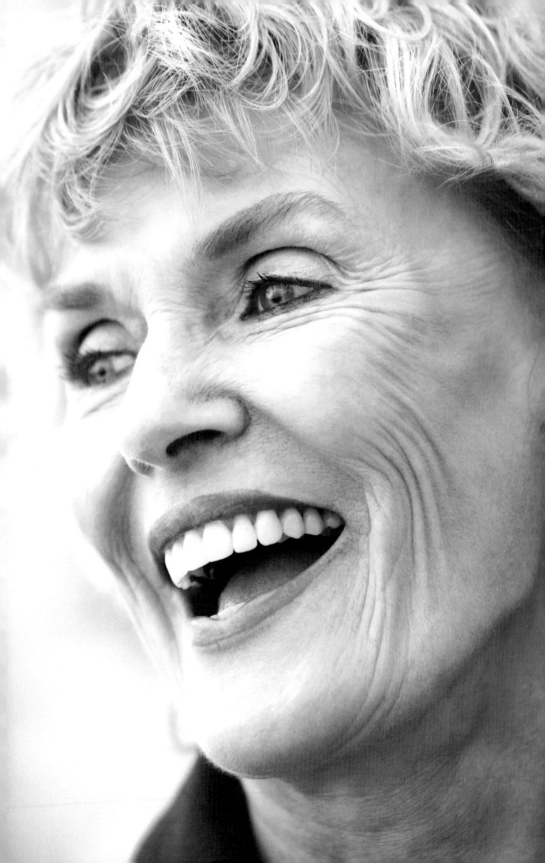

CHAPTER 13

* * *

TURNING BACK THE CLOCK:
WHY SURGERY OFFERS
THE BIGGEST BANG FOR YOUR BUCK

"Everything will be okay in the end. If it's not okay, it's not the end."
—*John Lennon*

After months (or perhaps years) of thinking about it, you've finally decided to have surgery. It's a big decision. The best thing you can do at this point is to take the proper steps to ensure that you're prepared both for the surgery and for your recovery.

Let me reassure you that if you have done your research, chosen a great surgeon, and have realistic expectations, you're going to be happy with the decision you've made. No product — no injectable, no cream, no magic tincture — is going to offer the dramatic results and satisfaction of surgery.

On the run-up to childbirth, parents anxiously plan for and await their newborn's arrival. They decorate the nursery, shop for baby clothes, and read *What to Expect When You're Expecting*, overlooking no detail in preparing for the arrival of their child. But often when the baby arrives, they're flummoxed. While they've prepared for the immediate realities of a baby crib and tiny onesies, they haven't prepared for longer-term issues, and all the little surprises that come along down the road.

The same is often true with surgery. We put all of our time and effort into the front end, doing months of late-night research on our desired procedure. But we can often neglect the important back-end details — proper nutrition, rest, recovery — that are so essential.

This chapter is intended to prepare you for both sides of the surgery equation: the prep work and also the follow-through, both of which will make a sizeable difference in how you heal and recover.

PLANNING AHEAD

Below are a number of steps you should take before you walk into that hospital room or surgical suite, to ensure that you have everything in place for a comfortable and speedy recovery. You shouldn't have to race to Walgreens with your face covered in gauze to refill a prescription or to suddenly realize that there are no easy meals to prepare in your kitchen at home. Follow this checklist and you will go into surgery feeling confident and ready for any contingency.

• See your Primary Care Physician (PCP) to ensure that you are physically fit to undergo surgery.
• Divulge all previous surgeries, medical conditions, medications or supplements; and any drug, cigarette or alcohol usage to your doctor. All of these factors can complicate your surgery and need to be accounted for by your doctor.
• Understand any potential risks, both extreme (like infection or death) and minor (including scarring or the need for further surgery).
• Be especially mindful of your health in the weeks leading up to surgery. Eat plenty of fruits and vegetables and drink lots of water.
• Make sure you discuss the anticipated recovery time with your doctor, and understand any possible complications or warning signs to look for during your recovery. An educated patient can avoid surprises.
• Two weeks before surgery, if you aren't already taking a multivitamin, begin doing so. After surgery, your doctor may recommend supplements such as selenium, vitamins A, B, C, D, and K, bromelain, iron, and zinc.
• Do not take aspirin products, vitamin E, or alcohol two weeks prior to surgery.
• Ask your doctor about any herbal supplements you take and whether they should be discontinued during the surgery preparation and recovery time.
• If you are a smoker, avoid smoking for at least two weeks prior to surgery and for at least two weeks after surgery. Smoking seriously impedes blood flow, increases inflammation, and inhibits healing. Smoking increases the risk of cardiac arrest, stroke, and heart attack during surgery and creates a higher post-surgery infection rate. If you can make it all that time without a cigarette, consider quitting in the long term. You will see a remarkable improvement not just in your overall health, but in your looks.
• Check with your health insurance company if you are expecting full or partial coverage for your surgery to ensure that they've received any information or paperwork they require. There's nothing worse than having to deal with insurance-company red tape while you're trying to recover from surgery.

- Have a responsible adult on hand to provide overnight care for the first 24 hours after your surgery. And beyond those 24 hours, it's recommended that you have a family member or friend on hand for the first few days to aid in your recovery. If your caregiver will be helping you with medication, make sure they understand the instructions for its use.
- Make a list of tasks for your caregiver, such as pet feeding, bill paying and children's activity schedules.
- Program your phone with a list of emergency numbers for yourself and your caregiver.
- Arrange for someone to help with children and pets during your early recovery days to avoid stressing yourself, or them.
- Fill prescriptions for any postoperative medications your doctor has prescribed. Place them in a dated pill caddy for easy access on your bedside table.
- Prepare your home for recovery. If your caregiver needs to leave after 24 hours, have plenty of healthy prepared foods on hand.
- Equip your bedside with tissues, cold compresses, Tylenol, bottled water, bendable straws for drinking, crackers, a towel to protect your pillow, and any other supplies you might need.
- If your surgery is extensive and you are unable to have friends or family assist you, consider an in-home post-operative health-care professional. Your doctor should be able to provide you with a list of qualified home-care providers.
- Two weeks prior to your surgery, check with your doctor to find out if any current medications or supplements should be discontinued.
- Have your house cleaned before your surgery, so you aren't tempted to straighten up when you should be recovering, and so that you return to a neat, welcoming space after your surgery.
- Plug in a night-light to help you find your way to the bathroom.
- Stock up on easily prepared, soothing foods such as protein shakes, yogurt, juice, oatmeal, applesauce, Jell-O, and soup.
- While the temptation may be there, especially for women, the period following a procedure is *not* the time to tackle a weight-loss program. Your body needs proper nutrition as it heals.

Avoid smoking for at least two weeks prior to surgery and for at least two weeks after surgery. Smoking seriously impedes blood flow, greatly increases inflammation, and inhibits the healing process.

- Buy several bags of frozen peas or berries to use as an ice pack.
- Make sure your TV remote and cell phone are charged and within easy reach of your bedside table.
- Stock up on DVDs, audio books, magazines, and other entertainment to help pass the time during your recovery.
- Put fresh sheets on your bed, extra pillows for support, and a comfortable blanket close by.
- Make sure you are stocked up on paper towels, toilet paper, and other staples you need for daily life.
- If you will need to change your bandages, stock up on supplies such as gauze and antibiotic creams.
- If you don't have some already, invest in a comfortable pair of slippers with non-slip soles.
- Have hair colored. For some facial procedures, such as brow lifts, you won't be able to color your hair for a month after surgery.
- Prepare for transportation following surgery.

THE COUNTDOWN

As you count down the hours until your surgery, you will want to take certain precautions. You will also need to follow these instructions to make sure your doctor can perform your surgery safely.

- Avoid food and drink eight hours before your scheduled surgery.
- Try to get a good night's sleep before the day of your surgery.
- If you take medication for high blood pressure or a heart condition, you may take this medicine the morning of the surgery with only a small sip of water to wash it down.
- Avoid taking water pills or diuretics the day of your surgery.
- Do not take any kind of oral anti-diabetic medication or inject insulin on the day of your surgery.
- Wash your hair the night before surgery, since it may be several days before you're able to shower again.
- Do not apply deodorant or perfume near the surgery site.
- Do not wear makeup or nail polish.
- Wear a button-down shirt so you won't need to pull your shirt over your head following the procedure.
- Leave all valuables and jewelry at home.

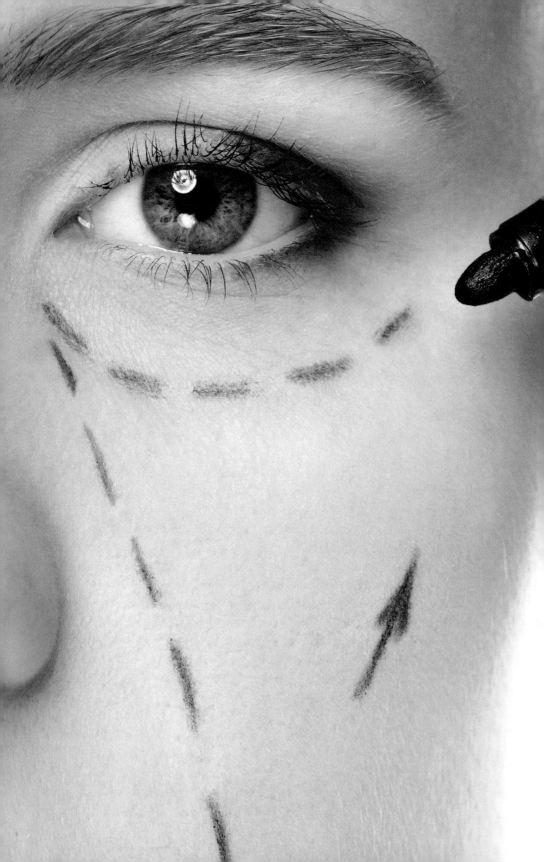

RECOVERY

As I've said again and again, surgery is serious business. Despite how youthful, healthy and rarin' to go you may feel, your body needs time to recover from the trauma of surgery. Be sure to follow your doctor's advice to the letter. And this is the perfect opportunity to take a little break. We all tend to lead overstressed, busy lives, but this is a time to slow down and take it easy. Look on the bright side: what better excuse will you have to read, watch movies, and nap whenever you like?

I'll be completely honest with you: surgery is often not a bed of roses. The healing process for the human body is a miraculous one but it can also be associated with pain. In the end, however, you're going to end up loving both yourself and your surgeon. These reactions aren't limited to lay people either. Recently, I had an ear, nose, and throat plastic surgeon as a patient. He came to me to have his eyes done and to have a face lift. He's been in this business for 30 years. For the first month following the procedure, he was quite upset. He regretted doing it. He was angry with me. A month later, though, he came into the office with a bottle of wine, truffles, candy, and lunch for my entire staff, along with an apology. He told me: "You did an A-1 perfect job."

Everyone, even doctors in the industry, will have the same basic human emotions and psychological reactions following surgery. But the key to maximizing healing after a procedure is to be strategic partners with your doctor in the endeavor.

Before I ever schedule a procedure with any patient, I always educate them up front, in writing, about the specifics of what they're about to go through. This helps both of us a lot. Everyone goes through what I call a love/hate/love relationship with their plastic surgeon. Many patients have come back to me and said, "This was actually so much easier than you told me it would be."

That's gratifying to hear. I always want my patients to be prepared, though. I want them to know the realities about the bruising, how they're going to feel, and how the surgery affects their endorphins. I'll discuss the mind/body connection with them and highlight the importance of positive thinking. I'll tell you: "We're a team, walking through this together, and I'll do everything I can to support you."

We live in such an instant-gratification society these days. Everything is "On Demand." However, there is no "On-Demand Healing" button on your TV remote.

Another obstacle docs deal a lot with these days is the proliferation of disclaimers being slapped on everything. Look at the drug ads on television. Fifty percent of the advertising time is spent on content. And the other 50 percent? It's spent on disclaimers. You can't order a cup of coffee without getting a disclaimer nowadays. As a result, we've become a society that tunes them out. We know the risks are there but we don't want to pay attention to them. We've become desensitized to the dangers stated in disclaimers.

For example, nobody thinks twice about taking a baby aspirin daily. The next time you take out that aspirin bottle, take a look at all the side-effects warnings on the back label. When you Google the words "aspirin side effects," 3 million results pop up. Potential side effects are so extensive that many aspirin manufacturers have taken to using peel-back, double-sided labels to fit them all on the bottle!

When you come to me as a patient, you're going to receive all the information you need about the risks associated with your procedure, along with a realistic idea about healing and recovery time frames. A lot of communication and some hand-holding, along with a great support staff, help immensely.

But we still have what I call the "frustration period" to get through: that hurry-up-and-wait period directly after surgery. It's important to have realistic expectations. Even with laser resurfacing, there's a stretch of about a week where you'll probably want to take some time off work. You'll want to use a little makeup on your face to camouflage what is going to resemble a sunburn. And expectations and recovery times are going to be different for each person, depending on age and gender.

When women have a major procedure, most approach it proactively, so they know to book an at-home nurse for two nights. But a lot of men think they can still make that dinner reservation the same night. Chances are good that you're not going to even be in the mood to eat, let alone be up for socializing in public at a restaurant. Sometimes, I have to tell the men, "No golf for two weeks (unless it's *miniature* golf)."

We live in such an instant gratification society these days. Everything is "On Demand." But, you have to remember there is no "On-Demand healing" button on your TV remote.

I'm always grateful when a wife comes in with the husband following a procedure; she can become an important ally in his healing. The wives end up telling their husbands: "Did you hear that, honey? You can't jog for a week. You can't lift weights for two weeks." They're helping me look out for him.

My staff is always available for any questions following a procedure, and they'll follow up with you as you recover, as well, just to make sure you're applying that ice pack and taking your antibiotics. I'm also available, 24/7/365, and I mean that.

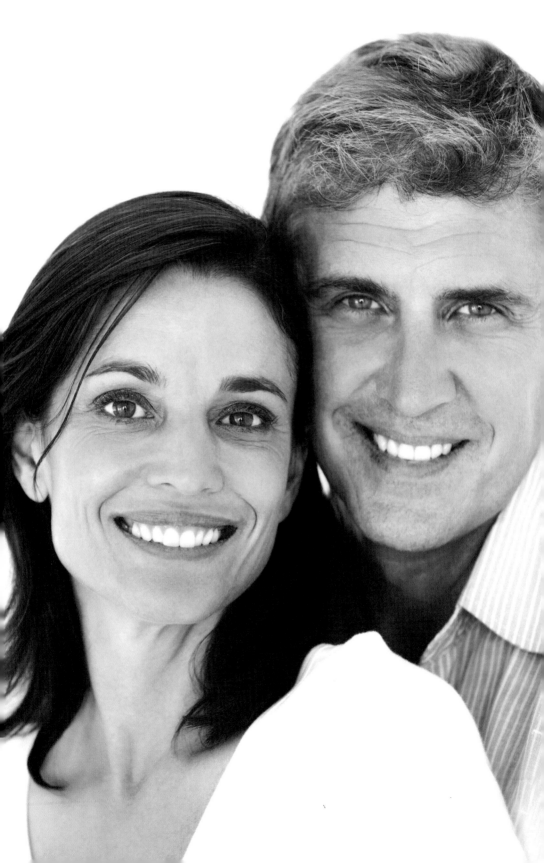

The general rule with most of us in the industry is this: If you're still a little mad at your plastic surgeon, it's because you haven't finished healing yet. Healing takes time and there's just no rushing it. Of course, that's not always going to be easy in our fast-paced, instant-gratification culture. But it's crucial that you prepare for some downtime. And by downtime, I don't mean cleaning out the closets or straightening up the garage. It's not the time for at-home busy work. I don't want you bringing a pile of work home from the office.

If you've had facial surgery, there will be swelling around the eyes. The cornea may also be swollen, causing light rays to bend differently. Your eyesight may be a bit blurry at first. You're probably OK to answer e-mails, but you need to avoid detailed reading. As much as you might want to, I wouldn't recommend sitting down with that stack of novels you've been meaning to get to. Rest and recovery means resting the entire mind-body.

In other words, put your butt on the couch or in the bed. Line up some movies or TV shows on demand or listen to those audio books you've been meaning to get to. Catch up with friends via speaker phone or headset. (If you've had facial surgery, I don't want you spending a lot of time leaning to one side while on the phone).

I've also had groups of girlfriends, or husbands and wives, who've had procedures at the same time. It's actually a lot of fun to recover together and go through the experience with someone. You'd be amazed at the number of couples, friends, mothers and daughters who book their procedures together. They support one another throughout the process.

Oftentimes when you step away from your routine, co-workers or friends will want to know the details. It's up to you to decide how much you want to tell people. I always recommend just to spool out a few tidbits of information — you don't need to feel like you're going to confession. It's OK to be general, and using certain buzz words can be helpful. You can say, "I had a little laser work done." People won't know how to react, and therefore will be more likely to let it go at that.

Patients can sometimes get very creative when they don't necessarily want to reveal to the world that they've had some work done. They tell their friends: "I had a precancerous skin lesion removed." As soon as they mention the word "cancer," people automatically change the subject, and they're in the clear. Other patients who have experienced some facial swelling tell friends they had sinus surgery, or they blame it on a wisdom-tooth removal. Some have also been known to shop for a new set of glasses or a new hairstyle or cut. When their friends or co-workers see them, they're giving them something else to focus on. It's a bit of a fun decoy.

It surprises me that the social stigma about having plastic surgery or a youth-enhancing procedure persists today. It may go back to how we were raised. Many of us grew up in the generation where we didn't realize our parents argued. They only had disagreements behind closed doors, away from the kids. Consequently, we grew up and were surprised when we got into open disagreements with each other, until our parents let us in on their little secret.

It's the same with cosmetic surgery. Nobody discusses it but everyone's doing it. I always joke, nobody ever knows about my best work. Except for the person who matters most: the patient.

It might also help to know that some patients experience depression in the days following surgery. They may be anxious about their surgery results or fearful about complications, worried about finances, or have trouble adjusting to their new look. This is normal, and like the bruising and the discomfort, this too shall pass. Let your loved ones and your partner know if you're worried and need their support. I also recommend keeping a "before" photo at your bedside. You may need reminding of the real reason you're lying in your bed and eating nothing but soup and Jell-O for a few days (remember how much you hated those jowls, drooping eyelids, and descending features?). Also remember that bruising and swelling are only temporary. You may look bad initially, as the stress of surgery on your body begins to subside. But don't panic: you made the right decision. And don't worry about this hiccup in your routine following surgery. It can be hard to adjust, especially if you're one of those high-powered, type-A personalities. Instead, look at your recovery as an opportunity — a chance to watch last year's Academy Award–winning films. Make recovery a pleasure and you'll be surprised how quickly the time will pass.

I know I've done my job when my patients come back in following a procedure acting differently. They walk with more confidence, a little spring in their step, a sparkle in their eye. I can notice a physical shift, not only in their appearance but also in their attitude. There's been a life change. That's when I know for certain that I've gotten my patient closer to the ultimate goal: achieving inner beauty.

THINGS TO REMEMBER AS YOU RECOVER

1   Ask your doctor about supplements that may aid in your healing and recovery.
2   Drink plenty of fluids.
3   Don't stress your body with heavy lifting, exercise or housecleaning.
4   Men: avoid shaving until your doctor gives you the go-ahead.
5   Feed your body the right foods to promote healing.
6   Limit visitors. Too many friends or neighbors stopping by to check on you can be exhausting and add to your stress level.
7   Avoid the sun.
8   Don't diet. Your body heals best when it is properly nourished.
9   Avoid salt, alcohol, smoking and spicy foods.

Complaint: Denise and Thomas are husband-and-wife physicians who came from Kentucky to see me. Thomas was interested in cosmetic enhancement, primarily around the eye region. He volunteered that he had worked very hard throughout his career but had begun receiving comments from his patients that he always looked tired and didn't seem as jovial as he had a decade earlier.

Upon examination, he showed prolapse of the fatty cushions to the upper and lower lids, giving him a shadowed appearance and a look of fatigue around the eyes. He had contour changes to both lower lids and had downward descent of his cheek region. He also had loss of contour to his neckline and jawline, and a chin that doubled over onto his shirt collar.

When I consulted with Denise, she told me she was primarily concerned about her lower face region. Upon examination, she showed midfacial descent of the cheek pad and loss of volume in the lower eyelid region. She experienced loss of definition to her lower jawline with extensive jowling, contour changes and shadowing. She also had periorbital rhytides (wrinkles), along with chronic sun damage to the eye region.

The Restoration Rx: For Thomas, we did upper and lower eyelid blepharoplasty, combined with a lower face lift and tightening of his platysma muscle and jawline. He underwent his surgical procedures and stayed over at a local hotel, along with his recovering wife and a nurse, for the first several days postoperatively.

Finding it difficult to be the patient, Thomas took off only a minimal amount of time from his medical practice. We did extensive educating and counseling on the postoperative healing events. But in typical male fashion, he felt that he would heal more quickly than the time frame we had established for him. Consequently, he deviated from his postoperative schedule and returned to a full surgical inpatient load the second week after surgery. In week three, he even entered and won a significant local golf tournament. Later, he realized this had been a mistake. While Tom won the first-place trophy for his mantel, he suffered a setback in swelling and fatigue. He told me it took him four weeks to recover from that one overdone weekend!

For Denise, I recommended that she undergo an endoscopic midface lift, lower face lift with platysmal tightening, and laser resurfacing of the eye region.

Outcome: Denise and Thomas both had an excellent result. While they were pleased from a surgical standpoint, we also discussed that they both had drastically underestimated their recovery process. But Denise remained good-natured about it and continues to joke about it. She even uses her experience as a cautionary tale to stress proper preparation and recovery planning for her patients. She conceded that she used to get frustrated by patients who did not listen to her. And here she was — *becoming* that patient who had often frustrated her in her own practice.

It was quite a "pair-o'-docs": even people in the medical field need to be educated about realistic expectations regarding recovery time. We all like to think we're super human, busy people who can bounce right back. But any time you have a surgical procedure, your body has been through a traumatic experience and requires time to heal itself. You mustn't underestimate the healing process.

While many wives attempt empathy when their husbands are feeling under the weather, Denise knew *precisely* how Thomas felt when he awakened recently, following laser resurfacing and a neck lift, because she was in the bed across from him in their hotel suite, recovering from similar procedures. Apparently, the familiar adage is true:

"*Doctors do make the absolute worst patients!*" Denise now concedes with a laugh. "*We were horrible. I don't like being down and being sick. I don't respond well to taking medications. I much prefer taking care of others to being taken care of myself.*"

Taking my advice, the couple booked a two-night post-procedure stay in a hotel suite where an around-the-clock nurse stayed on the other side of the living room, along with Denise's parents.

Denise cautions other prospective patients to take into account their loved one's personalities before asking them to play nurse. Often, it's better to hire an impartial medical professional.

"*My father was helpful with creating a meds chart for us to follow, since we were taking a lot of antibiotics, antifungals, steroids, and even anti-herpes medications, with all that raw exposed skin you have following a laser resurfacing procedure,*" she recalls.

Denise and Thomas also developed acute cases of buyer's remorse in the days following their procedures. "*I'll be completely honest,*" she recalls. "*My face felt like it had been sandblasted. It was a burned, beet-red, oozing, weeping and scabby mess. We both had to keep a thick Vaseline-like goo on our face so the exposed skin wouldn't dry out. I looked over and Thomas looked exactly the same way. I remember asking him, 'Do I look as grotesque as you do?' He told me, 'You actually look a little worse!' We're both doctors and we couldn't believe we chose to have these elective surgeries on ourselves. I was so angry and so frustrated.*"

Thomas and Denise allotted themselves only the minimum two-week window for recovery, as well. That decision, she says, was a mistake. "*You really need to give*

Denise and Tom Facial Rejuvenation

This physician couple, ages 49 and 52, decided to undergo facial rejuvenation together — at the same time. They were both very pleased with their results but underestimated the recovery process. They joked how they went from the 4 chin to a 2 chin family.

BEFORE ▼   ▼ AFTER

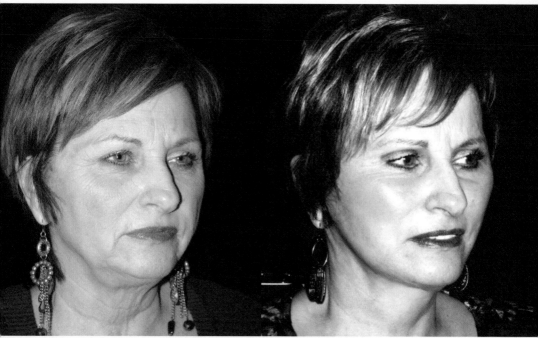

BEFORE ▼   ▼ AFTER

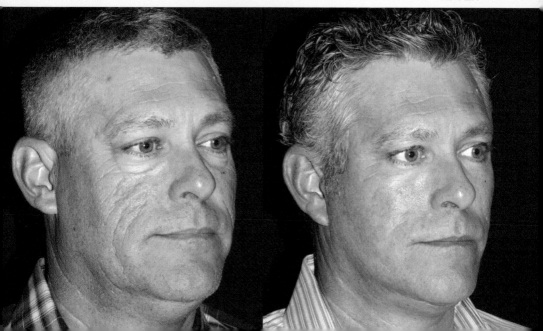

yourself more time for recovery than we did," she admits. *"The human body is tricky. There were days when we would feel pretty good in the morning, and by 5 p.m., we had completely crashed and were in a lot of pain. As a doctor, I always wondered why the patient calls would come in late in the day. Now, I know. You need to plan for way more downtime. We were just dumb doctors."*

Still, Denise says, going through the medical misery with her husband was therapeutic. *"In the end, it actually helped that we were both doctors,"* she says. *"It was good to know the science behind the procedures, the recovery process, and the meds. It also helped to have the insight into how the other person was feeling. You have a much deeper level of sympathy when you're on the same road. It was definitely a test of our relationship. But I have to say, most days we made a pretty good team."*

Eighteen months after their procedures, Denise and Thomas are reaping the youthful benefits of all that discomfort. The bags under Thomas's eyes are gone, and so is that tired, middle-aged doctor who used to disdainfully diagnose his appearance in the mirror.

As for Denise, the lines around her eyes and mouth, and the excess skin and fat under her chin and neck, have vanished.

"We've gone from a four-chin family to a two-chin family," she jokes. "We were at a party together recently and an old friend asked us how we can look so good working such crazy hours. Naturally, I lied and said, 'Oh, just good genes I guess.' Doctors are just as vain as everyone else!"

CHIP'S TIPS

1 If you're preparing for surgery, plan on taking the recommended time off. Healing is science and goes through defined stages.

2 Although you may consider yourself a fast healer, don't assume your body will respond accordingly. Healing is a process, not an attitude. Everyone heals differently.

3 Remember, the full results of cosmetic surgery are not immediate. It takes patience and time to reach your final destination.

4 You may "hate me" for a little while after your procedure, but I promise it won't last forever. I call it the "love-hate-love" relationship with your doctor.

5 Avoid smoking for at least two weeks prior and two weeks after surgery. Smoking significantly impedes blood flow, increases inflammation and inhibits the healing process.

6 Risks are real. Percentages are real. However, if you have a 5 percent chance of a healing complication before surgery and then have one after surgery, it is now 100 percent. Same for everything in life.

7 If you are still mad at the medical office after surgery, you are still healing. Final healing is variable but will occur — remember love-hate-love.

8 Each side of your face has different, but very similar, nerves and muscle tissue. You will always start off healing with asymmetry. The two sides will catch up and reach the finish line "holding hands."

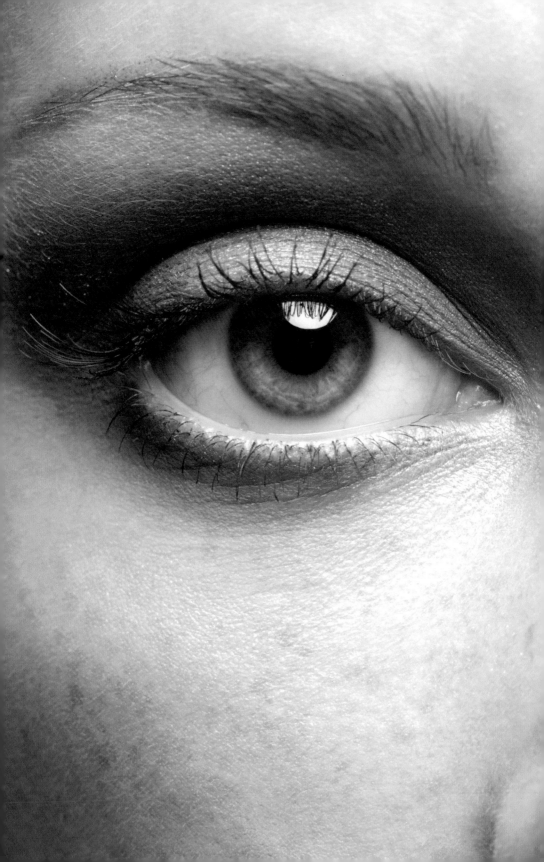

CHAPTER 14

* * *

COMMENCEMENT:
TIME TO FACE CHANGE

"Beauty is not in the face; beauty is a light in the heart."
— Kahlil Gibran

Throughout this volume, I've given you the tools to make informed decisions about your appearance — not only with regard to choosing the right surgical procedure, but also the right products and approaches to daily maintenance that will keep you looking your best at every age.

But just as important, I hope I've imparted something about what it means to be a fulfilled and balanced person, inside and out. As we learn again and again, all the money and material objects in the world can never duplicate the true radiance that comes from a contented life.

And even if you skipped around from chapter to chapter (or passed the book to your husband at Chapter 7… wink, wink), I hope you've culled something valuable from these pages on your journey into beauty, wellness, and optimal health.

I've emphasized the importance of good nutrition; of limiting indulgences like sugar, dairy, and gluten (after all, surface beauty is really a function of what's happening deep down inside). For as vital as outside-in measures are — such as skillful cosmetic surgery, good skin products and regular massage — it's equally critical to work from the inside-out, to replenish and nourish our skin by drinking plenty of water and juice, exercising regularly, and eating consciously: regional, seasonal, sustainable. If it was good enough for our great-grandparents, it should be good enough for us.

I've touched on the importance of philanthropy — of doing what we can for the benefit of humanity. The sense of contribution and belonging that comes from serving the underserved, lending a voice to the voiceless, giving company to the lonely, cannot be overestimated. It connects us to God in ways that cannot be measured, and it ensures a good night's sleep and long life in ways that cannot be bought.

In short, I have experienced that true beauty extends from a healthy, engaged life — from having family, friends, and adoring pets around us. From folding activity and movement into our daily routine, to finding our passion and pursuing it to the ends of the earth.

And so, like students on graduation day percolating with possibility, it's time to throw that graduation cap high in the air, go out into the world and start putting this into practice. And remember, as you navigate the waters of optimal health and beauty, I'm always here as a resource and a sounding board, to serve as a confidant and friend.

Yours truly, in everything you do,

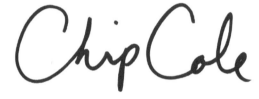

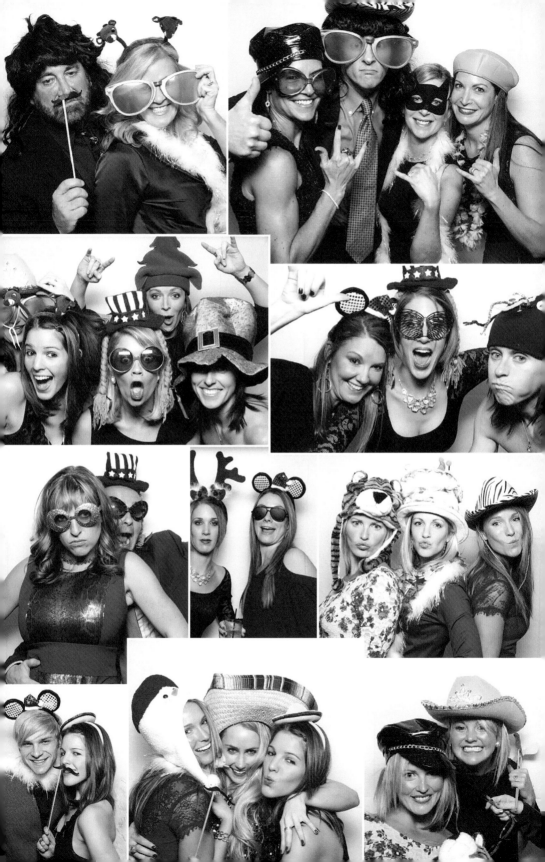

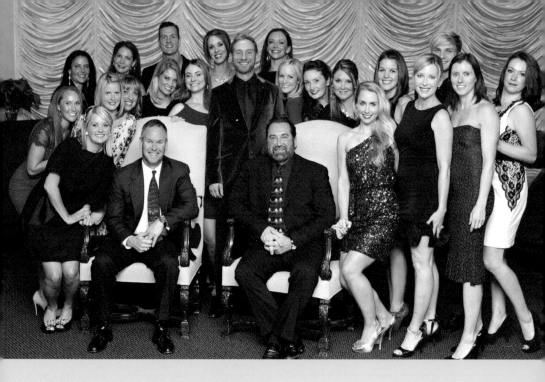

From myself and all of our family at
Oculus Plastic Surgery and Oculus Skin Care Center,
we wish you the best in your pursuit of better health
and greater happiness through all of life's journeys.

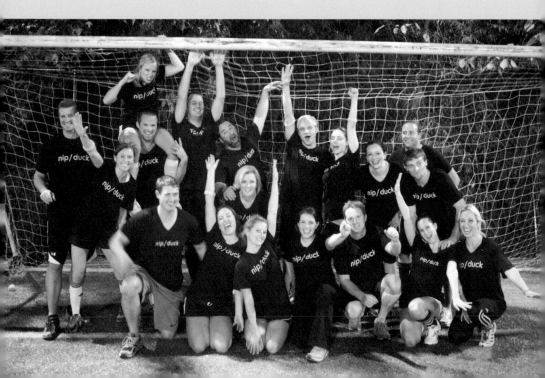

CHIP'S TIPS GREATEST HITS

1 Love yourself. A positive and healthy inside makes the outside radiate with beauty and energy.

2 Life by the inch is a cinch. Life by the yard is hard. Life by the mile is wile[d]. Live each day inch by inch.

3 Make sure your surgeon is not only board certified by the ABMS, but is a specialist in the type of surgery you are contemplating.

4 Risks are real. Percentages are real. However, if you have a 5 percent chance of a healing complication before surgery and then have one after surgery, it is now 100 percent. Same for everything in life.

5 You may "hate me" for a little while after your procedure, but I promise it won't last forever. I call it the "love-hate-love" relationship with your doctor.

6 With age comes wisdom and wrinkles. Physician-prescribed skin care will reduce the wrinkles. Laser surgery will essentially eliminate the wrinkles. Both allow you to keep the wisdom.

7 Human growth factors are the most significant advancement in skin cell architecture. These gel products are pricey but worth the investment.

8 The most natural appearing rejuvenation is achieved by undergoing several smaller procedures as you age. Sow as you go, and no one will know.

9 Remember to address the two "tattletale areas" when undergoing facial rejuvenation: the neck and ears. Not only are most phone cameras HD, but your "attentive" girlfriends are, too.

10 Stay close to your family, especially your siblings. Friends will come and go, but your family will be there for you forever.

11 Final thought: Go forth each day and try to be at least half the person your dog thinks you are.

NOTES

CPSIA information can be obtained
at www.ICGtesting.com
Printed in the USA
LVIC04n1505210714
395332LV00005B/9